The Structured Oral Examination in Clinical ANAESTHESIA

Practice examination papers

Cyprian Mendonca, Car
Josephine James, GS /

tfm Publishing Limited, Castle Hill Barns, Harley, Nr Shrewsbury, SY5 6LX, UK. Tel: +44 (0)1952 510061; Fax: +44 (0)1952 510192 E-mail: nikki@tfmpublishing.com; Web site: www.tfmpublishing.com

Design & Typesetting: Nikki Bramhill BSc Hons Dip Law
First Edition: © May 2009
Background cover image © Comstock Inc., www.comstock.com

ISBN: 978 1 903378 68 7

Printed by Gutenberg Press Ltd., Gudja Road, Tarxien, PLA 19, Malta. Tel: +356 21897037; Fax: +356 21800069.

Contents

Preface

This book consists of ten complete sets of structured oral examination (SOE) papers. Each set is subdivided into two sections: clinical anaesthesia and clinical science. Each clinical anaesthesia section is composed of one long case and three short cases. For each long case clear candidate information and relevant clinical material have been presented. The clinical science section is composed of four key topics, one each from applied anatomy, applied physiology, applied pharmacology and the physics of equipment used in anaesthetic practice. In order to provide additional breadth and depth of knowledge, a further tutorial on the key topic is included.

The aim of this book is to help trainees who are sitting their anaesthetic examinations. The book enables candidates to assess their knowledge and skills within certain time limits. A thorough revision of the book should enable the trainee to understand their strengths and weaknesses in areas of clinical knowledge, clinical skills, technical skills, problem solving, organisaton and planning.

We are grateful for the feedback and suggestions provided by trainees who attended the examination preparation courses at Coventry. We sincerely hope that the information in this book will be beneficial to trainees in their preparation for postgraduate examinations and competency assessments.

We wish you good luck with your revision and the exam.

Cyprian Mendonca MD, FRCA, Consultant Anaesthetist
University Hospitals Coventry and Warwickshire, Coventry, UK
Carl Hillermann FRCA, Consultant Anaesthetist
University Hospitals Coventry and Warwickshire, Coventry, UK
Josephine James FRCA, Consultant Anaesthetist
Heart of England Foundation Trust, Birmingham, UK
GS Anil Kumar FCARCSI, Specialist Registrar
Warwickshire School of Anaesthesia, UK

Acknowledgements

We are indebted to Dr Shyam Balasubramanian, Consultant Anaesthetist, University Hospitals Coventry and Warwickshire, who critically reviewed the entire manuscript and also for permission to use some of the illustrations from *The Objective Structured Clinical Examination in Anaesthesia - Practice papers for Teachers and Trainees* (ISBN 978-1-903378-56-4).

We are grateful to Mr Jason McAllister, Graphic Designer, University Hospitals Coventry and Warwickshire, for his help with the illustrations, to Dr Madhu Varma Chittari, Specialist Registrar in Cardiology, University Hospitals Coventry and Warwickshire, for his help with ECG interpretation, and to Dr Vandana Gaur, Consultant Radiologist, for her assistance with chest X-rays. We also thank Nikki Bramhill, Director, tfm publishing, for critically reviewing the manuscript and for permission to use some of the illustrations from *The Objective Structured Clinical Examination in Anaesthesia - Practice papers for Teachers and Trainees*.

We also extend our thanks to the following who contributed questions and case scenarios to the various sections on this book:

Dr Billing John
Dr Mohan Ranganathan
Dr Seema Quasim
Dr Priya Kothare
Dr Sridhar Gummaraju
Dr Parag Shastri
Dr Raja Lakshmanan
Dr Rathinavale Shanmugam
Dr Janardhan Baliga

Dr P Sathya Narayanan
Dr Soorly Sreevathsa
Dr Nicholas Crombie
Dr Vanessa Hodgetts

We are grateful to all the trainees who attended the examination preparation courses at Coventry and who provided their suggestions and feedback to improve the manuscript.

Abbreviations

AAA	Abdominal aortic aneurysm
AAI	Atlanto-axial instability
AAS	Atlanto-axial subluxation
AAT	Alpha-1 antitrypsin
ACA	Anterior cerebral artery
ACE	Angiotensin-converting enzyme
AChR	Acetylcholine receptors
ACS	Abdominal compartment syndrome
ACTH	Adrenocorticotrophic hormone
ADH	Anti-diuretic hormone
ADP	Adenosine diphospate
AEP	Auditory evoked potential
AF	Atrial fibrillation
AHI	Apnoea/hypopnoea index
AICD	Automated implantable cardioverter-defibrillator
AKI	Acute kidney injury
ALI	Acute lung injury
ALS	Advanced life support
ALT	Alanine transaminase
AMP	Adenosine monophosphate
AMPA	α-amino-3-hydroxyl-5-methyl-4-isoxazole-propionate
ANP	Atrial natriuretic peptide
AP	Anteroposterior
APACHE	Acute Physiology and Chronic Health Evaluation
APL	Adjustable pressure limiting
APLS	Advanced Paediatric Life Support
APTT	Activated partial thromboplastin time
ARDS	Acute respiratory distress syndrome
ASA	American Society of Anesthesiologists
AT	Anaerobic threshold
ATN	Acute tubular necrosis
ATP	Adenosine triphospate
AV	Atrioventricular
AVA	Aortic valve area

BD	Twice a day
BE	Base excess
BIS	Bispectral Index Score
BP	Blood pressure
BSE	Bovine spongiform encephalopathy
BURP	Backward, upward and right-sided pressure
CABG	Coronary artery bypass grafting
CBF	Cerebral blood flow
CCB	Calcium channel blocker
CCK	Cholecystokinin
CGRP	Calcitonin gene-related peptide
CI	Cardiac index
CICV	Cannot intubate, cannot ventilate
CK	Creatine kinase
Cl	Chloride
$CMRO_2$	Cerebral metabolic rate for oxygen
CNS	Central nervous system
CO	Cardiac output
COAD	Chronic obstructive airway disease
COMT	Catechol-O-methyl transferase
CPAP	Continuous positive airway pressure
CPET	Cardiopulmonary exercise testing
CPK	Creatinine phosphokinase
CPP	Cerebral perfusion pressure
CPR	Cardiopulmonary resuscitation
CSF	Cerebrospinal fluid
CT	Computer tomography
CTZ	Chemoreceptor trigger zone
CVA	Cerebrovascular accident
CVP	Central venous pressure
DES	Drug-eluting stents
DI	Diabetes insipidus
DIC	Disseminated intravascular coagulation
DINAMAP	Device for indirect non-invasive automated mean arterial pressure
DIT	Diiodotyrosine
DVT	Deep vein thrombosis
ECF	Extracellular fluid
ECG	Electrocardiogram
ECT	Electroconvulsive therapy
EDV	End-diastolic volume
EEG	Electroencephalogram

EMG	Electromyography
EMI	Electromagnetic interference
EMLA	Eutectic mixture of local anaesthetic
EOG	Electro-oculogram
ERV	Expiratory reserve volume
ESR	Erythrocyte sedimentation rate
ETCO$_2$	End-tidal CO$_2$
ETT	Endotracheal tube
EVAR	Endovascular aneurysm repair
FEF	Forced expiratory flow
FEV	Forced expiratory volume
FFP	Fresh frozen plasma
FGF	Fresh gas flow
FID	Functional iron deficiency
FID	Foot impulse device
FRC	Functional residual capacity
FVC	Forced vital capacity
GA	General anaesthesia
GABA	Gamma aminobutyric acid
GCS	Glasgow Coma Scale
GFR	Glomerular filtration rate
GH	Growth hormone
H	Hydrogen
Hb	Haemoglobin
HBO	Hyperbaric oxygen therapy
HCO$_3$	Bicarbonates
Hct	Haematocrit
HDU	High dependency unit
HIV	Human immunodeficiency virus
HOCM	Hypertrophic obstructive cardiomyopathy
HPA	Hypothalamic-pituitary adrenal
HPV	Hypoxic pulmonary vasoconstriction
HR	Heart rate
5-HT	5-hydroxytryptamine
IAP	Intra-abdominal pressure
IBD	Inflammatory bowel disease
ICA	Internal carotid artery
ICP	Intracranial pressure
ICU	Intensive care unit
IDDM	Insulin-dependent diabetes mellitus
IHD	Ischaemic heart disease

IJV	Internal jugular vein
ILMA	Intubating laryngeal mask airway
INR	International normalised ratio
INVCT	*In vitro* contracture testing
IOP	Intra-ocular pressure
IPP	Inspiratory plateau pressure
IPPV	Intermittent positive pressure ventilation
IV	Intravenous
JVP	Jugular venous pressure/pulse
K	Potassium
KCl	Potassium chloride
LA	Local anaesthesia
LAD	Left anterior descending
LBBB	Left bundle branch block
LCA	Left coronary artery
LDH	Lactate dehydrogenase
LFT	Lacrimal, frontal and trochlear nerves
LGL	Lown-Ganong-Levine
LiDCO	Lithium indicator dilution cardiac output
LMA	Laryngeal mask airway
LMWH	Low-molecular-weight heparin
LOS	Lower oesophageal sphincter
LVEDP	Left ventricular end-diastolic pressure
LVH	Left ventricular hypertrophy
MAC	Minimum alveolar concentration
MAO	Monoamine oxidase
MAP	Mean arterial pressure
MCA	Middle cerebral artery
MCHC	Mean corpuscular haemoglobin concentration
MCV	Mean corpuscular volume
MEAC	Minimum effective analgesic concentration
MEN	Multiple endocrine neoplasia
MEP	Maximal expiratory pressure
MET	Metabolic equivalent
$MgSO_4$	Magnesium sulphate
MH	Malignant hyperthermia
MIBG	Meta-iodo-benzyl guanidine
MIP	Maximal inspiratory pressure
MIT	Monoiodotyrosine
MOI	Monoamine oxidase inhibitor
MPAP	Mean pulmonary artery pressure

MRA	Magnetic resonance angiography
Na	Sodium
NASCET	North American Symptomatic Carotid Endarterectomy Trial
nCPAP	Nasal continuous positive airway pressure
NDNMB	Non-depolarising neuromuscular blocker
NIBP	Non-invasive blood pressure
NICE	National Institute for Health and Clinical Excellence
NIDDM	Non-insulin dependent diabetes mellitus
NMDA	N-methyl-D-aspartate
NMJ	Neuromuscular junction
NMS	Neuroleptic malignant syndrome
N_2O	Nitrous oxide
NO	Nitric oxide
NO_2	Nitrogen dioxide
NRTI	Nucleoside reverse transcriptase inhibitors
NSAID	Non-steroidal anti-inflammatory drugs
NSTEMI	Non-ST elevation myocardial infarction
OD	Once a day
OSA	Obstructive sleep apnoea
OSAHS	Obstructive sleep apnoea hypopnoea syndrome
PA	Postero-anterior
PAOP	Pulmonary artery occlusion pressure
PAP	Pulmonary artery pressure
PAWP	Pulmonary artery wedge pressure
PCA	Patient-controlled analgesia
PCC	Prothrombin complex concentrate
PCI	Percutaneous coronary intervention
PCT	Proximal convoluted tubule
PCWP	Pulmonary capillary wedge pressure
PDPH	Post-dural puncture headache
PE	Pulmonary embolism
PEEP	Positive end expiratory pressure
PEFR	Peak expiratory flow rate
PEP	Post-exposure prophylaxis
PET	Positron emission tomography
PHN	Post-herpetic neuralgia
PI	Protease inhibitors
PMH	Past medical history
PNMT	Phenyl-ethanolamine-N-methyltransferase
PONV	Postoperative nausea and vomiting
PPF	Plasma protein fraction

PPH	Primary postpartum haemorrhage
PPM	Parts per million
PSG	Polysomnography
PT	Prothrombin time
PVR	Pulmonary vascular resistance
PVRI	Pulmonary vascular resistance index
QDS	Four times a day
RAP	Right atrial pressure
RAST	Radio-allergosorbent testing
RBBB	Right bundle branch block
RBC	Red blood cell
rEPO	Recombinant erythropoietin
rFVIIa	Recombinant activated factor VII
rhAPC	Recombinant human activated protein-C
RSBI	Rapid shallow breathing index
RV	Residual volume
SA	Sino-atrial
SAB	Subarachnoid block
SAH	Subarachnoid haemorrhage
SAYGO	Spray as you go
SBP	Systolic blood pressure
SBT	Spontaneous breathing trial
SC	Subcutaneous
SCM	Sternocleidomastoid
SF	Serum ferritin
SNRI	Serotonin and norepinephrine reuptake inhibitor
SPECT	Single photon emission computed tomography
SSRI	Selective serotonin reuptake inhibitor
STEMI	ST-segment elevation myocardial infarction
SVI	Stroke volume index
SVR	Systemic vascular resistance
SVRI	Systemic vascular resistance index
TBSA	Total body surface area
TBW	Total body water
TCA	Tricyclic antidepressant
TCI	Target controlled infusion
TDS	Three times a day
TENS	Transcutaneous electrical nerve stimulation
TF	Tissue factor
TFPI	Tissue factor pathway inhibitor
TIBC	Total iron binding capacity

TIVA	Total intravenous anaesthesia
TLC	Total lung capacity
TLCO	Transfer factor for carbon monoxide
TNF	Tumour necrosis factor
TOE	Transoesophageal echocardiography
TPN	Total parenteral nutrition
TRALI	Transfusion-related acute lung injury
TSAT	Transferrin saturation
TSH	Thyroid stimulating hormone
TURP	Transurethral resection of the prostate
VAS	Visual Analogue Score
VC	Vital capacity
vCJD	Variant Creutzfeldt-Jakob disease
VF	Ventricular fibrillation
VIP	Vasoactive intestinal peptide
VMA	Vanillyl mandelic acid
VT	Ventricular tachycardia
WBC	White blood cell
WFNS	World Federation of Neurosurgeons
WPW	Wolff-Parkinson-White

Structured oral examination 1

Long case 1

Information for the candidate

History

A 70-year-old male patient underwent elective abdominal aortic aneurysm repair 24 hours ago. His past medical history includes hypertension and ischaemic heart disease. His medications up to the day of surgery included simvastatin 30mg o.d., enalapril 10mg o.d., atenolol 50mg o.d. and aspirin 75mg o.d. He smoked 20-30 cigarettes until 6 months ago, after which he completely stopped.

The intra-operative blood loss was 1.2 litres with an aortic cross-clamp time of 65 minutes. The average urine output during the intra-operative period was 90ml/hour. Following the release of the aortic clamp, he required inotropic support for a brief period. He was transferred to the intensive care unit and ventilated overnight. Postoperative pain relief is still provided with epidural infusion of 0.125% bupivacaine and fentanyl 2µg/ml. He was weaned off the ventilator and extubated 4 hours ago.

You have been called to see the patient as he has developed shortness of breath.

Clinical examination

He is conscious, breathless, sweaty and clammy. His peripheral oxygen saturation is 94% whilst breathing spontaneously 60% oxygen. On examining the chest there is bilateral equal air entry with crackles at both bases.

Table 1.1 Clinical examination.

Weight	78kg
Height	170cm
Heart rate	120 bpm
Blood pressure	95/65mmHg
Temperature	36.9°C

Investigations

Table 1.2 Biochemistry.

		Normal values
Sodium	138mmol/L	135-145mmol/L
Potassium	3.2mmol/L	3.5-5.0mmol/L
Urea	14.5mmol/L	2.2-8.3mmol/L
Creatinine	123µmol/L	44-80µmol/L
Blood glucose	8.5mmol/L	3.0-6.0mmol/L

Table 1.3 Haematology.

		Normal values
Hb	11.3g/dL	11-16g/dL
Haematocrit	0.24	0.4-0.5 males, 0.37-0.47 females
RBC	2.75×10^{12}/L	$3.8-4.8 \times 10^{12}$/L
WBC	7.5×10^9/L	$4-11 \times 10^9$/L
Platelets	296×10^9/L	$150-450 \times 10^9$/L
INR	1.4	0.9-1.2
PT	14.4 seconds	11-15 seconds
APTT ratio	1.4	0.8-1.2

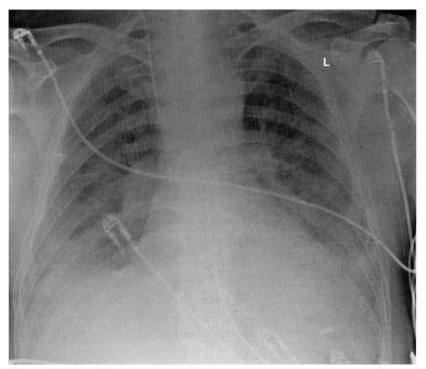

Figure 1.1 Chest X-ray.

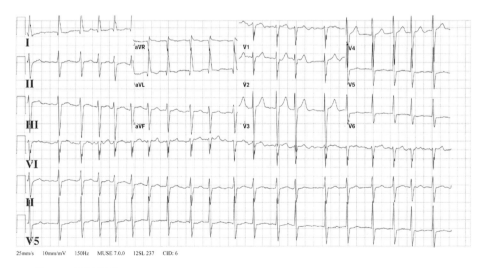

Figure 1.2 ECG.

Examiner's questions

Please summarise the case

A 70-year-old male patient, known to have hypertension and ischaemic heart disease, recovering in intensive care following AAA repair, has developed hypotension and hypoxia at 24 hours postoperatively following tracheal extubation. His biochemistry results suggest impaired renal function and hypokalaemia.

What is the differential diagnosis?

The important causes of postoperative hypotension and hypoxia in this patient can be listed systematically as follows.

Cardiovascular system

◆   Myocardial infarction.
◆   Left ventricular failure or congestive cardiac failure.
◆   Arrhythmias such as atrial fibrillation (AF).

Respiratory system

◆   Pulmonary embolism.
◆   Pleural effusion.
◆   Pneumothorax.
◆   Transfusion-related acute lung injury (TRALI).

Metabolic causes

◆   Electrolyte imbalance.

Infection

◆   Severe systemic infection (sepsis).

Analgesia-related

◆   High level of epidural blockade.

What are the abnormal findings in the ECG?

The ECG shows atrial fibrillation as the rhythm is irregularly irregular with absent P waves and the heart rate is approximately 120 bpm. There is left ventricular hypertrophy and left axis deviation suggesting longstanding hypertension.

What are the causes of atrial fibrillation (AF)?

Cardiac causes

- Ischaemic heart disease.
- Mitral valve disease.
- Hypertension.
- Cardiomyopathy.

Non-cardiac causes

- Hypoxia.
- Acute hypovolaemia.
- Sepsis.
- Electrolyte disturbances - potassium, magnesium and phosphate.
- Pulmonary thromboembolism.
- Thyrotoxicosis.

In this patient the cause of AF is likely to be ischaemic heart disease, pneumonia and an electrolyte imbalance (low potassium).

How would you treat fast atrial fibrillation?

- Ensure adequate airway and breathing, and administer 100% oxygen.
- Establish continuous ECG, blood pressure and pulse oximetry monitoring.
- Correct any precipitating factors where possible.
- Determine if the patient is stable or not.

If the patient is unstable, he should be treated with synchronised DC cardioversion with shocks up to three attempts. If there is no response, intravenous amiodarone 300mg should be administered over 10-20 minutes and the shock repeated if needed, followed by an amiodarone 900mg IV infusion over 24 hours.

In stable patients the rate should be controlled with a beta-blocker or digoxin administered intravenously.

If the onset of AF is within 48 hours, consider amiodarone 300mg IV over 20-60 minutes followed by amiodarone 900mg over 24 hours. In general, patients who have been in AF for more than 48 hours should not be treated by cardioversion (electrical or chemical) until they have been fully anticoagulated for at least 3 weeks, or unless transoesophageal echocardiography has shown the absence of atrial thrombus.

How would you determine whether the patient is stable or not?

Signs of instability include:

◆ A reduced level of consciousness.
◆ Chest pain.
◆ Systolic BP <90mm Hg.
◆ Heart failure.

Signs of instability are uncommon at rates less than 150 bpm.

How would you correct hypokalaemia and hypomagnesaemia?

Potassium

◆ IV via peripheral venous access: maximum concentration is 40mmol KCl/litre over 4-6 hours.
◆ IV via central venous access: maximum 40mmol KCl in 100ml of 0.9% saline, with ECG monitoring, in the ICU/HDU/theatre environment (usually at a rate of 20mmol/hour).
◆ Recheck plasma potassium at least hourly during the rapid replacement phase.

Magnesium

◆ 5g of magnesium sulphate (20mmol of Mg^{++}) should be administered intravenously over 20 minutes followed by 1g/hour as an IV infusion.

What are the clinical features of hypermagnesaemia?

The effects are essentially those of a calcium channel blocker combined with a membrane stabiliser. Magnesium binds to many calcium binding sites and therefore blocks the effect of calcium in a number of enzyme systems. A serum concentration of at least 2mmol/L is necessary to produce clinical effects.

Cardiovascular effects

- ECG:
    - <5mmol/L - delayed interventricular conduction, prolonged QT interval;
    - >5mmol/L - first and second-degree atrioventricular (AV) block;
    - >12.5mmol/L - complete AV block and asystole.

Hypotension is usually only transient. Except in severe toxicity or following rapid parenteral administration of $MgSO_4$, hypermagnesaemia does not usually produce a profound reduction in systemic vascular resistance (SVR).

Neurological effects

- Varying degrees of neuromuscular block by decreasing impulse transmission across the neuromuscular junction.
- A decrease in post-synaptic membrane responsiveness and an increase in the threshold for axonal excitation also occur.
- One of the earliest clinically noticeable signs of magnesium toxicity is diminution of deep tendon reflexes. Hypoventilation may occur due to respiratory muscle paralysis. High levels of magnesium may lead to somnolence and coma.

How would you manage hypermagnesaemia?

Stop administration of magnesium. If the patient is haemodynamically stable, with no evidence of respiratory depression and reflexes are present, simply observe for further symptoms and maintain urine output. If there are signs of severe systemic effects, the effect of magnesium can be antagonised by IV calcium gluconate in bolus doses of 2.5-5mmol.

In life-threatening complications or in patients with renal impairment, magnesium excretion may also be enhanced by dialysis with magnesium-free dialysate.

Can you comment on the chest X-ray?

The chest X-ray shows cardiomegaly with signs of congestive cardiac failure (hilar congestion and upper lobe diversion of blood vessels). There is a central line inserted via the right internal jugular vein which is correctly positioned. There is haziness at both costophrenic angles.

How would you manage cardiac failure in this patient?

- Check the airway, breathing and circulation.
- Keep the patient in a head-up position and administer 100% oxygen.
- Administer morphine 5-10mg or diamorphine 2.5-5mg, as an IV slowly. This relieves anxiety and pain, and also produces transient venodilation and reduces myocardial oxygen demand.
- Administer furosemide 40-80mg IV slowly; this produces transient venodilation and subsequent diuresis.
- Check blood gases.
- Non-invasive ventilation with continuous positive airway pressure (CPAP).
- Invasive ventilation by reintubation and ventilation.
- Monitor the patient in a critical care environment.
- Monitor central venous pressure (CVP), invasive blood pressure, cardiac output, fluid balance and urine output.
- Vasodilatory/inotropic support may be required.

After 2 hours of resuscitation, the urine output has fallen to 10ml over the past 2 hours. The CVP is 15mm Hg, BP is maintained at a mean arterial pressure (MAP) of 80-90mm Hg, the heart rate is 90 bpm and there is sinus rhythm.

What are the causes of renal failure?

The causes of renal failure can be classified as pre-renal, renal and post-renal.

Pre-renal

Pre-renal failure is caused by renal hypoperfusion, e.g. blood loss, hypovolaemia, cardiac failure, renal artery stenosis or due to decreased renal perfusion as a result of increased intra-abdominal pressure (abdominal compartment syndrome).

Renal

Renal failure causes can be of glomerular or tubular origin. Glomerular causes include glomerulonephritis, amyloidosis and diabetes mellitus.

Tubular and interstitium-related causes include acute tubular nephritis, drugs (NSAIDs, aminoglycosides, acyclovir, radio contrast dyes) and tubular obstruction, e.g. myeloma.

Nearly 90% of intrinsic acute kidney injury (AKI) cases are caused by ischaemia or toxins, both of which lead to acute tubular necrosis (ATN). Ischaemic acute renal failure is associated with reduced blood flow to the kidneys (renal hypoperfusion), which leads to tissue death and irreversible kidney failure.

Post-renal

Post-renal failure causes include obstruction in the urinary collection system, such as bladder outlet obstruction due to an enlarged prostate gland or a bladder stone and renal stones in both ureters. A neurogenic bladder (over-distended bladder) is caused by an inability of the bladder to empty. Retroperitoneal fibrosis can cause obstruction of the ureters and result in renal failure. When there is complete absence of urine, mechanical obstruction of the catheter should be ruled out.

This patient has a tense distended abdomen. Is there anything else which may result in acute kidney injury?

This patient is at risk of developing abdominal compartment syndrome.

What is the pathophysiology of acute kidney injury in abdominal compartment syndrome?

The mechanism for renal failure with an elevated intra-abdominal pressure (IAP) is multifactorial. There is a decrease in renal plasma flow and glomerular filtration rate and an increase in renal vascular resistance which may lead to low urine output and subsequently cause acute kidney injury.

Magnesium therapy in critically ill patients

To maintain normal serum magnesium levels in critically ill patients, serum magnesium and creatinine levels should be measured daily. The table below incorporates the volume and delivery for infusion via a central venous catheter.

Magnesium can be administered according to the chart below once daily until the serum level of magnesium is ≥1.0mmol/L. Magnesium can be diluted either with sodium chloride 0.9% or 5% glucose.

Table 1.4 Magnesium therapy.

Serum magnesium	Serum creatinine		
	<150µmol/L	150-250µmol/L	250-400µmol/L
>1.0mmol/L	None	None	None
0.55-0.99mmol/L	5g in 50ml over 1 hour	2.5g in 50ml over 1 hour	None
0.40-0.5mmol/L	7.5g in 50ml over 2 hours	5g in 50ml over 1 hour	2.5g in 50ml over 1 hour
<0.40mmol/L	10g in 50ml over 2 hours	7.5g in 50ml over 2 hours	5g in 50ml over 1 hour

Each 10ml vial of magnesium sulphate contains 5g of magnesium sulphate which equals approximately 20mmol of magnesium (2mmol/ml).

Abdominal compartment syndrome

Abdominal compartment syndrome (ACS) can be defined as an increased intra-abdominal pressure associated with organ dysfunction. It is associated with significant morbidity and mortality. An intra-abdominal pressure greater than 25mm Hg leads to respiratory, cardiovascular and renal dysfunction. Prompt recognition and management by abdominal decompression and fluid resuscitation is likely to improve the prognosis.

The risk factors for the development of ACS include:

◆ Severe penetrating and blunt abdominal trauma.
◆ Ruptured abdominal aortic aneurysm.
◆ Retroperitoneal haemorrhage.
◆ Pneumoperitoneum.
◆ Neoplasm.
◆ Pancreatitis.
◆ Massive ascites.
◆ Liver transplantation.

The exact incidence of ACS in critically ill patients is not known. Among the trauma population, the reported risk is approximately 14%. Patients undergoing 'damage control' laparotomy, especially with intra-abdominal packing are at a greater risk. The incidence following primary closure following repair of a ruptured abdominal aortic aneurysm is reported in one series at 4%.

Pathophysiology

Increased intra-abdominal pressure exerts adverse physiological effects on the cardiovascular, respiratory and renal system. It reduces cardiac output by the following mechanisms:

◆ A decrease in venous return (compression of inferior vena cava causing a reduction in venous return from the lower portion of the body).
◆ An increase in afterload (direct compression of blood vessels and vascular beds).
◆ Changes in ventricular compliance (diaphragmatic elevation which causes distortion of ventricular compliance).

Transmission of IAP to the vena cava and vascular beds causes an increase in CVP and pulmonary artery occlusion pressure (PAOP) and hence CVP and PAOP are not good indicators of fluid status in these patients. There is also an increased risk of venous thrombosis due to venous stasis. These derangements are exacerbated by concomitant hypovolaemia.

An increased intra-abdominal pressure decreases respiratory compliance with a progressive reduction in residual volume, functional residual capacity (FRC) and total lung capacity (TLC). Pulmonary vascular resistance increases due to hypoxia and increased intrathoracic pressure.

An increase in IAP is transmitted to the central nervous system via CVP and results in an increased intracranial pressure (ICP).

An increased IAP results in reduced gut perfusion, mucosal ischaemia and bacterial translocation.

Measurement of intra-abdominal pressure

Intra-abdominal pressure can be measured either directly or indirectly:

- Direct - direct measurement at laparoscopy.
- Indirect - transduction of pressure from the femoral vein, stomach, rectum and bladder.

The most commonly used method is measurement of intravesical pressure via a Foley catheter.

Abdominal compartment syndrome is graded into four grades depending on the intra-abdominal pressure (Table 1.5).

Table 1.5 Grades of abdominal compartment syndrome.

Grade	Bladder pressure (mmHg)	Recommendation
I	10-15	Maintain normovolaemia
II	16-25	Hypervolaemic resuscitation
III	26-35	Decompression
IV	>35	Decompression and re-exploration

The principle of management includes early surgical decompression and aggressive fluid resuscitation.

Key points

♦ Postoperative hypotension and hypoxia are common following major intra-abdominal surgery.
♦ Pre-operative blood loss, hypotension, hypoxia and electrolyte imbalance can predispose to cardiac arrhythmias in patients with pre-existing ischaemic heart disease and subsequently lead to cardiac failure.
♦ There is a risk of acute kidney injury and abdominal compartment syndrome following repair of an abdominal aortic aneurysm.

Further reading

1. Bailey J, Shapiro MJ. Abdominal compartment syndrome. *Critical Care* 2000; 4: 23-9.
2. Flesher ME, Archer KA, Leslie BD, *et al.* Assessing the metabolic and clinical consequences of early enteral feeding in the malnourished patient. *Journal of Parenteral and Enteral Nutrition* 2005; 29: 108-17.
3. Hopkins D, Gemmell LW. Intra-abdominal hypertension and the abdominal compartment syndrome. *British Journal of Anaesthesia CEPD review* 2001; 1: 56-9.

Short case 1.1: Pyloric stenosis

A 4-week-old male child presents with projectile vomiting for the past 5 days and has generally been unwell since birth. The mother gives a history of vomiting from very early on after birth which now has progressed to being projectile in nature. The baby also has constipation.

What do you think is the most likely diagnosis?

Infantile (congenital) pyloric stenosis.

What is the incidence of pyloric stenosis?

- The worldwide incidence is 3 per 1000 live births.
- Male preponderance with a male: female ratio of 4:1.
- Usually presents between the 3rd and 5th week of life.

What is the metabolic disturbance expected in this condition?

The classical metabolic picture is hypochloraemic, hypokalaemic, hyponatraemic metabolic alkalosis. The urine is initially alkaline which later on becomes acidic (paradoxical aciduria).

Describe the pathophysiology of these biochemical changes

As a result of vomiting, gastric acid (H^+ and Cl^-), water, Na^+ and K^+ are lost. Normally gastric acid is neutralised by pancreatic HCO_3^- as it crosses the duodenum. In the case of vomiting with an intact stomach and duodenum, both acid and HCO_3^- are lost. However, in cases of pyloric stenosis, only H^+ is lost, resulting in a net increase in $HCO3^-$. Increased HCO_3^- reaches the proximal convoluted tubule (PCT) of the kidney and overwhelms the reabsorptive capacity, resulting in a loss of HCO_3^- in urine (alkaline urine of early stages).

Extracellular fluid (ECF) volume depletion causes the kidney to conserve Na^+ by stimulating aldosterone secretion and causing kaliuresis (loss of K^+ ions in the urine). Loss of K^+ in vomiting and an extracellular to intracellular shift of K^+ due to plasma alkalosis causes significant hypokalaemia. Hypokalaemia forces Na^+ absorption in exchange for H^+, resulting in acidic urine (paradoxical aciduria). Cl^- loss occurs as a result of vomiting.

Therefore, the final metabolic derangement is hypochloraemic, hypokalaemic, hyponatraemic metabolic alkalosis.

How would you assess fluid loss?

The severity of dehydration is assessed with clinical examination. The severity can be graded as mild, moderate and severe (Table 1.6). The fluid deficit in millilitres can be calculated following an estimation of the degree of dehydration expressed as a percentage of body weight, e.g. a 10kg child who is 5% dehydrated has a water deficit of 500ml.

Table 1.6 Severity of fluid loss.			
Severity	Mild	Moderate	Severe
Fluid loss (% of body wt.)	5%	10%	15%
Anterior fontanelle	Normal	Sunken	Markedly depressed
Skin turgor	Normal	Decreased	Greatly decreased
Mucous membrane	Moist	Dry	Very dry
Eyes	Normal	Sunken	Markedly sunken
Pulse	Normal	Increased	Greatly increased
Respiration	Normal	Tachypnoea	Rapid and deep
Urine output (ml/kg/hour)	<2	<1	<0.5

How would you resuscitate this patient?

Ensure that the dehydration and electrolyte imbalance are corrected prior to surgery. Venous access should be secured and the baseline haemoglobin and electrolytes should be measured. Serum HCO_3^- is measured from a capillary blood sample. A nasogastric tube should be inserted and gastric washouts performed at least 4-hourly using saline until the aspirate is clear. Metabolic targets for resuscitation include:

◆ Serum Cl^- - >100mmol/L.
◆ Serum Na^+ - >135mmol/L.
◆ Serum HCO_3^- - <26mmol/L.
◆ Urine Cl^- - >20mmol/L.
◆ Urine output - >1ml/kg/hour.

Intravenous fluids

For moderate to severe dehydration with hypochloraemic alkalosis, a fluid bolus of 20ml/kg (0.9% sodium chloride) is administered to correct intravascular fluid deficits. Further fluid replacement should be continued with 0.45% sodium chloride in 5% dextrose at a rate of 6-8ml/kg/hour.

Once urine output is established, potassium chloride 20mmol/L can be added to the replacement fluid. Once the metabolic targets are nearly achieved, maintenance fluid is administered at a rate of 4ml/kg/hour.

Nasogastric losses should be replaced with 0.9% sodium chloride (normal saline) ml for ml. Serum electrolytes should be checked every 6-12 hours until the resuscitation target is achieved, and then every 24 hours for the duration of fluid therapy.

How would you anaesthetise this patient?

Ensure that the child has been appropriately resuscitated to correct the electrolyte and acid base imbalance, and that senior help is available.

Intra-operative management

Monitoring includes peripheral oxygen saturation (pulse oximetry), ECG and non-invasive blood pressure. The stomach should be emptied using nasogastric suction. To prevent hypothermia, operating room temperature should be maintained at 20-22°C and a warming mattress should be used along with skin temperature monitoring.

Induction

In the presence of pre-existing patent intravenous access, following pre-oxygenation, intravenous induction is performed with thiopentone 5-7mg/kg and succinylcholine 2mg/kg. Tracheal intubation is performed with an uncuffed tube (3-3.5mm size). Anaesthesia is maintained with oxygen, sevoflurane (or isoflurane), nitrous oxide and a non-depolarising muscle relaxant (e.g. atracurium 0.3-0.5mg/kg). Atropine 20µg/kg can be used at induction to obtund vagal reflexes.

IV fluids

0.45% saline in 5% dextrose at 4ml/kg/hour is used as maintenance fluid.

Analgesia

Paracetamol at a rectal loading dose of 30-40mg/kg, then 15-20mg/kg orally, 4-6 hourly, up to a maximum of 90mg/kg/day. The surgical wound is infiltrated with 0.25% bupivacaine at a dose not exceeding 2mg/kg. At the end of the procedure the muscle relaxant is reversed with neostigmine (50µg/kg) and glycopyrrolate (10µg/kg) and the child is extubated when fully awake.

Postoperative management

- Supplemental oxygen.
- Apnoea monitor for 6-12 hours.
- Gradual feeding commenced 12 hours postoperatively.
- Maintenance intravenous fluids continued until feeding is established to prevent hypoglycaemia.

Anatomy and physiology of neonates and infants

Infants differ from adults both anatomically and physiologically.

The respiratory system

Anatomically, infants have a large head, a short neck, a large tongue and a small mouth. They have narrow, easily blocked nasal passages. They are obligatory nose breathers, so that maintaining patency of nasal air passage is important. The epiglottis is floppy and U-shaped. The larynx is positioned higher than in the adult (at the level of C4 in a child, C5 in an adult). The narrowest part of the airway is at the level of the cricoid cartilage in children. In adults it is at the level of the vocal cords. The mucosal lining at the cricoid cartilage is pseudostratified ciliated epithelium which is loosely bound to areolar tissue. Any trauma can easily result in oedema. The trachea is short and this predisposes to endobronchial intubation. Infants have a limited ability to increase tidal volume because of a horizontal rib cage. In adults the bucket handle effect of the rib cage allows significant increase in the anteroposterior diameter. Children have a more compliant chest wall and relatively low FRC. They have a high metabolic rate. Oxygen consumption is two to three times higher in infants. On a ml/kg bodyweight basis, tidal volume is about the same as an adult, so the respiratory rate is two to three times faster. Due to a low FRC, they have less oxygen reserve, resulting in hypoxia and bradycardia during airway obstruction. The closing volume is relatively larger in infants and encroaches on the tidal volume. Atelectasis and hypoxia develop more easily than in an adult.

Cardiovascular system

The stroke volume is relatively fixed, therefore, cardiac output is dependent upon the heart rate. The cardiovascular response to hypoxia in neonates is bradycardia with pulmonary and systemic vasoconstriction.

Renal system

Renal blood flow and glomerular filtration rate are low in infants. Both fluid overload and dehydration is poorly tolerated in children.

Temperature control

Children have a large body surface area to weight ratio. The shivering mechanism is poorly developed. Peri-operative hypothermia is more likely and measures should be taken to prevent hypothermia.

Fluid management in infants

Fluid therapy can be divided into three parts:

◆ Replacement of any fluid deficit.
◆ Administration of maintenance fluid.
◆ Replacement of any losses.

The fluid used to replace the deficit should be isotonic fluid - such as 0.9% sodium chloride or Ringer lactate (Hartmann's) solution. Hypovolaemia should be corrected with an initial fluid bolus of 10-20ml/kg of an isotonic fluid or colloid, repeated as necessary as per the Advanced Paediatric Life Support (APLS) guideline. In severe blood loss, transfusion will be required.

The hourly requirement of maintenance fluid can be calculated using the 4-2-1 rule.

Table 1.7 Maintenance fluid: 4-2-1 rule.	
Weight	**Rate of intravenous fluid infusion**
10kg	4ml/kg/hour
11-20kg	40+ 2ml/kg/hour for every 1kg of weight over 10kg
>20kg	60+ 1ml/kg/hour for every 1kg weight over 20kg

During the intra-operative period the majority of children should be given fluids without dextrose. Blood glucose should be monitored if no dextrose is given. The maintenance fluid used during surgery should be isotonic, such as 0.9% sodium chloride or Ringer lactate/Hartmann's solution. Neonates in the first 48 hours of life should be given dextrose during surgery.

Third space loss is difficult to quantify and normally an estimate is made with 1-2ml/kg/hour given for superficial surgery, 4-7ml/kg/hr given for thoracotomy and 5-10ml/kg/hour given for abdominal surgery. Clinical signs such as heart rate, blood pressure and capillary refill time should be assessed to ensure adequate fluid replacement.

All losses during surgery should be replaced with an isotonic fluid such as 0.9% sodium chloride, Ringer lactate or Hartmann's solution, a colloid or a blood product, depending upon the child's haematocrit. In stable, critically ill children, a haemoglobin threshold of 7g/dl for red cell transfusion can decrease transfusion requirements without increasing adverse outcomes.

Key points

♦ Infantile pyloric stenosis usually presents at the 3rd to 5th week of life.
♦ The classical metabolic derangement is hypochloraemic, hypokalaemic, hyponatraemic metabolic alkalosis.
♦ All measures should be taken to correct acid base and electrolyte abnormalities prior to surgery.

Further reading

1. Fell D, Chelliah S. Infantile pyloric stenosis. *British Journal of Anaesthesia CEPD review* 2001; 1: 85-8.
2. APA consensus guideline on preoperative fluid management in children, 2007. http://www.apagbi.org.uk/docs/Perioperative_Fluid_Management_2007.pdf.

Short case 1.2: Difficult airway

You are asked to anaesthetise a patient for an elective laparoscopic cholecystectomy. After induction, initial laryngoscopy reveals an unexpectedly poor view of the larynx.

How would you grade the laryngoscopic view?

By using the Cormack and Lehane grading of laryngoscopic views:

♦ Grade 1: complete visualisation of vocal cords.
♦ Grade 2: only posterior portion of laryngeal aperture seen.

- Grade 3: only the epiglottis seen.
- Grade 4: not even the epiglottis seen.

You have a grade 3 view of the larynx in this patient. What can be done to improve the view?

Optimising the head and neck position, use of an optimum external laryngeal manoeuvre and use of an alternate laryngoscope blade can be helpful in improving the laryngoscopic view. The optimum head and neck position is achieved by extension of the neck at the atlanto-occipital joint and slight flexion of the neck on the chest.

The procedure of direct laryngscopy involves alignment of three anatomic axes: the laryngeal axis, the pharyngeal axis and the oral axis for the successful visualisation of glottic opening. The pharyngeal and laryngeal axes are brought into alignment with each other by flexion of the neck. The oral axis is brought into alignment with others by extension of the head. Flexion of the neck is achieved by elevating the head by about 10cm

Optimum external laryngeal manipulation or the BURP (backward, upward and right-sided pressure on the thyroid cartilage) manoeuvre should be applied to improve the laryngeal view. This is more successful when the laryngoscopist himself applies the pressure to determine the optimal direction, and then asks the assistant to perform the same manoeuvre. If these measures fail, a different laryngoscope should be used. The McCoy laryngoscope or a laryngoscope with a straight blade has been proven to help.

What properties would an 'ideal pillow' have for aiding intubation?

The pillow should elevate the head approximately 10cm above the table, should extend down to support the shoulders, and provide a 'sniffing the morning air' position; it should be mouldable to maintain stability.

Describe the McCoy laryngoscope

It is a long Macintosh blade with a distally hinged tip, operated by a lever adjacent to the laryngoscope handle. The lever when operated will provide vertical force to the epiglottis, lifting it out of the way of the vocal cords. This is of use when a large epiglottis obscures the cords. It can convert a Cormack and Lehane grade 3 view into a grade 2 view. It will not improve a grade 4 view.

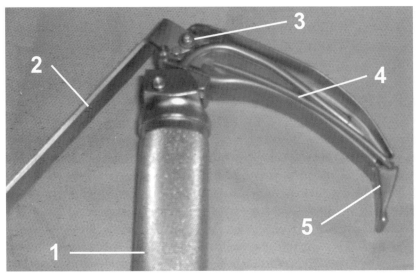

Figure 1.3 McCoy laryngoscope.
1. Laryngoscope handle; 2. Lever; 3. Spring-loaded drum; 4. Connecting shaft; 5. Hinged tip.

After optimum positioning and with a McCoy laryngsocope you have a grade 3 view. What adjunct would you choose to facilitate tracheal intubation?

A gum elastic bougie can be passed under the edge of the epiglottis into the trachea and the endotracheal tube is railroaded over the bougie. Presence of clicks as the bougie slides down the trachea over the tracheal rings or distal hold up and slight resistance at a distance of 45cm or coughing (if the patient is not fully paralysed) indicate the correct position of the bougie in the trachea.

With all of the above measures there is no improvement in the view. What would you do?

This is an unexpected failed intubation and it is important to summon for senior help. In the mean time, the primary aims should be:

◆   To provide oxygenation.
◆   To ensure hypnosis until the muscle relaxant effect wears off.

A bag and mask ventilation with 100% oxygen should be attempted. Inserting an oropharyngeal airway would be helpful. Having two persons, one to hold the mask and another to squeeze the bag, can make the ventilation more effective.

Plan B is then attempted with secondary tracheal intubation, which firstly involves insertion of a laryngeal mask airway (LMA) or intubating laryngeal mask airway (ILMA). After confirming adequate ventilation and oxygenation, tracheal intubation is attempted preferably guided through a fibreoptic scope. Intubation should only be attempted once.

You have inserted an ILMA and are able to ventilate but you have failed to intubate. What would you do next?

In this scenario surgery should be postponed, ventilation and oxygenation continued and anaesthesia should be maintained until the muscle relaxation wears off.

What would you do if you failed to oxygenate via an ILMA?

Revert back to face mask ventilation, preferably as a two-person technique using the oropharyngeal or nasopharyngeal airway and then the patient should be woken up.

What options are available at this stage if you are not able to ventilate and the patient desaturates?

This is a 'cannot intubate, cannot ventilate scenario'. If the patient continues to desaturate, resort to an emergency cricothyroidotomy.

How would you predict a difficult airway?

The possibility of a difficult airway can be predicted by the history, clinical examination and investigations:

◆ History: a previous history of a difficult airway, surgery or injury to the head and neck region, radiotherapy, history of snoring and obstructive sleep apnoea.

◆ Examination: anatomical abnormalities around the head and neck region, a short neck and obesity.

◆ Inter-incisor gap: with the mouth maximally open, the gap between the incisors. If this is <3cm, a difficult laryngoscopy is likely.

◆ Mandibular protrusion:
  - Class A - able to protrude the lower incisors anterior to the upper incisors;
  - Class B - lower incisors just reach the margin of the upper incisors;
  - Class C - lower incisors cannot protrude to the upper incisors.
  Classes B and C are associated with more risk of a difficult laryngoscopy.

◆ Thyromental distance (Patil test): the distance between the tip of the thyroid cartilage to the tip of the mandible, with the neck fully extended. If <6cm, this predicts a difficult laryngoscopy.

◆ Sternomental distance: the distance between the upper border of the manubrium to the tip of the mandible, with the neck fully extended and mouth closed. If <12.5cm, this predicts a difficult laryngoscopy.

◆ Movement of the cervical spine: flexion and extension movements of the cervical spine. With a finger on the patient's chin and the other one on the occipital protuberance, the head is extended maximally and the position of the chin in relation to the occipital protuberance is noted. If the chin is higher than the occipital protuberance, there is normal cervical spine mobility. If the two fingers are at the same level, there is moderate limitation of cervical spine mobility. If the chin is lower than the occipital protuberance, there is a severe limitation of cervical spine mobility.

What scoring systems do you know for predicting a difficult airway?

There are several scoring systems to assess a difficult airway, but none are reliable in predicting this and so they should be used in combination, as this provides a better overall assessment of the airway.

Modified Mallampati (with Samson and Young's modification)

The test is performed with the patient sitting opposite to the anaesthetist with their mouth open as wide as possible and the tongue protruded. Depending on the pharyngeal structures visualised, four classes are described:

◆ Class 1: faucial pillars, soft palate and the uvula are visible.
◆ Class 2: faucial pillars and soft palate are visible, but the base of the tongue masks the uvula.
◆ Class 3: only soft palate is visible.
◆ Class 4: even soft palate is not visible.

Classes 3 and 4 are associated with difficult intubation. The test is prone to inter-observer variation. The modified test has a sensitivity of 68% and specificity of 53% in predicting difficult intubation (laryngoscopic view of grades 3 or 4).

Wilson risk sum score

The Wilson risk sum score includes five risk factors (Table 1.8).

The total possible score is 10; a total score of >3 predicts 75% of difficult intubations; a total score of >4 predicts 90% of difficult intubations.

A combination of the above tests has a better predictive value. The modified Mallampati test, thyromental distance, ability to protrude the mandible and movement of the cervical spine are commonly used.

Table 1.8 Wilson risk sum score including five risk factors.

Risk factor		Score
Weight (kg)	<90	0
	90-110	1
	>110	2
Head and neck movement (degrees)	>90	0
	~90	1
	<90	2
Jaw movement	Incisor gap >5cm or subluxation >0	0
	Incisor gap <5cm and subluxation = 0	1
	Incisor gap <5cm and subluxation <0	2
Receding mandible	Normal	0
	Moderate	1
	Severe	2
Buck teeth	Normal	0
	Moderate	1
	Severe	2

What are the predictors of difficult bag and mask ventilation and oxygenation?

The five predictors of difficult bag and mask ventilation and oxygenation can be summarised in the word 'OBESE':

◆ Obese (body mass index >26kg/m^2).
◆ Bearded.
◆ Elderly.
◆ Snorers.
◆ Edentulous.

Guidelines for the management of unanticipated difficult intubation

The Difficult Airway Society guidelines for an unanticipated difficult intubation include a series of plans that can be implemented when a primary technique fails. The basic structure of flow charts contains:

◆ Plan A: initial tracheal intubation plan.
◆ Plan B: secondary tracheal intubation plan, when plan A has failed.
◆ Plan C: maintenance of oxygenation and ventilation, postponement of surgery and awakening the patient when earlier plans fail.
◆ Plan D: rescue techniques for a cannot intubate, cannot ventilate (CICV) scenario.

The progress of the above plans depends upon the nature of the clinical scenario. During initial tracheal intubation, optimum head and neck position, appropriate laryngoscopic technique and external laryngeal manipulation should be considered. The secondary tracheal intubation plan involves use of a dedicated airway device such as LMAs or ILMAs. When both plan A and plan B fail, ventilation and oxygenation should be continued with a dedicated airway device. It is important to avoid trauma to the airway. Elective surgery should be cancelled. If ventilation is impossible and serious hypoxaemia is developing, then plan D should be implemented.

Emergency cricothyroidotomy

Emergency cricothyroidotomy is performed in a CICV scenario to oxygenate the patient. The following are the three different techniques for emergency cricothyroidotomy.

Needle cricothyroidotomy and transtracheal jet ventilation

A 13G cricothyroidotomy cannula or a 14G venflon is commonly used. The small cannula (2-3mm internal diameter) has a high resistance, and needs a high pressure oxygen source to ventilate. A jet injector at 1-4 bar pressure (Sanders injector or VBM Manujet) is used. Exhalation is passive and must occur through the pharynx and larynx. Some degree of upper airway patency is essential to facilitate exhalation. In the case of complete airway obstruction, a second cannula through the cricothyroid membrane may be required to facilitate exhalation.

Large purpose made cannula with an internal diameter of 4mm or more

The lungs can be ventilated using an anaesthetic breathing system. Both cuffed and uncuffed versions of cannula-over-needle-type devices are available.

Surgical cricothyroidotomy: rapid four-step technique

This involves:

- Palpation of the cricothyroid membrane.
- Horizontal stab incision over the cricothyroid space.
- Traction with a tracheal hook. A scalpel handle inserted through the skin incision is then rotated 90°.
- Downward traction with a tracheal hook and intubation with a 6mm cuffed tracheostomy tube.

The early complications of cricothyroidotomy include bleeding, posterior tracheal wall perforation, pneumothorax, vocal cord injury, oesophageal perforation and failure of the procedure. The late complications are tracheal or subglottic stenosis, tracheo-oesophageal fistula, infection and tracheomalacia.

Key points

- History and clinical examination are important components of prediction of difficult intubation.
- Successful airway management requires a careful primary plan with an adequate back-up plan when the primary plan fails.
- During initial tracheal intubation, optimum head and neck position, the BURP manoeuvre and an alternate laryngoscope blade should be considered.
- A secondary tracheal intubation plan involves intubation through an LMA or ILMA, preferably using fibreoptic-assisted intubation.
- Failed intubation with increasing hypoxaemia and difficult mask ventilation requires an emergency cricothyroidotomy for rapid reoxygenation of the patient.

Further reading

1. Henderson JJ, *et al.* Difficult Airway Society guidelines for management of the unanticipated difficult intubation. *Anaesthesia* 2004; 59: 675-94.
2. Yentis SM. Predicting difficult intubation: worthwhile exercise or pointless ritual. *Anaesthesia* 2002; 57: 106-9.
3. Frerk CM. Predicting difficult intubation. *Anaesthesia* 1991; 46: 1005-8.
4. Samson GLT, Young JRB. Difficult tracheal intubation: a retrospective study. *Anaesthesia* 1987; 42: 487-90.
5. Wilson ME, *et al.* Predicting difficult intubation. *British Journal of Anaesthesia* 1988; 61: 211-6.
6. Patel B, Frerk C. Large-bore cricothyroidotomy devices. *British Journal of Anaesthesia CEACCP* 2008; 8: 157-60.

Short case 1.3: Tension pnuemothorax

A 56-year-old trumpeter collapsed while playing at a concert. On arrival at the emergency department he appears pale and breathless. A chest X-ray has been taken. His pulse is 110/minute, BP is 82/61mm Hg, SpO_2 is 89% and the GCS is 14/15.

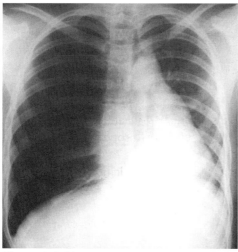

Figure 1.4 Chest X-ray.

What is your diagnosis?

The patient is tachycardic, hypoxic and hypotensive. The chest X-ray shows a right-sided tension pneumothorax with a shift of the mediastinum to the left side.

How would you classify pneumothoraces?

Free gas, usually air, within the pleural cavity is called a pneumothorax. It can be classified based on whether the gas is under tension or not.

A simple pneumothorax occurs where gas is not under tension, which can be an open simple pneumothorax (the communication between the gas source and pleura still persists) or a closed simple pneumothorax (the communication between the gas source and the pleura has closed off).

A tension pneumothorax occurs where gas is under tension as the flow of gas within the pleural cavity is unidirectional and a valve effect prevents its release. The tension may cause a mediastinal shift.

What are the possible mechanisms by which a pneumothorax can occur?

There are three possible mechanisms by which a pneumothorax can occur:

◆ Damage to the parietal pleura: chest trauma causing an open chest wound, during central venous cannulation and during operative procedures such as nephrectomy, tracheostomy, laparoscopy.
◆ Damage to the visceral pleura: fractured ribs, spontaneous rupture of the emphysematous bullae, during central venous cannulation, during regional anaesthetic procedures such as interscalene supraclavicular, intercostal and paravertebral nerve blocks.
◆ Intrapulmonary rupture: high inflation pressures during positive pressure ventilation or high pressure jet ventilation, severe cough and in chronic lung diseases such as asthma.

Explain the pathophysiology underlying a tension pneumothorax

Lung, chest wall injury or rupture of an emphysematous bulla, may result in a one-way valve effect. With each breath, more gas moves into the pleural cavity which ultimately results in an increase in intrathoracic pressure and compression of structures. Compression of the great veins leads to reduced venous return and cardiac filling, resulting in tachycardia and hypotension. Collapse of one lung will also create a large shunt with a percentage of blood passing through the lung without taking up oxygen. This leads to decreased oxygen saturation as the deoxygenated blood mixes with oxygenated blood. Hypotension and hypoxaemia may lead to a reduced conscious level.

How would you treat a tension pneumothorax?

It is a life-threatening emergency and the gas under tension in the pleural cavity needs to be released urgently.

Treatment of a tension pneumothorax involves:

- Circulatory support with intravenous fluid and vasopressor drugs.
- Decompression of the pneumothorax by inserting a large-bore cannula at the second intercostal space in the mid-clavicular line.
- A chest drain must be inserted following needle thoracocentesis.

Once the intrathoracic pressure is reduced, venous return increases which increases cardiac output and improves gas exchange.

Describe how you would insert a chest drain

The patient is positioned in the supine position with their arm on the side of the lesion behind the patient's head to expose the axillary region.

The drain insertion site is in the mid-axillary line through the 'safe triangle'. This is a triangle bordered by the anterior border of latissimus dorsi, the lateral border of the pectoralis major muscle, a line superior to the horizontal level of the nipple, and the apex below the axilla.

An aseptic technique should be employed and local anaesthetic should be infiltrated into the site of insertion of the drain. The skin should be incised over the upper border of the lower rib to avoid injury to the neurovascular bundle which runs along the inner aspect of the lower border of the rib. Although a rigid trochar is provided along with the chest drain tube, its use should be avoided as it increases the likelihood of injury to the lung. After incising the skin and deep tissues, blunt dissection is achieved using artery forceps. Once the pleura is punctured, a finger tip should be inserted to sweep the lung away from the insertion site. The chest drain tubes have side holes to facilitate drainage and a radio-opaque line so that the position can be checked using a chest X-ray.

The tip of the chest drain should be aimed apically for a pneumothorax and basally for fluid. Two sutures are usually inserted: a closure suture to assist later closure of the wound after the drain removal and a stay suture to secure the drain. The drain should be connected to a drainage system which allows unidirectional flow, e.g. an underwater seal bottle or a flutter valve. A chest X-ray should be performed post-insertion.

What are the physical principles of draining air or fluid from the pleural cavity?

Air in the pleural space is moist and flow is turbulent. Flow depends on the Fanning equation:

$$Flow = \pi r^5 P / fl$$

where r = radius, P = pressure gradient, f = frictional factor, l = length.

What pressure gradient decides the flow?

$$Flow = P/R$$

where R = resistance and P = pleural pressure - pressure in the underwater seal collection system. It is the pressure gradient between pleural pressure and pressure in the underwater seal device.

What are the features of an underwater seal device?

The chest drain is usually attached to a drainage system which allows only one direction of flow. This is usually the underwater seal bottle (Figure 1.5) and it should have the following features:

♦ The tube must be wide enough to minimise resistance.
♦ The total volume of the water in the bottle should be more than the volume of the drainage tube so that with maximum negative pressure, despite water being sucked in the tube, there is enough in the bottle to maintain an underwater seal.
♦ The tube should be approximately 3cm below the surface of the water. If it is more than 5cm, it increases the resistance to air or fluid escaping from the pleural cavity.
♦ The bottle should be at least 45cm below the level of the patient's chest. Water may be drawn into the pleural cavity during maximal negative inspiratory effort if it is more close to the patient.
♦ The chest drain bottle should always be kept below the level of the patient. If suction is required, a low pressure high volume suction (-10 to -20cm H_2O) should be used. It should only be used for a non-resolving pneumothorax.

In a single-bottle system, as the chamber is filled with fluid or blood, the resistance increases. In haemopneumothorax, a two or three-bottle system is used. In a two-bottle system, the first bottle acts as a collection chamber and the second bottle acts as an underwater seal. The disadvantage of this system is that the air in the fluid trap forms an extension of the patient's pleural space and increases the total air dead space. This reduces the drainage efficiency and may impede re-expansion of the lung. Applying negative pressure to the collection chamber will increase the pressure difference between the pleural space and the collection chamber. The safest method of regulating suction pressure is to add a control bottle between the underwater seal and suction device. In a three- bottle system, the first bottle acts as a collection chamber, the second bottle acts as an underwater seal and the third bottle is used for suction control.

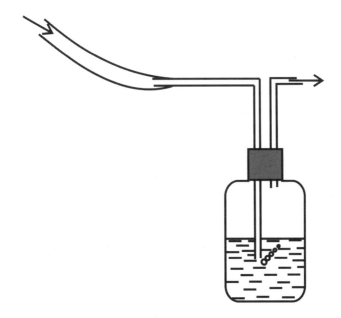

Figure 1.5 Single-bottle underwater seal system.

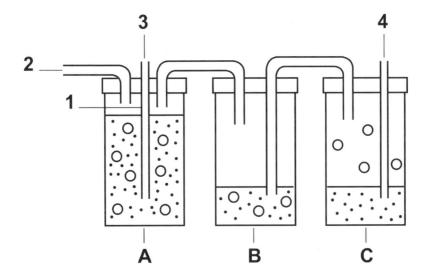

Figure 1.6 Three-bottle underwater seal system.
A. Suction control bottle; B. Underwater seal bottle; C. Fluid trap.
1. Control tube; 2. Suction attachment; 3. Air inlet; 4. Chest drain tube inlet.

Indications for insertion of a chest drain

According to British Thoracic Society (BTS) guidelines, a chest drain may be helpful in the following settings:

◆ Pneumothorax in any ventilated patient.
◆ Tension pneumothorax after initial needle thoracocentesis.
◆ Persistent or recurrent pneumothorax after simple aspiration.
◆ Large secondary spontaneous pneumothorax in patients over 50 years.
◆ Malignant pleural effusion.
◆ Empyema and complicated parapneumonic pleural effusion.
◆ Traumatic haemopneumothorax.
◆ Postoperative - thoracotomy, oesophagectomy, cardiac surgery.

Complications of chest drain insertion

◆ Visceral injury: laceration of lung, liver, pericardium, heart.
◆ Injury to intercostal vessels and nerve.
◆ Haemothorax.
◆ Subcutaneous emphysema.
◆ Infection.
◆ Incorrect tube position, kinking of tube, tube blockage.

Key points

◆ A tension pneumothorax results in hypoxia and severe hypotension.
◆ Treatment of a tension pneumothorax includes immediate needle thoracocentesis followed by insertion of a chest drain.

Further reading

1. Kam AC, O'Brien M, Kam PCA. Pleural drainage systems. *Anaesthesia* 1993; 48: 154-61.
2. Laws D, Neville E, Duffy. BTS Guidelines for the insertion of a chest drain. *Thorax* 2003; 58: ii53.

Applied anatomy 1.1: Anatomy for ophthalmic anaesthesia

A 75-year-old lady is to undergo cataract surgery to her left eye. She has a past medical history of angina and insulin-dependent diabetes mellitus for which she is on appropriate therapy.

What types of regional anaesthetic blocks can you use to provide adequate anaesthesia for cataract surgery?

- ◆ Peribulbar block.
- ◆ Sub-Tenon's block.
- ◆ Retrobulbar block.
- ◆ Subconjunctival infiltration.
- ◆ Topical corneoconjunctival anaesthesia.

Describe the anatomy of the orbital cavity, extra-ocular muscles of the eye and their nerve supply

The bony orbit contains the eye and the extra-ocular muscles of the eye. It is pyramidal in shape with the base at the front and apex pointing towards the middle cranial fossa. The orbit is separated into two major compartments, the intraconal space and the extraconal space. The intraconal space is bounded by four rectus muscles, extends from the annulus of Zinn at the orbital apex to their penetration through the Tenon's capsule. The extraconal space is outside the muscle cone within the bony orbit.

The margins of the orbit are:

- ◆ Roof: orbital plate of the frontal bone.
- ◆ Floor: maxilla and zygoma.
- ◆ Medial: frontal process of the maxilla and lacrimal bone (anterior); orbital plate of the ethmoid and body of the sphenoid (posterior).
- ◆ Lateral: zygoma and greater wing of the sphenoid.

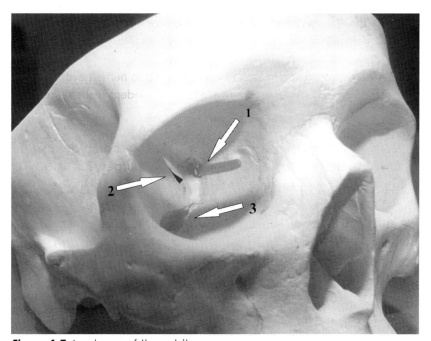

Figure 1.7 Anatomy of the orbit.
1. Optic foramen; 2. Superior orbital fissure; 3. Inferior orbital fissure.

The orbit has three openings: the superior and inferior orbital fissures and the optic canal.

The superior orbital fissure carries the lacrimal, frontal, nasociliary (branches of the ophthalmic division of the trigeminal nerve), oculomotor, trochlear, abducens nerves and superior ophthalmic vein. Lacrimal, frontal and trochlear (LFT) nerves lie outside the muscle cone.

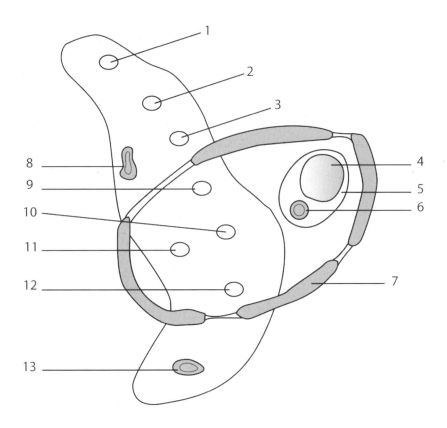

Figure 1.8 Contents of the superior orbital fissure.
1. Lacrimal nerve; 2. Frontal nerve; 3. Trochlear nerve; 4. Optic nerve; 5. Optic foramen; 6. Ophthalmic artery; 7. Ring formed by muscle tendons; 8. Superior ophthalmic vein; 9. Superior oculomotor nerve; 10. Nasociliary nerve; 11. Abducens nerve; 12. Inferior oculomotor nerve; 13. Inferior ophthalmic vein.

The contents of the inferior orbital fissure carries the maxillary division of the trigeminal nerve, inferior ophthalmic vein and infra-orbital artery.

The contents of the optic canal transmits the optic nerve and the ophthalmic artery.

The eye globe occupies the anterior part of the orbit and normally has an axial length of 24mm (20-25mm). In myopic individuals it is usually elongated (more than 26mm). The globe has three layers: the innermost is made up of neural tissue-retina; the middle layer is the vascular layer and contains choroid, ciliary body and the iris; and the outermost layer of cornea and sclera. Tenon's capsule is a thin layer which encapsulates the globe and extends all the way from the optic nerve to fuse with the conjunctiva anteriorly.

Tenon's capsule invests the globe and extra-ocular muscles in the anterior central orbit. It extends from the corneal limbus anteriorly to the optic nerve posteriorly. Anteriorly it is penetrated by the four rectus muscles and by two oblique muscles, prior to their insertion to the sclera.

Extra-ocular muscles

There are six extra-ocular muscles which help to control the movements of the eye: four rectus muscles (superior, inferior, lateral and medial) and two oblique muscles (superior and inferior obliques). The rectus muscles congregate at the apex of the orbit to form a fibrotendinous ring, the annulus of Zinn. Bands of connective tissues merge with the extra-ocular muscles to form the cone in which the sensory supply to the globe is embedded.

Nerve supply

- The motor nerve supply to the extra-ocular muscles is by the third, fourth and sixth cranial nerves.
- Lateral rectus is supplied by the abducens nerve (sixth cranial nerve).
- Superior oblique is supplied by the trochlear nerve (fourth cranial nerve).
- Superior, inferior and medial rectus, and inferior oblique are supplied by the oculomotor nerve (third cranial nerve).

N.B. A mnemonic is LR6 SO4.

- Sensory innervation to the eye is by supratrochlear and lacrimal branches of the ophthalmic division of the trigeminal nerve (fifth cranial nerve).
- Autonomic innervations are via the parasympathetic supply from the Edinger Westphal nucleus, accompanying the third cranial nerve to the synapse with the short ciliary nerves in the ciliary ganglion.
- The sympathetic fibres are from the first thoracic sympathetic outflow, synapses in the superior cervical ganglion before joining the long and short ciliary nerves.

Which nerve supplies levator palpebrae superioris?

Superior branch of the oculomotor nerve.

Describe the procedure of peribulbar block

- Preparation includes explanation to the patient, local anaesthetic agents, equipment check, intravenous access and monitoring (oxygen saturation, ECG and non-invasive blood pressure).
- Contraindications include anticoagulation with an INR >2.5, an axial length >26mm (sausage-shaped eyeball in severely myopic patients), infection of the eye and when the patient is unable to lie flat or still.
- A local anaesthetic mixture with 5ml of 0.75% bupivacaine, 75 units of hyaluronidase and 5ml of 1% lignocaine with 1:200,000 epinephrine is commonly used.
- Topical anaesthesia is achieved by applying benoxinate or amethocaine solution on the conjuctiva.
- With the patient lying supine ask the patient to look straight ahead and focus on a point on the ceiling.
- Inferolateral injection is performed at the junction of the medial two-thirds and lateral third of the inferior orbital rim. Just lateral to the groove on the inferior orbital rim and 1mm above the orbital rim, a needle (25G, 25mm) is inserted either through the conjunctival reflection or percutaneously. 5-6ml of local anaesthetic is injected after careful aspiration while trying to assess the globe tension by the other hand. Following injection, light pressure is applied to the eye with a soft pad or compression device (Honan balloon) to dissipate the local anaesthetic solution.

◆ Medial injection: at times a second injection is needed to provide a greater degree of akinesia. A needle is passed through the conjunctiva in the medial canthus, medial to the caruncle and directed straight back parallel to the medial wall of the orbit pointing 20° cephalad until the hub of the needle is at the level of the iris. 4-5ml of local anaesthetic is injected.

What nerves would you block with inferolateral injection?

This blocks the ophthalmic division branches (nasociliary, lacrimal, frontal, supra-orbital and supratrochlear branches) and the maxillary division branches (infra-orbital branch) of the 5th cranial nerve (trigeminal).

What nerves would you block with medial injection?

This blocks the nasociliary nerve, long ciliary nerve, infratrochlear and supra-orbital nerve.

Why is pressure applied and how much pressure is used?

After injecting the local anaesthetic solution, the eye is closed and pressure is applied for 10 minutes. This is to lower intra-ocular pressure by reducing aqueous humour production and increase its reabsorption and to dissipate the local anaesthetic

What are the signs of a successful block?

◆ Ptosis.
◆ Akinesia of the eye.
◆ Inability to close the eye once opened.

What are the complications of peribulbar block?

◆ Intravascular injection.
◆ Anaphylaxis.
◆ Haemorrhage.
◆ Penetration/perforation of the globe.
◆ Central spread of local anaesthetic via the dural cuff accompanying the optic nerve.

- Oculocardiac reflex.
- Penetration of the optic nerve sheath causing optic nerve atrophy.

Who is more likely to get a globe perforation?

Normally the eye has an axial length of 24mm (20-25mm). In myopic individuals it is usually elongated (more than 26mm) and they are predisposed to thin-walled protuberances of the scleral wall which can be perforated during the peribulbar block. Myopic patients are therefore more prone to perforation.

What is the oculocardiac reflex?

Bradycardia following traction on the eye, especially the medial rectus or due to pressure on the globe. It is particularly active in children. In some instances the bradycardia may cause asystole. It usually resolves immediately after the stimulus is removed

What is the mechanism for oculocardiac reflex?

Afferent impulses travel via the long and short ciliary nerves, via the ciliary ganglion, to the trigeminal (gasserian) ganglion through which the sensory fibres pass. Efferent impulses pass via the vagus nerve to the sino-atrial node.

How can it be treated?

- Stop the surgery.
- Relieve pressure on the globe and release traction on the extra-ocular muscles.
- Atropine or glycopyrrolate should be administered.

It may be prevented by avoiding pressure on the globe, the use of prophylactic anti-emetics, giving pre-operative anticholinergic drugs such as atropine, avoiding opioids and avoiding hypercapnia, hypoxia and light levels of anaesthesia.

Eye blocks

In retrobulbar block, the needle is inserted into the intraconal space behind the globe. As the local anaesthetic is deposited close to the motor and sensory nerves, a small volume (1.5-4ml) of local anaesthetic is adequate to produce a satisfactory block.

In peribulbar block, the needle is placed outside the muscle cone, further away from the apex. A larger volume of local anaesthetic (6-10ml) is required to produce satisfactory block.

In sub-Tenon's block, Tenon's capsule is elevated from the sclera and local anaesthetic is deposited into the sub-Tenon's space (episcleral space). The sub-Tenon's space is accessed by dissecting at the inferonasal quadrant. After topical anaesthesia to the conjunctiva using amethocaine or benoxinate, the patient is asked to look upwards and outwards. A fold of conjunctiva is drawn upwards at the inferonasal quadrant with forceps. A small incision at the base of the fold with surgical scissors creates access to the sub-Tenon's space. A blunt cannula is then inserted into the space and directed backwards following the contour of the globe. 3-5ml of local anaesthetic solution is injected.

Complications related to ophthalmic regional block are:

- Retrobulbar haemorrhage.
- Subconjuctival haemorrhage.
- Subconjuctival oedema (chemosis).
- Optic nerve damage.
- Globe perforation.
- Intravascular injection.
- Central spread of local anaesthetic with clinical features including drowsiness, vomiting, convulsions and cardio-respiratory arrest.
- Oculocardiac reflex due to traction on the eye, rapid distension of tissues by local anaesthetic or by haemorrhage.

Key points

- The optic nerve, ophthalmic artery and central retinal vein pass through the optic foramen.
- The lacrimal, frontal and trochlear (LFT) nerves pass through the superior orbital fissure and lie outside the muscle cone.
- The inferior orbital fissure transmits the infra-orbital nerve, infra-orbital artery and infra-orbital vein.
- The motor nerve supply to the extra-ocular muscles is by the third, fourth and sixth cranial nerves. A mnemonic is LR6 SO4.

Further reading

1. Johnson RW. Anatomy for ophthalmic anaesthesia. *British Journal of Anaesthesia* 1995; 75: 80-7.
2. Hamilton RC. Techniques of orbital regional anaesthesia. *British Journal of Anaesthesia* 1995; 75: 88-92.
3. Varvinski AM, Eltringham R. Anaesthesia for ophthalmic surgery. *Update in Anaesthesia* 1996; 6(3). (http://www.nda.ox.ac.uk/wfsa/html/u06/u06_012.htm).

Applied physiology 1.2: Pulmonary vascular resistance

A 52-year-old male patient is admitted to undergo elective cholecystectomy. He has been a heavy smoker in the past. His lung function tests are suggestive of moderate to severe obstructive airway disease. On cardiac catheterisation his pulmonary vascular resistance (PVR) is calculated to be at 320 dynes.s.cm^{-5}.

Can you comment on the pulmonary vascular resistance of this patient?

The normal PVR is 100-200 dynes.s.cm^{-5}. This patient has a high PVR. This could be due to hypoxia, hypercapnia and acidosis associated with his chronic obstructive airway disease.

What are the factors affecting pulmonary vascular resistance?

Pulmonary vascular resistance is the relationship between the pulmonary driving pressure and cardiac output:

$$PVR = 80 \times (MPAP - PCWP) / CO$$

where MPAP = mean pulmonary arterial pressure, PCWP = pulmonary capillary wedge pressure, CO = cardiac output.

Table 1.9 Vascular resistance range.	
Measurement	**Reference range**
Systemic vascular resistance	900-1200 dynes.s.cm^{-5}
Pulmonary vascular resistance	100-200 dynes.s.cm^{-5}

Factors affecting PVR

There are passive and active factors that control PVR. Pulmonary vascular resistance is influenced by passive factors such as alveolar pressure and volume.

Effect of lung volume
PVR is lowest at lung volume close to FRC and increases with low or high lung volumes. At high lung volumes, the alveolar capillaries are compressed and PVR increases. At low lung volumes, compression of corner capillaries (the capillaries that lie within the junction between three or more alveoli) and extra-alveolar capillaries results in increased PVR.

Active factors
There are several mechanisms that control PVR. Pulmonary vasculature is normally kept in a state of active vasodilatation:

♦ Hypoxia increases PVR.
♦ Acidosis and hypercapnia increase PVR.

- Alkalosis and hypocapnia reduce PVR.
- Vasodilator drugs such as nitric oxide, prostacyclin, ACE inhibitors and phopshodiesterase inhibitors decrease PVR.
- Sympathetic stimulation increases PVR.
- Parasympathetic stimulation decreases PVR.
- Catecholamines such as epinephrine and related inotropes such as dopamine increase PVR.
- Histamine relaxes the pulmonary vascular smooth muscle, whereas serotonin (5-HT) is a potent vasoconstrictor.

What is hypoxic pulmonary vasoconstriction (HPV) and what is the mechanism?

Reduced partial pressure of oxygen in the alveoli (PAO_2 <9kPa) causes reflex vasoconstriction of pulmonary arterioles. It occurs rapidly, within seconds of a decrease in PAO_2. It is significant during one lung ventilation. In left ventricular failure it may cause vasoconstriction in the bases and divert the blood flow to upper lobes away from the hypoxic basal area. It is a biphasic phenomenon: in the first phase there is return of the pulmonary vascular resistance to baseline and the second phase which is usually slower and is characterised by a much sustained vasoconstriction.

The exact mechanism is unknown but it may involve the release of chemical mediators. It is not neurally mediated since it occurs in denervated isolated lungs. Nitric oxide contributes to the normal vasodilatation of pulmonary vasculature; reduced nitric oxide production secondary to hypoxia will lead to vasoconstriction. Hypoxia may stimulate production of endothelin, a vasoconstrictor peptide. Hypoxia may alter the response of oxygen-sensitive potassium channels and lead to opening of calcium channels which results in smooth muscle contraction. Cyclo-oxygenase activity is inhibited by hypoxia, which may diminish the effects of vasodilator products such as prostacyclin.

The mechanism of hypoxic pulmonary vasoconstriction is multi-factorial and most likely results from a combination of the direct effect of hypoxia on smooth muscle modulated by endothelium-dependent factors.

Are there any benefits of HPV?

Hypoxic vasoconstriction is beneficial as it improves the match between perfusion and ventilation by diverting flow from poorly ventilated areas to better ventilated areas. It maintains this balance of ventilation to perfusion on a breath to breath basis.

What happens to PVR in a neonate soon after birth?

During transition from fetal to neonatal circulation, the first breath increases alveolar PO_2 and is partially responsible for the decreased PVR at birth.

What are the effects of general anaesthesia on HPV?

Intravenous anaesthetics have generally been found to have no effect on HPV, except for ketamine which increases the PVR.

Inhaled anaesthetics have been reported to inhibit HPV in a variety of *in vitro* experimental preparations. For example, in isolated rat lungs, *in vitro*, halothane, enflurane, and isoflurane inhibit HPV. In more intact animal preparations and in patients, a concentration of more than one minimal alveolar concentration (MAC) is needed to inhibit HPV.

Which pulmonary vessels (size of the vessel) are responsible for HPV?

Hypoxic vasoconstriction mainly occurs in small pre-capillary arterioles but small pulmonary veins also constrict in response to hypoxia, although not more than 20% of the total change in PVR.

What is the clinical application of pulmonary vasodilatotors?

Pulmonary vasodilators, such as nitric oxide and prostacyclin, are used for correction of hypoxaemia in patients with acute respiratory distress syndrome (ARDS) to vasodilate the most healthy well ventilated lung regions.

What is the dose of nitric oxide?

It is usually started at a dose of 5-6ppm. If no response is recorded, the dose may be increased gradually to a maximum dose of 80ppm. The normal dose used throughout treatment is between 5-20ppm. When the maximum dose is achieved and no response is noted, then the patient is discontinued from this course of therapy and is considered a non-responder to inhaled nitric oxide.

What are the complications of inhaled nitric oxide?

Nitric oxide in the presence of oxygen will, in most instances, combine to become nitrogen dioxide (NO_2). High levels of NO_2 have produced pulmonary oedema when extremely high doses of inhaled nitric oxide are used. For this reason the monitoring of NO/NO_2 is very important. Nitric oxide has been found to have an affinity for haemoglobin that is 280 times greater than carbon monoxide; therefore, continuous monitoring is essential. High levels of methaemoglobin can potentially interfere with tissue oxygen delivery and result in hypoxia. One other potential complication is the possible effect on coagulation caused by decreased platelet aggregation.

Pulmonary vascular resistance (PVR)

PVR is controlled by both passive and active factors. Lung volume is one important passive factor that determines pulmonary vascular resistance. PVR is lowest at lung volume close to FRC and increases both at low and high lung volumes. If alveolar pressure rises, capillaries tend to be squashed and their resistance increases. At high altitude, hypoxic pulmonary vasoconstriction increases PVR.

There are several substances that act on various receptors in the pulmonary vasculature to control the vascular tone. Substances known to increase pulmonary vascular resistance include serotonin and

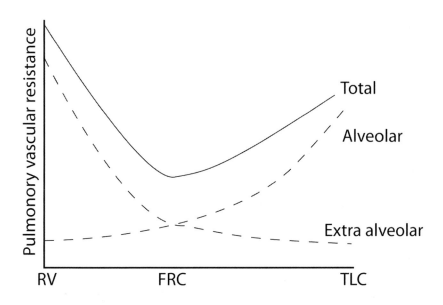

Figure 1.9 Pulmonary vascular resistances in relation to lung volume.

norepinephrine. Substances known to relax pulmonary vascular smooth muscle include isoproterenol, nitric oxide, prostacyclin and acetylcholine. Inhaled nitric oxide and prostacyclin (PGI$_2$) reduce PVR and increase alveolar perfusion in the ventilated regions of the lung. This improves the VA/Q (VA = alveolar ventilation, Q = perfusion) matching by a redistribution of perfusion to the lung regions with better ventilation and increases the PaO$_2$.

Table 1.10 Effects of various substances on pulmonary vascular resistance.

Substance	Receptor group	Effect
Epinephrine	Beta 2	Dilatation
Norepinephrine	Alpha 2	Dilatation
Acetylcholine	M3 cholinergic	Dilatation
Histamine	H2	Dilatation
Prostacyclin	-	Dilatation
Substance P	NK1	Dilatation
Vasopressin	V1	Dilatation
Bradykinin	B2	Dilatation
Angiotensin	AT	Constriction
Neurokinin A	NK2	Constriction
Norepinephrine	Alpha 1	Constriction
Thromboxane A_2	-	Constriction

Key points

- PVR is lowest at lung volume close to FRC.
- Hypoxia, hypercapnia and acidosis associated with chronic obstructive airway disease, increase PVR.
- Hypoxic vasoconstriction is beneficial as it improves the match between perfusion and ventilation in the lungs.
- The mechanism of hypoxic pulmonary vasoconstriction is multifactorial; a combination of the direct effect of hypoxia on smooth muscle and modulation by endothelium-dependent factors.

Further reading

1. Yuan JXJ. *Hypoxic pulmonary vasoconstriction: cellular and molecular mechanisms.* Springer, 2004.

Applied pharmacology 1.3: Calcium channel blockers

A 65-year-old male patient, scheduled for an inguinal hernia repair, was diagnosed to be hypertensive at the pre-operative assessment clinic. He has never been on any medication. His blood pressure is 180/100mm Hg.

What is the drug of choice for initiating antihypertensive therapy?

The NICE guidelines state that a calcium channel blocker (nifedipine or amlodipine) or a thiazide diuretic is the drug of choice for initial therapy.

What are the other indications for the use of calcium channel blockers?

- Angina.
- Migraine.
- Prevention of vasospasm in subarachnoid haemorrhage.
- Arrhythmias (certain supraventricular arrhythmias).
- Raynaud's syndrome.
- Pulmonary hypertension.

How do they work and what is the mechanism of action?

There are numerous calcium channels across the cell and other membranes. They are either triggered by chemical mediators (ligand-gated calcium channels) or voltage changes (voltage-gated calcium channels). Calcium channel blockers (CCBs) work by blocking L-type voltage-gated calcium channels while leaving T-, N- and P-type calcium channels unaffected. There is variable affinity of CCBs for the L-type channels in myocardial, vascular smooth muscle and nodal tissue and this results in variable effects. This reduces calcium levels in the cells, leading to less muscle contraction.

In the heart, a decrease in calcium causes slowing of the conduction of action potentials at the sino-atrial (SA) and atrioventricular (AV) nodes, resulting in reduced heart rate and contractility.

In the blood vessels, a decrease in calcium results in less contraction of the vascular smooth muscle and therefore an increase in vasodilation.

Vasodilation decreases total peripheral resistance, while a decrease in cardiac contractility decreases output. Since blood pressure is determined by cardiac output and peripheral resistance, blood pressure drops. With a relatively low blood pressure, the afterload on the heart decreases; this decreases the amount of oxygen demand. This can help ameliorate symptoms of ischaemic heart disease such as chest pain.

How do they differ from beta-blockers?

Unlike beta-blockers, calcium channel blockers do not decrease the responsiveness of the heart to input from the sympathetic nervous system. Since moment-to-moment blood pressure regulation is carried out by the sympathetic nervous system (via the baroreceptor reflex), calcium channel blockers allow blood pressure to be maintained more effectively than by beta-blockers.

How are calcium channel blockers classified?

There are three main groups of calcium channel blockers:

- Dihydropyridine - nifedipine and amlodipine. Dihydropyridine calcium channel blockers are often used to reduce systemic vascular resistance (SVR) and hypertension. They are not used to treat angina because vasodilation and hypotension can lead to reflex tachycardia.
- Phenylalkylamine - verapamil. Phenylalkylamine calcium channel blockers are relatively selective for myocardium, reducing myocardial oxygen demand and reversing coronary vasospasm, and are often used to treat angina. They have minimal vasodilatory effects compared with dihydropyridines.
- Benzothiazepine - diltiazem. Benzothiazepine calcium channel blockers are an intermediate class between phenylalkylamine and dihydropyridines in their selectivity for vascular calcium channels. They have both cardiac depressant and vasodilator actions. They are able to reduce arterial pressure without producing the same degree of reflex cardiac stimulation caused by dihydropyridines.

Table 1.11 Cardiovascular effects of calcium channel blockers.

	Nifedipine	Verapamil	Diltiazem
Reduction in SVR	+ + +	+ +	+
Coronary vasodilatation	+ +	+ +	+
Reduction in contractility	+	+ +	0
Reduction in blood pressure	+ +	+	0
Reflex increase in sympathetic tone	+ +	+	0
Slowing of AV nodal conduction	0	+ + +	+ +

What are the side effects of calcium channel blockers?

Calcium channel blockers have the following four cardiovascular effects:

◆ Peripheral vasodilatation.
◆ Negative chronotropy (decreased heart rate).
◆ Negative inotropy (decreased cardiac contractility).
◆ Negative dromotropy (decreased cardiac conduction).

Because of these actions it can lead to various degrees of heart block or cardiac failure.

Other side effects include:

◆ Flushing.
◆ Headache.
◆ Palpitations - reflecting the reflex tachycardia in response to vasodilatation.
◆ Pedal oedema - dilatation of the precapillary 'sphincters' and not generally a reflection of worsening heart failure.

Name some other drugs that may interact with calcium channel blockers

Calcium channel blockers may interact with a number of other drugs:

◆ Diuretics may cause enhanced hypotensive effects when given with calcium channel blockers.
◆ Beta-blockers taken along with calcium channel blockers may increase the effects of both drugs; they can cause worsening of cardiac failure and may cause severe hypotension.
◆ Digoxin with calcium channel blockers may increase the plasma concentration of digoxin.
◆ Carbamazepine may cause a reduction in the effect of calcium channel blockers.
◆ Cyclosporine may increase the plasma concentration of some calcium channel blockers.
◆ Grapefruit juice may increase the effects of some calcium channel blockers by increasing its plasma concentration.

Antihypertensive drugs

Antihypertensive drugs can be classified based on their site and mechanism of action:

◆ Thiazide and loop diuretics reduce the extracellular fluid volume. Thiazide diuretics also produce peripheral vasodilatation.
◆ Vasodilators act on the smooth muscle either directly or indirectly. Direct acting vasodilators include hydralazine and sodium nitroprusside. Beta-blockers with selective properties (acebetalol, atenolol, metoprolol) bind to beta1 receptors in the heart and non-selective beta-blockers (propranolol, labetolol) bind both to beta1 receptors in the heart and beta2 receptors in the vascular and bronchial smooth muscles. Calcium channel blockers produce arteriolar vasodilatation.
◆ Angiotension-converting enzyme inhibitors, such as captopril, enalapril and lisinopril, prevent the conversion of angiotensin I to angiotensin II.
◆ Angiotensin II receptor antagonists, such as valsartan and irbesartan, block the angiotensin1 (AT1) receptors.

◆ Alpha1 adrenergic receptor antagonists, such as prazosin, terazocin and doxazocin, produce vasodilatation of both arterial and venous vasculature by inhibiting the activation of alpha adrenoreceptors by catecholamines.

◆ Centrally acting drugs include methyldopa and clonidine, reduce sympathetic activity.

NICE guidance on antihypertensive therapy

In hypertensive patients aged 55 or older or black patients of any age, the first choice for initial therapy should be either a calcium channel blocker or a thiazide-type diuretic. For this recommendation, black patients are considered to be those of African or Caribbean descent, not mixed-race, Asian or Chinese.

In hypertensive patients younger than 55, the first choice for initial therapy should be an angiotensin-converting enzyme (ACE) inhibitor (or an angiotensin-II receptor antagonist if an ACE inhibitor is not tolerated).

Key points

◆ Calcium channel blockers have wide clinical application, most important of which is use as an antihypertensive agent.

◆ They exert their action by blocking L-type calcium channels.

◆ They cause peripheral vasodilatation, decrease heart rate, decrease cardiac contractility and decrease cardiac conduction.

Further reading

1. NICE clinical guideline 34: Hypertension: management of hypertension in adults in primary care. http://www.nice.org.uk/nicemedia/pdf/CG034NICEguideline.pdf.

2. British Hypertension Society recommendations for combining blood pressure lowering drugs. Better blood pressure control: how to combine drugs. *Journal of Human Hypertension* 2003; 17: 81-6.

Equipment, clinical measurement and monitoring 1.4: Ayre's T-piece

An 8-month-old boy weighing 9kg is scheduled for a herniotomy.

What breathing systems would you use?

In an infant weighing 9kg the following breathing systems can be used:

◆ The most commonly used breathing system is an Ayre's T-piece with a Jackson-Rees modification (Mapleson F breathing system).

Other breathing systems that can be used include:

◆ Ayre's T-piece (Mapleson E).
◆ Humphrey ADE system - the E mode is similar to the T-piece.
◆ Paediatric circle system (suitable for children over 5kg).

What are the components of an Ayre's T-piece?

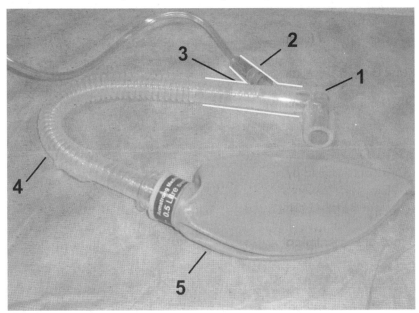

Figure 1.10 Ayre's T-piece system.
1. Patient end; 2. FGF inlet; 3. Expiratory limb; 4. Reservoir tube; 5. Breathing bag.

Dr Philip Ayre first used this in infants in 1937. It is a T-piece with three components:

◆ Fresh gas flow (FGF) inlet from the anaesthesia machine.
◆ Reservoir tube, the length of which decides re-breathing or waste of FGF.
◆ The patient end decides the amount of dead space.

The original T-piece consisted of a straight metal tube with a sidearm, forming the shape of a T. Later in 1950 it was modified by Jackson-Rees. He added a double-ended bag at the end of the reservoir tube so that respiration could be better monitored, intermittent positive pressure ventilation (IPPV) could be delivered more effectively and CPAP could be applied.

What are the advantages of this system?

◆ It is a compact, valveless and low resistance system.
◆ Can be used both for spontaneous and assisted ventilation.
◆ Can be used as a monitor of spontaneous respiration (rate and tidal volume).
◆ Can be used for applying CPAP.

How does it work and can you describe the mechanism?

◆ During inspiration: the patient inspires fresh gas from the reservoir tube.
◆ During expiration: the patient expires into the reservoir tube. Although fresh gas is still flowing into the system at this time, it is wasted as it is contaminated by expired gas.
◆ Expiratory pause: fresh gas washes the expired gas out of the reservoir tube, filling it with fresh gas for the next inspiration.

What are the clinical uses of this system?

◆ In children up to 25-30kg body weight, it can be used for spontaneous or assisted and mechanical ventilation.
◆ It can be used for applying CPAP (CPAP to the non-dependent lung during one lung ventilation).

What FGF is required for this system?

The FGF for it depends on the mode of ventilation. If spontaneously ventilating then the FGF required to prevent rebreathing is 2-3 times minute ventilation. If there is evidence of rebreathing, then the FGF can be increased. If used with controlled ventilation with an expiratory pause then the recommended FGF is equal to the patient's minute ventilation.

What should be the volume of the reservoir tube?

The volume of the reservoir tube should be equal to the tidal volume. If a small reservoir tube is used then there can be air entrainment; if a large reservoir tube is used then rebreathing of expired gases may occur.

What are the disadvantages of the Ayre's T-piece?

◆ Scavenging is not always possible, so air pollution can occur.
◆ If a small reservoir tube is used then there can be air entrainment.
◆ If a large reservoir tube is used then rebreathing of expired gases can occur.
◆ It requires high FGF during spontaneous respiration to prevent rebreathing.

Anaesthetic breathing systems

Breathing systems deliver oxygen and gases to the patient and help to eliminate carbon dioxide from the alveolar gas. They are broadly classified into rebreathing and non-rebreathing systems. In a rebreathing system, rebreathing is normally prevented by use of high FGF. A non-rebreathing system either uses a carbon dioxide absorber or a unidirectional valve to prevent rebreathing.

An ideal breathing system:

◆ Should be easy to use, fail safe and reliable.
◆ Should have low dead space.
◆ Should not impose any additional inspiratory or expiratory resistance.
◆ Should be efficient both for spontaneous and controlled ventilation.
◆ Should be economical in using FGF and volatile agents.
◆ Should be efficient for both adults and children.

The main components of breathing systems include a reservoir bag, flexible hosing, an adjustable pressure limiting (APL) valve and a face mask.

In the Mapleson A system, the APL valve is located close to the face mask and the reservoir bag is situated near the machine end. A corrugated tube with a minimum length of 110cm (with an internal tidal volume of 550ml) connects the machine end to the mask. This system was designed by Sir Ivan Magill and hence is known as the Magill system. An FGF rate equal to 70-90% of minute volume is needed to prevent rebreathing during spontaneous ventilation. It is less efficient for controlled ventilation. The Lack system is a coaxial Mapleson A system in which exhaled gases travel through the inner tube and FGF is delivered through the outer tube.

The Bain system is a co-axial Mapleson D system. Fresh gas flow is delivered through the inner tubing, and expiratory gases carried through the outer tubing. The APL valve is located close to the reservoir bag. It is less efficient for spontaneous ventilation than the Mapleson A system but it is more efficient for controlled ventilation. In adults, a FGF of 70-80ml/kg/minute is required to maintain normocapnia. Mapleson E and F systems perform similarly to the Mapleson D system.

Key points

- ◆ The T-piece is a Mapleson E breathing system; the Jackson-Rees modification is a Mapleson F breathing circuit.
- ◆ The T-piece system is a valveless and low resistance system for children weighing up to 25-30kg.
- ◆ When using the T-piece system a FGF rate of 2-3 times the minute ventilation should be used during spontaneous ventilation and a flow rate equal to the minute ventilation during IPPV.
- ◆ The Mapleson A system is an efficient system for spontaneous ventilation; the Mapleson D is very efficient for controlled ventilation.

Further reading

1. Mapleson WW. Anaesthetic breathing systems - semi-closed systems. *British Journal of Anaesthesia CEPD review* 2001; 1: 3-7.

2. Brooks W, Stuart P, Gabel PV. The T-piece technique in anesthesia; an examination of its fundamental principle. *Anesthesia Analgesia* 1958; 37: 191-6.

Structured oral examination 2

Long case 2

Information for the candidate

History

A 68-year-old male patient presents on the trauma list for hemi-arthroplasty. He had an episode of loss of consciousness 3 days ago, and sustained a fracture to the neck of the femur.

His past medical history includes the following:

He suffered from rheumatic heart disease as a child and had an aortic valve replacement 5 years ago. Postoperatively, he developed a stroke from which he has made a good recovery. Before this recent episode he was able to walk for about 100 metres using a stick before getting breathless.

His current medication includes bumetanide 1mg o.d., spironolactone 25mg o.d., digoxin 62.5µg o.d. and dihydrocodeine 30mg q.d.s. for pain in his knees. He also takes a variable dose of warfarin.

Clinical examination

He is a frail 68-year-old man, fully conscious and not confused. He has numerous bruises and is complaining of pain from his fractured femur.

Table 2.1 Clinical examination.

Weight	~50kg
Height	~170cm
Heart rate	60 bpm
Blood pressure	130/65mmHg
Resp rate	22/minute
SpO$_2$ on air	94%
Temperature	37.2°C

Chest expansion is bilaterally symmetrical. Breath sounds are vesicular with crackles heard over both lung bases. The apex beat is palpable in the 6th intercostal space. His first heart sound is faint but he has an audible 'clicking' second heart sound. No murmurs are audible. Neurological examination reveals a weakness in the right arm, which the patient is not aware of.

Investigations

Table 2.2 Biochemistry.

		Normal values
Sodium	128mmol/L	135-145mmol/L
Potassium	4.2mmol/L	3.5-5.0mmol/L
Urea	12.4mmol/L	2.2-8.3mmol/L
Creatinine	132μmol/L	44-80μmol/L
Blood glucose	8.6mmol/L	3.0-6.0mmol/L
LDH	310 IU/L	70-250 IU/L
CK	190 IU/L	25-170 IU/L
Troponin T	1.5μg/L	<0.01μg/L

Table 2.3 Haematology.

		Normal values
Hb	10.3g/dL	11-16g/dL
Haematocrit	0.34	0.4-0.5 males, 0.37-0.47 females
RBC	2.75 x 10^{12}/L	3.8-4.8 x 10^{12}/L
WBC	6.5 x 10^9/L	4-11 x 10^9/L
Platelets	296 x 10^9/L	150-450 x 10^9/L
MCV	88.4fL	80-100fL
MCHC	33.2g/dL	31.5-34.5g/dL
INR	3.6	0.9-1.2
PT	11.4 seconds	11-15 seconds
APTT ratio	1.1	0.8-1.2

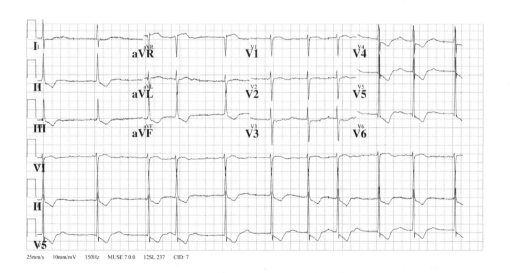

25mm/s   10mm/mV   150Hz   MUSE 7.0.0   12SL 237   CID: 7

Figure 2.1 ECG.

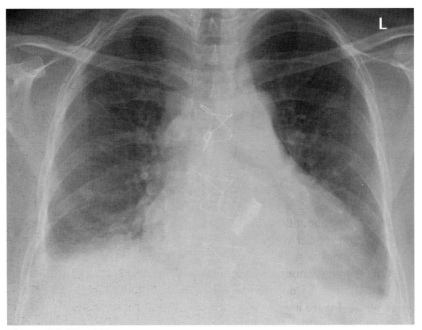

Figure 2.2 Chest X-ray.

Examiner's questions

Please summarise the case

This is a frail elderly man with cardiac problems. In the past he has suffered a cerebrovascular accident. His ECG shows ischaemic changes and atrial fibrillation; he is probably suffering from congestive cardiac failure. He has renal impairment as suggested by blood results. Prior to his surgery he needs optimisation of his cardiac function and control of his coagulation status.

Comment on his chest X-ray

The abnormal findings in the chest X-ray are:

◆ Cardiomegaly.
◆ Presence of sternal wires and prosthetic valve (aortic).
◆ Haziness of both costophrenic angles.

Can you interpret this ECG?

Confirm the patient's name, age and the date of the ECG.

◆ Heart rate: about 60 bpm.
◆ Rhythm: irregular with absence of P waves; atrial fibrillation.
◆ Axis: normal axis.
◆ QRS complex: normal duration, <0.12 seconds.
◆ ST segment: ST depression in leads II, III, V4-V6.
◆ T wave: T-wave inversion in leads II, III, avF, V4-V6.

The ECG shows atrial fibrillation (rate controlled) and ischaemic changes in the lateral leads. The abnormal findings in the ECG along with the history of loss of consciousness and elevated troponin T suggests that this patient might have had non-ST elevation myocardial infarction (NSTEMI) 3 days ago.

Describe the ECG changes following myocardial infarction

Classically, the following ECG changes are seen after a myocardial infarction:

◆ Hyperacute changes (within minutes): tall T waves and progressive ST elevation.
◆ Acute changes (minutes to hours): obvious ST elevation and gradual loss of R wave.
◆ Early changes (hours to days) within 24 hours: the T wave inverts as the ST elevation begins to resolve and within days the pathological Q wave begins to form.
◆ Indeterminate changes (days to weeks): Q waves and persistent T wave inversion.

- Old changes (weeks to months): persisting Q waves and normalised T waves.

In acute coronary syndrome, ST depression, T-wave inversion, new left bundle branch block (LBBB) formation and non-specific changes may occur. In 20% of myocardial infarctions, the ECG may initially be normal.

Comment on his blood results

The blood results show elevated cardiac enzymes, hyponatraemia, elevated urea and creatinine, anaemia and abnormal clotting.

His cardiac enzymes, lactate dehydrogenase (LDH), creatine kinase (CK) and troponin T are elevated.

Why are these cardiac enzymes elevated?

These enzymes are elevated when cardiac muscle is damaged and these substances are released into the bloodstream.

The cardiac causes of elevated cardiac enzymes are:

- Acute coronary syndromes - STEMI and NSTEMI.
- Myocardial contusion.

Which of these enzymes are the most specific to cardiac damage?

Troponins I and T.

What is troponin?

Troponin is a calcium binding protein present in thin filaments of myofibrils. It consists of three subunits: troponin I, troponin T and troponin C.

Following myocardial damage troponin T is slowly released into the blood stream; it peaks after 12 hours of myocardial infarction and is highly specific for cardiac injury. Troponin T may remain elevated for 7-10 days following a cardiac event.

What are the other causes of elevated troponin levels?

The causes of troponin elevation:

◆ Cardiac failure.
◆ Arrhythmias.
◆ Renal failure.
◆ Pulmonary embolus.

What is creatine kinase?

Creatine kinase (creatine phosphokinase; CK or CPK) is an enzyme which catalyses the conversion of creatine to phosphocreatine consuming adenosine triphospate (ATP) and generating adenosine diphospate (ADP). There are three iso-enzymes: CK-MM, CK-MB, and CK-BB. They are non-specific cardiac markers and are elevated within 2-4 hours of myocardial damage.

Which iso-enzymes of creatine kinase are expressed in the myocardial muscle?

◆ Myocardial muscle expresses 60-70% CK-MM and 30-40% CK-MB.
◆ Skeletal muscle expresses 99% CK-MM.

What are the causes of an elevated CK?

◆ Muscle injury.
◆ Rhabdomyolysis.
◆ Myocardial infarction.
◆ Muscular dystrophy.
◆ Myositis.
◆ Myocarditis.
◆ Malignant hyperthermia.

Hyponatraemia

The serum sodium is low: 128mmol/L. In this patient the causes of hyponatraemia include diuretic therapy, cardiac failure or osmolar diuresis due to raised glucose.

How would you treat hyponatraemia?

The presence of symptoms, duration of the hyponatraemia and the state of hydration will influence treatment. In chronic hyponatraemia, fluid restriction should be considered. In a hypovolaemic patient, isotonic saline should be administered to correct dehydration.

Acute hyponatraemia may be treated with normal saline. A symptomatic patient with acute hyponatraemia is in danger of developing cerebral oedema.

In a patient with chronic hyponatraemia, correction of serum sodium that is too rapid may precipitate severe neurologic complications, such as central pontine myelinosis, which can produce spastic quadriparesis, a swallowing dysfunction, pseudobulbar palsy, and mutism. In chronic severe symptomatic hyponatraemia, the rate of correction should not exceed 0.5-1mmol/L/hour, with a total increase not to exceed 10-12mmol/L per day.

Haemoglobin

He is anaemic with a haemoglobin of 10.3g/dL. Since mean corpuscular volume (MCV) and mean corpuscular haemoglobin concentration (MCHC) are within normal limits, this is normocytic normochromic anaemia.

What could be the cause of his anaemia?

The anaemia could be due to acute blood loss from the fractured femur or due to a chronic condition with a normal MCV:

♦ Anaemia of chronic disease.
♦ Renal failure.
♦ Hypothyroidism.
♦ Haemolysis.

Abnormal clotting

This patient has a high INR of 3.6 due to his oral anticoagulation therapy; this level increases the risk of moderate to high intra-operative blood loss.

Would you correct his INR?

He is receiving warfarin to prevent thrombosis from the mechanical aortic valve. Because of this, the peri-operative management of patients with prosthetic cardiac valves should be discussed with the patient's cardiologist prior to surgery. As a general rule, mechanical mitral valves should be considered a high thrombotic risk and patients should receive bridging heparin. Aortic valves are considered lower risk; bridging heparin may not be required and stopping anticoagulation for a short period during the peri-operative period will not increase the risk of thrombosis.

What other information should you elicit from the patient?

A medical history:

◆ Cardiovascular system: previous history of chest pain/angina, palpitations, orthopnoea; more information concerning the valve replacement such as the type of valve and cardiology follow-up; any recent echocardiograms and ECGs.
◆ Nervous system: previous strokes and recovery from those and any special investigations which have been performed in this respect, e.g. CT scans, carotid Doppler studies. Liaise with his primary care physician to determine whether the right-sided weakness is new, or residual from a previous cerebral event.
◆ History of previous anaesthetics.
◆ Drug allergy.
◆ Any other injuries sustained during his current fall: head injury with loss of consciousness, c-spine injury and other fractures.

What further investigations would you conduct?

Echocardiography.

Why an echocardiography?

The use of a 2-D echocardiography can:

◆ Quantify the global and regional left ventricular function, and can measure end-diastolic function, and it can detect focal and global regional wall motion abnormalities.

♦ Detect valve disease: evaluation of the prosthetic valve and detection of stenotic or regurgitating valve lesions. The valve areas and pressure gradients across the valve can also be measured.

♦ Detect endocarditis, identifying vegetations on the prosthetic and other valves.

Would you transfuse blood to this patient?

No, with his current Hb of approximately 10g/dL, the risk of transfusion would outweigh any benefit. Should his haemoglobin fall below 9g/dL, blood should be transfused to maintain adequate oxygen carriage, especially in view of his acute MI.

Would you anaesthetise this patient for hemi-arthroplasty of the hip?

Ideally the operation should be postponed and he should be optimised, especially in view of his cardiac condition as he has clinical signs of cardiac failure.

A detailed discussion with the surgical team, the patient and his relatives is essential during which the risks of the proposed surgery need to be clearly conveyed. This discussion should also entail the possibility of non-surgical treatment of his fracture.

How would you optimise him prior to surgery?

In view of his current clinical condition and his recent myocardial infarction he should be optimised in the High Dependency Unit, and his care should be guided by a cardiologist.

An outline of therapy is as follows:

♦ Oxygen supplementation.
♦ Analgesia.
♦ Aspirin.
♦ Improvement of cardiac function with the aid of beta-blockers, nitrates or inotropes. Invasive monitoring of arterial blood pressure and central venous pressure, and cardiac output monitoring would be beneficial.

◆ Hydration and correction of electrolyte imbalance.
◆ Correction of abnormal coagulation status.

Would you consider coronary artery reperfusion?

This therapy would be guided by the cardiologist but since there is a delay of more than 24 hours since his cardiac event, this may be of limited benefit to the patient.

What are the options for coronary artery reperfusion?

◆ Thrombolysis, but this is contraindicated in this case as the benefit is outweighed by the risk of an intracerebral bleed and peri-operative bleeding.
◆ Percutaneous coronary intervention using balloon angioplasty or a stent.
◆ Coronary artery bypass graft surgery.

How would you provide analgesia during his pre-operative optimisation?

The following techniques, along with immobilisation of the limb, should provide adequate analgesia:

◆ Opioid-based analgesia, either oral or intravenous (IV).
◆ Regional anaesthesia; this can be done with a continuous peripheral nerve block using a catheter technique to block the femoral nerve or lumbar plexus.
◆ Regular simple analgesia, e.g. paracetamol should always be prescribed.

Management of postoperative myocardial infarction in non-cardiac surgical patients

Peri-operative myocardial infarction is a major cause of mortality and morbidity in patients undergoing non-cardiac surgery. Major abdominal, thoracic and head and neck surgery is associated with a high risk of cardiovascular complications. The risk peaks within the first 3 postoperative days.

The joint task force of the American College of Cardiology and European Society of Cardiology recommends the definition of myocardial infarction to include all patients who have elevation of cardiac biomarkers in the presence of clinical presentation consistent with acute ischaemic heart disease. ECG evidence of myocardial ischaemia includes ST elevation >1mm in more than two contiguous leads, ST segment depression, T-wave inversion and evidence of new Q waves. Cardiac wall motion abnormalities on an echocardiogram may indicate myocardial ischaemia.

Peri-operative myocardial infarction can be categorised into non-ST segment elevation myocardial infarction (NSTEMI) and ST-segment elevation myocardial infarction (STEMI). Most patients with peri-operative MI have NSTEMI, manifesting as ST-segment depression on the ECG. The aggressive treatment of postoperative MI with antiplatelet and antifibrinolytic agents is limited by the increased risk of surgical site bleeding. For non-surgical patients, the treatment of STEMI includes acute coronary perfusion therapy with fibrinolytic agents or percutaneous coronary intervention (PCI). In the postoperative period, urgent angiography and PCI are reserved for STEMI and haemodynamically unstable NSTEMI.

Medical therapy in postoperative patients who have suffered an acute MI consists of aspirin, a beta-blocker, nitrates and anticoagulants (if not contraindicated). Angiotensin converting enzyme inhibitors and lipid lowering agents (hydroxyl-3-methylglutaryl coenzyme A reductase inhibitors) have been shown to be beneficial in reducing the mortality associated with MI.

Peri-operative management of patients on anticoagulation

In patients with a metallic heart valve prosthesis, although the risk of thromboembolism over a few days is low, the period of sub-therapeutic anticoagulation is kept to a minimum. Patients with a mechanical mitral valve, however, may require bridging heparin therapy. The decision should be taken following discussion with a consultant cardiologist and the consultant surgeon. For elective surgery warfarin can be stopped 4 days prior to the surgery and intravenous heparin can be commenced once the INR falls below 2.0. Alternatively, a therapeutic dose of subcutaneous low-molecular-weight heparin (enoxaparin) may be used.

Heparin should be given as a bolus of 100 units/kg followed by approximately 1000 units/hour intravenous infusion, titrated to achieve an APTT of 1.5 to 2.5 times the control value. At the time of surgery the effects of heparin can be reversed if required by using protamine, or by stopping the infusion which is usually adequate to minimise the action of heparin, as the half-life of heparin is less than 1 hour. The usual dose of warfarin should be restarted as soon as the risk of surgical haemorrhage is minimal. If there is any delay with re-introduction of warfarin, either intravenous heparin or a therapeutic dose of subcutaneous enoxaparin should be commenced on the first postoperative day.

Patients with atrial fibrillation who are already on warfarin should have it stopped 4 days pre-operatively. Warfarin should be recommenced on the evening of the day of surgery or as soon as the risk of surgical haemorrhage is minimal.

Reversing the effect of the oral anticoagulant

Patients with a high INR due to oral anticoagulant therapy are at risk of increased bleeding during the peri-operative period. If the INR is very high (>3.5), warfarin should be stopped on admission or as soon as surgery is indicated. If the surgery can be delayed, phytomenadione (vitamin K) can be used to reverse the effect of warfarin but this may take 6 to 24 hours to be effective:

- If the INR is >6: phytomenadione injection 2mg IV.
- If the INR is 2-6: phytomenadione injection1g IV.

The INR should be repeated 6 hours later; if it remains high further advice should be obtained from the haematologist.

If surgery cannot be delayed, prothrombin complex concentrate (PCC) or fresh frozen plasma can be used.

Regional anaesthesia for fixation of a fracture of the neck of the femur

Regional anaesthesia for the management of patients with a fracture of the neck of the femur may confer several benefits. These include a decrease in the incidence of postoperative complications such as venous thromboembolism, myocardial infarction, pneumonia, respiratory depression and renal failure. The suggested mechanisms include altered coagulation, decreased surgical stress, improved blood flow and improved respiratory function due to superior analgesia. Spinal anaesthesia is preferred by most anaesthetists in the UK. The addition of morphine or diamorphine to the local anaesthetic solution injected into the subarachnoid space results in extended postoperative analgesia.

A Cochrane report published in 2004, based on 17 randomised controlled trials, involving 2035 patients receiving GA or RA for hip fracture, stated that there was only a borderline difference in mortality at the end of the first month, that this benefit disappeared by the third month, and there was no significant impact on postoperative outcome.

Key points

♦ A patient with a pre-operative myocardial infarction presenting for urgent surgery needs risk stratification, and optimisation of cardiovascular function.

♦ In a non-peri-operative setting, acute reperfusion therapy in the form of primary coronary intervention or fibrinolysis within the first 24 hours of onset, reduces mortality associated with STEMI.

♦ In the early postoperative period, fibrinolytic therapy increases the risk of surgical site bleeding.

♦ During the peri-operative period, the decision to administer an anti-coagulant and antiplatelet agent should be made in consultation with the operating surgeon and a cardiologist.

Further reading

1. Sheppard LP, Channer KS. Acute coronary syndrome. *British Journal of Anaesthesia CEACCP* 2004; 4: 175-80.

2. Oranmore-Brown C, Griffiths R. Anticogulants and the perioperative period. *British Journal of Anaesthesia CEACCP* 2006; 6: 156-9.

3. Sandby-Thomas M, Sullivan G, Hall JE. A national survey into the peri-operative anaesthetic management of patients presenting for surgical correction of a fractured neck of femur. *Anaesthesia* 2008; 63: 250-9.

Short case 2.1: Jehovah's Witness

A 15-year-old girl with ulcerative colitis is scheduled for an elective laparotomy for bowel resection. She is known to be a Jehovah's Witness. Her haemoglobin is 9.5g/dL pre-operatively.

What are the main issues in this case?

- Jehovah's Witness.
- Young patient.
- Major abdominal surgery with blood loss.
- Anaemia.

How will your pre-operative assessment differ in this patient compared with others?

As this child is a Jehovah's Witness, her parents are likely to refuse blood transfusion. This 15-year-old child may not be competent to give her own consent.

A full and frank discussion with the patient, parents, surgeon and the Jehovah's Witness local Hospital Liaison Committee regarding the possibility of a blood transfusion in a case of life-threatening blood loss must be held prior to the surgery.

In England and Wales, children younger than 16 years may be competent to give consent to a medical or surgical procedure if they demonstrate a clear grasp of the proposed treatment and the risks, benefits or consequences of acceptance or rejection of the proposed treatment. This is known as 'Gillick competence'.

If the child consents for an elective blood transfusion in the face of parental opposition, consent would be legitimate provided that the child can show evidence of Gillick competence.

How would you proceed if both the 15-year-old girl and the parents refuse a blood transfusion?

If consent for transfusion is refused and it is felt unreasonable to proceed with surgery without the freedom to transfuse, the anaesthetist and surgeon must approach the legal team of the Trust and seek advice from their solicitors.

The solicitors may contact CAFCASS (the Children and Family Court Advisory and Support Service). The CAFCASS will interview parents, the child and the medical staff and act on the child's behalf. The Trust may apply to the High Court for an Order giving consent for the proposed treatment.

The Court may grant an Order. The Court's paramount consideration will be the child's best interest. The Trust doctors can then proceed according to the Court ruling.

What type of anaemia is this patient likely to be suffering from?

Iron deficiency anaemia or anaemia of chronic disease.

What is the difference between iron deficiency anaemia and functional iron deficiency (FID) anaemia?

Absolute iron deficiency may be diagnosed when the transferrin saturation (TSAT) is <20% and serum ferritin (SF) is <100ng/ml:

$$TSAT = (SF/TIBC) \times 100$$

where TIBC = total iron binding capacity.

Patients with a functional iron deficiency have a TSAT <20% and normal SF levels (≥100ng/ml). They may experience an increase in haemoglobin/haematocrit after a course of intravenous iron therapy.

Functional iron deficiency occurs when there is an inadequate iron supply to bone marrow. It also must be differentiated from inflammatory iron block, which can occur in patients with chronic inflammatory conditions such as infections, certain malignancies, and autoimmune disorders. In these cases, both haemoglobin and haematocrit are reduced, and TSAT may be <20%. SF levels, on the other hand, may be 100-700ng/mL

How would you treat anaemia during the pre-operative period?

By ensuring that pre-operative haemoglobin is optimised. This can be done with the following and depends on the type of anaemia:

- Pre-operative iron supplementation.
- Pre-operative vitamin B12 supplementation if deficient.
- Recombinant erythropoietin (rEPO).

What time span is needed to optimise the haemoglobin with erythropoietin?

Four weeks allows sufficient time for rEPO to produce maximum erythropoiesis. The effects are first seen after 3 days. The equivalent of one unit of blood is produced within 7 days and five units are produced within 28 days.

What else needs to be given in conjunction with rEPO?

Intravenous iron supplementation should be given to all patients receiving rEPO, except those with elevated serum iron and transferrin saturation.

What problems are associated with rEPO?

- High cost of rEPO.
- An extensive infrastructure is required to monitor the effects of rEPO and administration of the intravenous iron supplementation, including support from consultant haematologists and the haematology laboratory.
- rEPO appears to be safe but there are reports of hypertension and seizures with its use.

What can be done intra-operatively in this patient to reduce the need for blood transfusion?

General measures

Surgical
◆ Thorough planning and staging of the surgical procedure and meticulous haemostasis help to minimise transfusion requirements.

Anaesthetic
◆ Reduction of transfusion triggers whilst ensuring adequate tissue oxygen delivery. Oxygen delivery should be optimised by using other components involved in the following equation:

Oxygen delivery = CO [(Hb × 1.34) x SaO_2 x 0.01 + (PaO_2 × 0.023)] where CO = cardiac output in dL, Hb = haemoglobin/dL, SaO_2 = arterial oxygen saturation, PaO_2 = partial pressure of oxygen in the arterial blood in kPa.

◆ The anaesthetist can manipulate the cardiac output with adequate fluid administration and the use of inotropes. Oxygen saturation can be improved by increasing the inspired oxygen concentration.
◆ Hypothermia and the associated coagulopathy should be prevented by adequate warming.
◆ Venous congestion and hypercapnia should be avoided.
◆ The use of hypotensive anaesthesia should be considered.
◆ Regional anaesthesia has been shown to reduce surgical blood loss and should be used if appropriate.

Drugs
◆ Antifibrinolytic drugs, e.g. tranexamic acid.
◆ Platelet-activating drugs, e.g. desmopressin (DDAVP).
◆ Non-steroidal anti-inflammatory drugs (NSAIDs) are best avoided.

Measures to minimise blood loss

◆ Acute hypervolaemic haemodilution: this involves the rapid transfusion of fluid to achieve haemodilution without the withdrawal of blood. This technique is unsafe in patients with cardiac compromise.
◆ Intra-operative red cell salvage.

What postoperative measures would you put in place?

HDU/ITU admission is mandatory, with invasive monitoring to help optimise tissue perfusion and oxygenation. There should be a high level of vigilance for the event of rebleeding, with early intervention/re-exploration. In cases of significant blood loss and ensuing anaemia:

- Electively ventilate the patient.
- Maintain cardiac output and oxygen flux if necessary with inotropes.
- Use total parenteral nutrition (TPN)/iron/erythropoietin early.
- Hyperbaric oxygen therapy can be used as a last resort.

Jehovah's Witnesses

In general, Jehovah's Witnesses will not accept the transfusion of blood or blood products, such as fresh frozen plasma, packed cells and platelets. Individual Jehovah's Witnesses may have different interpretations of the acceptability of blood transfusions. Some accept acute normovolaemic haemodilution and intra-operative cell salvaging as long as the blood continuously remains in contact with the patient's circulation. Cardiopulmonary bypass with non-haematogenous priming is usually acceptable. Some Witnesses are willing to accept the use of plasma protein fraction (PPF) or components such as albumin, immunoglobulins and haemophilic preparations, when asked individually. They may have varying opinions regarding the acceptability of organ transplantation, the use of epidural blood patches, and the use of haemoglobin-based oxygen-carrying solutions. Blood transfusion given against their wishes is unlawful and may lead to proceedings against the administering doctor.

Consent

Consent is a voluntary agreement or approval for a treatment or an investigation. In health care, consent is a competent person's agreement to a procedure after she/he has been informed of all the risks involved and the alternatives.

In England and Wales, 16- and 17-year-old children are presumed to be competent to consent to treatment. Parents can also give a valid consent on their behalf. Refusal for treatment by competent 16- and 17-year-olds can, however, be overruled by the Court, if the child is likely to suffer harm as a result of refusal. This rule does not apply in Scotland. In 2008, a 13-year-old girl was accepted as competent under the Gillick test when she refused a heart transplant.

Refusal of treatment by a competent adult is legally binding, even if the refusal is likely to result in a patient's death. The treatment of an incompetent adult is carried out in the patient's best interest. Competent patients, who anticipate future incompetence through illness, may indicate their preference for future treatment by completing an advance directive.

Making decisions about treatment and care for patients who lack capacity is governed in England and Wales by the Mental Capacity Act 2005, and in Scotland by the Adults with Incapacity (Scotland) Act 2000. This Act allows competent patients to appoint Lasting Powers of Attorney (LPA), permitting others to take decisions about their health care and welfare on their behalf if they lose their capacity in the future.

The functional test for decision making is as follows:

- The patient must be able to comprehend the information given.
- The patient must be able to retain the information.
- The patient must be able to use the information and weigh it up to arrive at a choice.

Key points

- All Jehovah's Witnesses must be consulted individually whenever possible, to ascertain what treatment they will accept.
- If it is unreasonable to proceed with the surgery without blood transfusion and if the parents refuse to consent for blood transfusion, a Court order should be obtained.
- In a life-threatening emergency in a child who is unable to give consent, all immediate life-saving treatment should be given, irrespective of the parents' wishes.

Further reading

1. Management of anaesthesia for the Jehovah's Witness. AAGBI, 2005.
2. Milligan LJ, Bellamy MC. Anaesthesia and critical care of the Jehovah's Witness. *British Journal of Anaesthesia CEACCP* 2004; 4: 35-9.
3. Consent: patients and doctors making decisions together. London: GMC, June 2008.

Short case 2.2: Aspiration under general anaesthesia

A 20-year-old patient undergoing a haemorrhoidectomy has been anaesthetised and has an LMA in place. He is positioned on the left lateral side for a caudal epidural. As you are about to perform the caudal epidural on the patient, you notice a copious volume of fluid in the LMA tube.

What is the immediate management?

- Stop the procedure and keep the patient in the left lateral position; if possible apply a head-down tilt.
- Administer 100% oxygen.
- Suction all the fluid through the LMA tube.
- If the laryngeal mask does not maintain the airway adequately, remove it and administer 100% oxygen via a tight-fitting face mask.

Further management depends on the degree of aspiration and whether or not the patient is breathing spontaneously:

- If the patient is breathing spontaneously, apply cricoid pressure.
- Apply mask CPAP and consider deepening anaesthesia. Avoid cricoid pressure if the patient is actively vomiting (risk of oesophageal rupture).
- Intubate the trachea with the aid of a muscle relaxant, and apply suction to the trachea. A bronchoscopy can be performed to visualise any signs of aspiration.

- ◆ If the regurgitation is minimal, the LMA is correctly placed, and the patient remains stable without desaturation, the tracheobronchial tree can be suctioned through the LMA using a fibreoptic scope, provided that the airway reflexes are adequately obtunded.
- ◆ If the patient is apnoeic, intubate immediately and commence ventilation. Treat as an inhaled foreign body by minimising excessive positive pressure ventilation until the endotracheal tube (ETT) and the airway have been suctioned and all aspirates are clear. A bronchoscopy could be performed to look for signs of aspiration.

How would you diagnose aspiration?

Diagnosis by:

- ◆ Clinical examination, which may reveal any of the following:
  - laryngospasm/airway obstruction;
  - bronchospasm/wheeze/crackles;
  - hypoventilation/dyspnoea/apnoea;
  - desaturation/bradycardia/cardiac arrest.
- ◆ Monitoring:
  - decreased oxygen saturation;
  - decreased lung compliance;
  - increased airway pressure;
  - increased slope of the capnograph trace.
- ◆ Investigations:
  - tracheal aspirate may be acidic (negative finding does not exclude aspiration);
  - chest radiograph: diffuse infiltration;
  - arterial blood gases: hypoxia, hypercarbia and acidosis;
  - bronchoscopy: visualisation of aspiration fluid.

What would be your subsequent management of this patient?

- ◆ Sedation, analgesia and intermittent positive pressure ventilation (IPPV) via an ETT.
- ◆ Suction of the airway.
- ◆ Optimisation of FiO_2 possibly with positive end expiratory pressure (PEEP).
- ◆ Bronchoscopy and bronchial lavage if necessary.
- ◆ Emptying of the stomach with a large-bore nasogastric tube before extubation.
- ◆ Monitoring respiratory function.

♦ Chest X-ray looking for evidence of pulmonary oedema, collapse or consolidation.

Further management depends on the clinical picture and results from the investigations:

♦ If the SPO_2 is >95% on minimal oxygen and the chest X-ray is normal, the patient can be extubated and monitored for signs of respiratory complications.
♦ If the SPO_2 remains at 95% and FiO_2 is <0.5, heart rate <100/min, respiratory rate <20/min and the patient remains apyrexial, the patient can be extubated and the oxygenation and atelectasis can be improved with CPAP (10cm H_2O) and chest physiotherapy.
♦ If SPO_2 remains 95% despite FiO_2 being >0.5, there may be solid food material obstructing part of the bronchial tree. The patient should be transferred to the ICU postoperatively for ventilatory support.
♦ Extubation should take place in the left lateral position with a head-down tilt.

Further management:

♦ Repeat the chest X-ray and blood gases.
♦ Sputum culture.
♦ Antibiotics are not routinely used.
♦ Explanation to patient and relatives.

What is the role of steroids and antibiotics?

Steroids may modify the inflammatory response early after aspiration but do not alter the outcome. They may potentially interfere with the normal immune response.

Prophylactic antibiotics are not routinely indicated but they may be required to treat subsequent secondary infections.

What are the risk factors for aspiration?

Patient factors

♦ Full stomach, fasting from food for less than 6 hours.
♦ Intra-abdominal pathology: intestinal obstruction, inflammation.

- Gastric paresis: drugs such as opiate analgesics, diabetes, uraemia, infection and trauma.
- Oesophageal disease: symptomatic reflux and motility disorders.
- Pregnancy.
- Obesity.
- Uncertainty about time of intake of food or drink.

Anaesthetic factors

- Insufficient depth of anaesthesia with airway reflexes (such as coughing, hiccoughs, or laryngospasm), or gastrointestinal motor responses (such as gagging or recurrent swallowing) being evoked and causing regurgitation/aspiration.
- During IPPV with a mask, anaesthetic gases may pass into the stomach and may increase the risk of regurgitation.

Surgical factors

- Upper gastrointestinal surgery.
- Increased intra-abdominal pressure, e.g. laparoscopic surgery.

Aspiration during anaesthesia

The LMA does not reliably protect the lungs from regurgitated stomach contents, although it may act as a barrier at the level of the upper oesophageal sphincter if it is correctly positioned. The incidence of clinically detectable regurgitation with the LMA is approximately 0.1%. The incidence of aspiration is low, approximately 0.02%, which is similar to the incidence of aspiration with tracheal intubation in elective patients.

The following are practical guidelines to minimise the risk of aspiration while using an LMA:

- Avoid use of an LMA in patients with an increased risk of aspiration.
- Ensure adequate anaesthesia during insertion of the LMA and during surgery.
- Avoid lubrication of the anterior surface, excessive lubrication, or use of lubricants containing non-aqueous solvents.

◆ Avoid gastric distension during positive pressure ventilation (minimise peak airway pressures, avoid inadequate paralysis).

Therapeutic strategies to prevent aspiration in patients with risk of aspiration

◆ Ensure that the patient is adequately fasted.
◆ Measures to increase gastric pH.
◆ Measures to reduce the volume of gastric secretion.
◆ Application of cricoid pressure.
◆ Protection of the airway by a cuffed ETT.
◆ Extubation in the lateral head-down position after suctioning the oropharynx.

The respiratory damage following aspiration depends on the acidity and volume of gastric content. 30ml 0.3M sodium citrate given 15-20 minutes prior to induction of general anaesthesia and H_2 receptor antagonists, such as ranitidine 150mg orally or 50mg intravenously, increase the pH of the gastric juice. Metoclopramide increases gastric motility and reduces the volume of gastric fluid.

Key points

◆ As soon as regurgitation is recognised, the airway should be thoroughly suctioned and 100% oxygen administered.
◆ Further management depends on the clinical condition of the patient as indicated by oxygen saturation and respiratory signs.
◆ Regurgitation and aspiration can be minimised by avoiding the use of an LMA in patients with an increased risk of aspiration.

Further reading

1. Brimacombe JR, Brain AIJ, Berry AM. *The laryngeal mask airway instruction manual*, 4th ed. Reading: Intavent Research Limited, 1999.
2. Brimacombe J, Keller C, Bittersohl J, *et al.* Aspiration and the laryngeal mask airway: three cases and a review of literature. *British Journal of Anaesthesia* 2004; 93: 579-82.

Short case 2.3: Emergency Caesarean section

You are called to the obstetric unit for an urgent Caesarean section on a 23-year-old pregnant patient who has fetal distress due to a cord prolapse.

How would you classify the urgency of Caesarean section?

The urgency of a Caesarean section can be classified according to categories described by the National Institute for Health and Clinical Excellence (NICE):

◆ Category 1: immediate threat to the life of the woman or fetus.
◆ Category 2: maternal or fetal compromise which is not immediately life-threatening.
◆ Category 3: no maternal or fetal compromise but needs early delivery.
◆ Category 4: delivery timed to suit woman or staff.

What are the implications of an umbilical cord prolapse?

Umbilical cord prolapse is an obstetric emergency and has been defined as the descent of the umbilical cord through the cervix alongside (occult) or past the presenting part (overt) in the presence of ruptured membranes. The only characteristic clinical sign is the finding of a palpable or visible umbilical cord in the vagina. It compromises the fetal circulation due to the occlusion of blood vessels within the cord. The overall incidence of cord prolapse ranges from 0.1% to 0.6%. It is an indication for a Category 1 Caesarean section.

What are the non-surgical ways to relieve the cord pressure?

The following measures can be taken to prevent the compression of the cord by the fetal head during contractions and to improve fetal perfusion while preparing for immediate delivery in theatre:

◆ The mother should be reassured, venous access should be established and a blood sample should be collected for a full blood count, electrolytes, blood group and save.
◆ Supplemental oxygen should be administered to the mother.

- If possible, the cord should be gently replaced into the vagina to keep it warm and prevent vasospasm. There should be minimal handling of loops of cord lying outside the vagina (to prevent vasospasm).
- Catheterising the urinary bladder and filling it up with 500-700ml of normal saline elevates the presenting part.
- The mother should be positioned in a knee-to-chest position with a head-down tilt (preferably in the left lateral position) to minimise cord compression.
- Any oxytocin infusion should be stopped.
- Tocolysis should be considered while preparing for Caesarean section if there are persistent fetal heart rate abnormalities and when the delivery is likely to be delayed.

The above mentioned methods are useful during preparation for delivery but they must not result in unnecessary delay.

What are the anaesthetic options available for Caesarean section for umbilical cord prolapse?

Traditionally, cord prolapse is managed with general anaesthesia. Regional techniques can be considered where there is time, when measures to reduce cord compression have been successful, but repeated attempts at regional anaesthesia should be avoided. If the foetal blood supply is compromised, then general anaesthesia may be the only option.

What advantages does spinal anaesthesia have over general anaesthesia?

The advantages of spinal anaesthesia are:

- Safer for mother and baby than general anaesthesia.
- Minimal risk of aspiration.
- Lower risk of anaphylaxis.
- Reduced passage of drugs crossing the feto-placental barrier.
- Early bonding of the mother and baby.
- Provides postoperative analgesia.
- Both mother and partner can be present at the delivery.

What types of spinal needle do you know of?

There are two different types of spinal needles:

◆ Cutting tip needle: Quincke.
◆ Non-cutting needles: Sprotte and Whitacre.

Both the Sprotte and Whitacre needles are designed to spread the dural fibres rather than cut them like cutting needles. The incidence of post-dural puncture headache is lower with these needles compared with cutting needles. The Sprotte needle has a smooth pointed tip with a wide lateral hole proximal to the tip. The Whitacre needle has a pencil-shaped tip with the hole just proximal to the tip. Needles are available in various sizes from 22G to 29G. The incidence of post-dural puncture headache is lower with the smaller needles. Small needles, such as 29G or 27G, may break or bend and it may be difficult to recognise the cerebrospinal fluid (CSF) back flow. As with intravenous cannulae, spinal needles are sized using the standard wire gauge. The bigger the number, the smaller the size of the needle.

General anaesthesia for Caesarean section

General anaesthesia is associated with increased maternal and fetal morbidity compared with regional anaesthesia. Nowadays, about 91% of elective and about 77% of emergency Caesarean sections are performed under regional anaesthesia. Even 41% of the Category 1 Caesarean sections are now performed under regional anaesthesia. General anaesthesia for Caesarean sections is associated with increased peri-operative blood loss and reduced neonatal Apgar scores. General anaesthesia is usually reserved for those women in whom regional anaesthesia is contraindicated, or when time is limited.

The following are specific problems associated with general anaesthesia.

Difficult airway

The incidence of failed intubation is approximately 1 in 300 in the obstetric population. The reasons include associated upper airway oedema, short neck, full dentition, increased breast mass preventing the insertion of the laryngoscope and application of cricoid pressure. An attempt at nasal intubation is likely to result in soft tissue injury and bleeding due to associated oedema and venous engorgement of nasal passages and upper airway.

Pulmonary aspiration

Pregnant women are more prone to aspiration due to reduced tone of the lower oesophageal sphincter. Reduction of gastric volume and pH of the gastric content is achieved by a combination histamine receptor (H_2) antagonist or proton pump inhibitor, and sodium citrate. To prevent aspiration, rapid sequence induction should be performed with pre-oxygenation and cricoid pressure. Cricoid pressure at 44N is likely to cause a difficult laryngoscopic view. Therefore, a force of 10N (equivalent to 1kg) should be applied while the patient is awake and increased to 30N when consciousness is lost. Prior to extubation, the stomach may be emptied using a large-bore orogastric tube.

Awareness

Although the risk of awareness during general anaesthesia is low, rapid sequence induction and associated difficult intubation may increase the risk.

Post-dural puncture headache (PDPH)

This headache develops following dural puncture associated with spinal anaesthesia or epidural anaesthesia. Its exact mechanism is not clear but it may be due to excessive leakage of CSF. This leads to intracranial hypotension and a demonstrable reduction in CSF volume, and may cause sagging of the intracranial structures. It is more common in pregnant patients. The reported incidence is very variable, being less than 1% with pencil-point spinal needles, but up to 75% with 16G epidural needles.

Spinal needles have undergone numerous modifications to reduce the incidence of dural puncture headache. The principal factor responsible for the development of a dural puncture headache is the size of the dural perforation. Headache and backache are the dominant symptoms that develop after accidental dural puncture. Ninety percent of headaches occur within 3 days of the procedure and last for 1-2 weeks. The headache is classically described as severe occurring over the frontal and occipital areas and radiating to the neck and shoulders. It is exacerbated by head movement and adoption of the upright posture, and relieved by lying down. It may be associated with nausea, vomiting, tinnitus, vertigo and hearing loss.

Diagnosis is made from a history of accidental or deliberate dural puncture and symptoms of a postural headache, neck ache and the possible presence of neurological signs.

The treatment of PDPH includes the following:

- Explanation and reassurance to the patient.
- Adequate hydration.
- Analgesics such as paracetamol and NSAIDs.
- Caffeine (produces cerebral vasoconstriction), dose: 300-500mg of oral or IV.
- Sumatriptan is a serotonin agonist which causes cerebral vasoconstriction. A few small case series have shown a benefit following a single subcutaneous dose of 6mg.
- Adrenocorticotrophic hormone (ACTH) has been used at a dose of 1.5 units/kg intravenously. There is no clear evidence demonstrating the benefit of the use of sumatriptan and ACTH in the treatment of PDPH.
- An abdominal binder (causes elevation of intra-abdominal pressure which is transmitted to the epidural space and may relieve the headache).
- Epidural blood patches are usually reserved when the headache is severe and persistent. Its success rate is 70-98% if carried out more than 24 hours after the dural puncture. If an epidural blood patch fails to resolve the headache, repeating the blood patch has a similar success rate. Some units use epidural injection of saline or blood at the time of dural puncture but this is a controversial technique. The use of a prophylactic blood patch is thought to be unnecessary.

Key points

◆ Cord prolapse is an obstetric emergency.
◆ Whilst preparing for emergency Caesarean section, measures should be taken to maintain placental circulation.
◆ Regional techniques should be considered where appropriate so long as there is no ongoing compromise to fetal blood supply.

Further reading

1. Guidelines for umbilical cord prolapse. Royal College of Obstetrics and Gynaecology. http://www.rcog.org.uk/resources/Public/pdf/ Greentop 50UmbilicalCordProlapse.pdf.
2. NICE guidelines for Caesarean sections. http://www.nice.org.uk/nice media/pdf/CG013fullguideline.pdf.
3. Turnbull DK, Shepherd DB. Post-dural puncture headache: pathogenesis, prevention and treatment. *British Journal of Anaesthesia* 2003; 91: 718-29.

Applied anatomy 2.1: Anatomy of the epidural space

You are requested to provide analgesia for a patient with multiple rib fractures. Which options are available?

The options of providing analgesia for rib fractures include:

◆ Epidural analgesia.
◆ Paravertebral analgesia.
◆ Extrapleural analgesia.
◆ Intrapleural analgesia.
◆ Intercostal block.
◆ Intravenous analgesia.

Clinical Science

Which modality provides the most effective analgesia for a patient with multiple rib fractures?

Epidural analgesia for pain control after severe blunt injury significantly improves subjective pain perception and critical respiratory function tests compared with intravenous opioids. Epidural analgesia is associated with less respiratory depression, sedation and gastrointestinal symptoms than IV opioids.

When you see a patient before inserting an epidural, what complications should you mention?

Complications associated with the procedure

◆ Inadvertent dural puncture, and subsequent PDPH (incidence 0.5%).
◆ Failure (1%).
◆ Unilateral, or patchy block (5-10%).
◆ Epidural haematoma.
◆ Risk of nerve damage: 1:10,000 risk of permanent neurological sequelae (usually minor, e.g. patch of residual numbness).

Complications of drugs injected

◆ Hypotension due to sympathetic block with associated nausea, light-headedness.
◆ High spinal block (inadvertent intrathecal injection): hypotension, dense motor block, respiratory weakness/distress.
◆ Local anaesthetic toxicity.
◆ Pruritus, nausea, vomiting and urinary retention associated with epidural opioids.

What precautions should you take to minimise the risks?

◆ Choice of technique: is it indicated?
◆ Pre-operative assessment to rule out any contraindications or risks (drug therapy: antiplatelets and anticoagulants).

What are the contraindications to an epidural block?

Absolute

- Patient refusal.
- Coagulopathy: insertion of an epidural needle or catheter into the epidural space may cause traumatic bleeding into the epidural space. Clotting abnormalities may lead to the development of a large haematoma leading to spinal cord compression.
- Therapeutic anticoagulation: as above.
- Skin infection at injection site: the insertion of an epidural needle through an area of skin infection may introduce pathogenic bacteria into the epidural space, leading to serious complications such as meningitis or an epidural abscess.
- Raised intracranial pressure (ICP): an accidental dural puncture in a patient with raised ICP may lead to brainstem herniation.
- Hypovolaemia.

Relative

- Unco-operative patients may be impossible to position correctly, and be unable to remain still enough to safely insert an epidural.
- Pre-existing neurological disorders, such as multiple sclerosis, may be a contraindication, because any new neurological symptoms may be ascribed to the epidural.
- Fixed cardiac output states: this includes aortic stenosis, hypertrophic obstructive cardiomyopathy (HOCM), mitral stenosis and complete heart block. Patients with these cardiovascular abnormalities are unable to increase their cardiac output in response to the peripheral vasodilatation caused by the epidural blockade, and may develop a profound circulatory collapse.
- Anatomical abnormalities of the vertebral column may make the placement of an epidural technically impossible.
- Prophylactic low-dose heparin.

Describe the anatomy of the epidural space

The epidural space is the area surrounding the dural sheath, within the vertebral canal. It extends from the foramen magnum to end by the fusion of its lining membranes at the sacrococcygeal membrane inferiorly. The dural sheath, comprising the dura mater, arachnoid mater, the sub-arachnoid space with CSF, the spinal nerves of the cauda equina, and filum terminale occupy most of the spinal canal. The remaining part of the spinal canal is occupied by fatty and fibrous tissues, and blood vessels. The epidural space is discontinuous and divided into segments where the dura mater comes into contact with the spinal canal. Normally this permits the easy passage of a catheter and solutions across the segments. In some, due to surgery or inflammation, the dura may be tethered to the spinal canal. This may result in a patchy epidural block or inadvertent dural puncture.

Boundaries of the epidural space

◆ Anterior: the vertebral bodies, and the intervertebral discs, with the overlying posterior longitudinal ligament.
◆ Lateral: the pedicles and intervertebral foramina. Through the lateral foramina, the epidural space is connected to the paravertebral space.
◆ Posterior: the vertebral laminae and the overlying ligamentum flavum.

The ligamentum flavum is 2-5mm thick and comprises two ligaments meeting in the midline connecting the laminae of adjacent vertebrae. They extend from the anterior and inferior aspect of the vertebral lamina above, to the posterosuperior surface of the vertebral lamina below.

The epidural space can be divided into anterior, lateral and posterior compartments. The anteroposterior dimension (depth) of the posterior epidural space is greatest at the mid-lumbar levels and decreases at the thoracic and cervical levels (cervical <thoracic <lumbar).

Contents (lumbar epidural space)

Spinal nerves, with an investing cuff of dura, loose fat, areolar connective tissue, lymphatics, and blood vessels.

Describe the veins of the epidural space

They run mainly in a vertical direction and form four main trunks: two lie on either side of the posterior longitudinal ligament and two lie posteriorly, in front of the vertebral arches.

They are valveless - 'the valveless vertebral venous plexus of Batson'. They receive the basivertebral veins, which emerge from each vertebral body on its posterior aspect. They communicate with branches from the vertebral, ascending cervical, deep cervical, intercostal, lumbar, iliolumbar and lateral sacral veins. These enter through the intervertebral and sacral foramina.

What is the pressure in the epidural space?

The pressure in the epidural space is subatmospheric. The epidural space is therefore identified by a loss of resistance technique. The advancement of the needle into the epidural space results in tenting of the dura mater, resulting in slight negative pressure. The transmission of subatmospheric thoracic pressure also contributes to the negative pressure of the epidural space.

Are there any differences between the thoracic and lumbar epidural spaces?

The lumbar epidural space is segmented and discontinuous. This is attributable to the dura being directly in contact with the lumbar bony canal and the predominance of epidural fat. The thoracic epidural space contains less fat and is less adherent to the bony canal.

What are your views on performing a thoracic epidural block in an anaesthetised patient?

Although serious nerve injury following epidural anaesthesia is rare, all measures should be taken to prevent nerve injury. In most centres epidurals are performed in an awake patient as standard practice.

Anaesthetised patient

As patients remain still during the procedure, there is less risk of the needle damaging the nerve roots due to patient movement. An epidural under general anaesthesia is often better accepted by the patients. It is easier to teach the procedure in an anaesthetised patient.

Awake patient

An awake patient can warn of impending nerve injury.

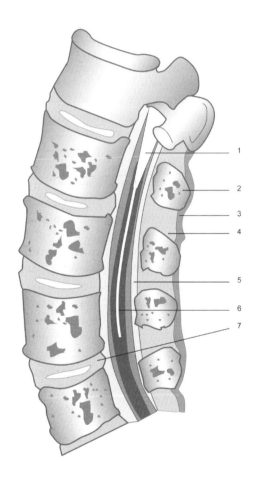

Figure 2.3 Anatomy of epidural space.

1. Spinal cord; 2. Spinous process; 3. Supraspinous ligament; 4. Interspinous ligament; 5. Ligamentum flavum; 6. Filum terminale; 7. Intervertebral disc.

Epidural analgesia for major abdominal surgery

The benefits of epidural analgesia for major abdominal surgery include:

◆ Respiratory function: there is a reduced incidence of postoperative atelectasis, pulmonary infection and improved oxygenation. Effective pain relief enables the patient to receive physiotherapy, and allows the patient to deep breathe and cough. There is a reduced risk of respiratory depression compared with opioids.
◆ Cardiovascular system: reduced sympathetic activity and improved respiratory function optimises myocardial oxygen supply/demand.
◆ Gastrointestinal tract: reduces opioid-related gastrointestinal side effects, the incidence of paralytic ileus, and promotes early postoperative feeding.
◆ Thromboembolic: there is a reduced incidence of DVT and reduced blood loss during the intra-operative period.

A multicentre, randomised control trial published in 2002 (Multicentre Australian Study of Epidural Anaesthesia, MASTER Anaesthesia trial) investigated the benefits of peri-operative epidural analgesia on outcome in 888 patients undergoing major abdominal surgery. This study revealed that epidural analgesia provides better postoperative analgesia and reduces postoperative respiratory complications. There was no significant difference, however, in the mortality or incidence of major morbidity. Further selected subgroup analysis of the MASTER trial found no difference in the outcome between epidural and control groups, even in a group of patents with increased risk of respiratory and cardiac complications.

Key points

◆ In patients with blunt chest injury, epidural analgesia significantly improves subjective pain perception and respiratory function tests compared with intravenous opioids.
◆ For major abdominal surgery, although epidural analgesia provides short-term benefits in the immediate postoperative period, there is no evidence to show that this reduces mortality compared with intravenous opioids.

Further reading

1. Macleod GA, Cumming C. Thoracic epidural anaesthesia and analgesia. *British Journal of Anaesthesia CEACCP* 2004; 4: 16-9.
2. Nimmo SM. Benefit and outcome after epidural analgesia. *British Journal of Anaesthesia CEACCP* 2004; 4: 44-7.
3. Rigg RJA, Jamrozik K, Myles PS, *et al.* Epidural anaesthesia and analgesia on peri-operative outcome of major abdominal surgery: A randomised trial. *Lancet* 2002; 359: 1276-82.
4. Ellis H, Feldman S, Harrop-Griffiths W. *Anatomy for anaesthetists*, 8th ed. Oxford: Blackwell Science Ltd, 2004.

Applied physiology 2.2: Arterial tourniquet

A 35-year-old male patient is undergoing arthroscopy of the right knee under general anaesthesia. The surgeon requests you to inflate the tourniquet.

What pressure would you use to inflate the tourniquet?

♦ For the lower limb tourniquet the pressure used is twice the systolic BP or a maximum of 150mm Hg above systolic blood pressure.
♦ For the upper limb it is 50mm Hg above systolic blood pressure.

What are the indications for using arterial tourniquets?

♦ To aid surgery: arterial tourniquets are commonly used to achieve a bloodless field during surgical procedures, aiding the identification of structures and reducing blood loss.
♦ Intravenous regional anaesthesia.

What are the contraindications to arterial tourniquets?

Absolute

♦ Suspected DVT - massive pulmonary embolism.
♦ Risk of dissemination of malignancy/infection.
♦ AV fistula.

Relative

◆ Peripheral arterial disease.
◆ Raynaud's disease.
◆ Severe crush injury.
◆ Sickle cell disease - may be used after full exsanguination, but should be used with caution for as short a duration as possible.
◆ Poor skin condition.
◆ Peripheral neuropathy.

List the effects and side effects of arterial tourniquet inflation

Cardiovascular system

Tourniquet inflation with exsanguination causes a central shift in blood volume and a theoretical increase in systemic vascular resistance. This leads to mild increases in central venous and systemic arterial pressures which are generally benign. These changes can be significant in patients with underlying cardiovascular disease and fluid overload can occur, which can lead to left ventricular failure in patients with cardiac disease. Exsanguination of the tourniquet to both legs increases the circulating blood volume by 15%.

Respiratory system

In patients with prolonged immobilisation and risk factors for DVT, emboli can be dislodged into the systemic circulation resulting in pulmonary embolism.

Central nervous system

Tumour embolism in the presence of malignancy.

Metabolic

When used for a prolonged duration of 1.5-2 hours, accumulation of metabolic products can cause acidosis. A localised infection may be disseminated into the systemic circulation during the process of tourniquet application.

Tourniquet pain

Inflation of the tourniquet results in vague dull pain in the limb with an increase in blood pressure. Prolonged tourniquet inflation causes an increase in heart rate and blood pressure.

Physical effects

Mechanical tourniquets cause unpredictably high pressure in underlying tissues, possible leading to skin trauma, arterial damage or nerve damage.

Tourniquet hypertension

Tourniquet-induced hypertension occurs in 11-66% of cases. Its onset is analogous to the onset of tourniquet pain, after approximately 30-60 minutes. The aetiology is unclear. It likely has the same origin as tourniquet pain, and requires a specific critical level of cellular ischaemia in the muscle or nerve. It is more common with general anaesthesia than with regional anaesthesia. The incidence is very low with spinal anaesthesia. Sympathectomy does not block its occurrence.

What is the maximum permissible time for tourniquet application?

The tourniquet should be used for the minimal duration possible. The upper limit in healthy patients is 2 hours. Elderly patients and patients with peripheral vascular disease are more susceptible to muscle injury. Most recommend limiting the total time between 1.5 to 2 hours. The surgeon should be alerted at 1 hour, 1.5 hours and at 2 hours, when the tourniquet should be deflated for at least 10 minutes to allow reperfusion of the muscles.

What are the effects of tourniquet deflation?

◆ Deflating a tourniquet leads to the release of blood with a low pH and high PCO_2, lactate, and K^+ into the systemic circulation. This leads to corresponding changes in systemic values: a decreased pH, decreased PO_2, increased PCO_2, increased K^+, and increased lactate.

◆ There is a transient fall in central venous oxygen tension (SvO_2) but systemic hypoxaemia is unusual (SaO_2 normal).

- There is a transient increase in $EtCO_2$, which increases by about 8mmHg after release of a thigh tourniquet with a corresponding increase in $PaCO_2$ of 10mmHg.
- These changes have been extensively studied and are generally mild and well tolerated.
- Several studies have shown that changes peak at approximately 3 minutes and return to baseline by 30 minutes.
- Transient fall in core temperature of 0.7°C within 90 seconds of deflation of a leg tourniquet.
- The deflation of a tourniquet is associated with an increase in cardiac output and release of CO_2 from the ischaemic limb into the systemic circulation. This leads to transient increases in end-tidal CO_2 concentration.
- Hypercapnia associated with tourniquet release increases cerebral blood volume which can have a significant adverse effect in patients with a head injury.
- Haemodynamics :
  - mild to moderate haemodynamic changes with a transient fall in central venous and systemic arterial pressures;
  - mean decreases in systolic BP of approximately 15-20mmHg;
  - mean increases in HR of approximately 5-10 bpm;
  - these changes are usually benign, but can be significant in patients with coexisting cardiovascular disease.

Local effects of a tourniquet

The pressure and duration of tourniquet application can result in injuries to underlying structures such as skin, nerves and muscles.

Nerve injury

Upper limb nerves are more prone to injury than lower limb nerves. The radial nerve is more vulnerable in the upper limb and the sciatic nerve is more vulnerable in the lower limb. The mechanism of nerve injury is most likely to be direct pressure rather than ischaemia. Most nerve injuries heal spontaneously in less than 6 months. Permanent nerve damage is very rare. Morbidly obese patients are more prone to peripheral nerve injuries.

Muscle injury

The mechanism includes a combination of ischaemia and mechanical deformation. Post-tourniquet syndrome is characterised by stiffness, weakness and pallor without paralysis. This is due to a combination of effects such as ischaemia, oedema and microvascular congestion of the muscle. The mechanical trauma to muscles is related to the pressure applied over the unit area. A wide and curved cuff designed to fit conical parts of the limbs enables the use of a lower inflation pressure.

Vascular injury

Vascular injury is most likely to occur in patients with peripheral vascular disease. The effect of the tourniquet may result in thrombosis of atherosclerotic vessels.

Arterial tourniquet and drug administration

Because the arterial tourniquet isolates the limbs, antibiotics should be administered at least 5 minutes before inflating the tourniquet to ensure that an adequate concentration of antibiotic is present at the site of surgery. If drugs are administered before inflation of the tourniquet they may be sequestrated in the limb distal to the tourniquet and become redistributed into the systemic circulation after release of the tourniquet. In the isolated forearm technique of Tunstall which monitors depth of anaesthesia, an arterial tourniquet is used to isolate the arm from neuromuscular blocking drugs.

Key points

- ◆ The use of an arterial tourniquet produces a bloodless field and improves the operating conditions.
- ◆ In healthy patients having a short duration procedure, when used with recommended pressures, the risks are minimal.
- ◆ Some patients are at an increased risk of developing complications.
- ◆ All tourniquet machines should be regularly checked for accuracy of the pressure gauge and integrity of the cuff and tubing.

Further reading

1. Kam PCA, Kavanaugh R, Yoong FFY. The arterial tourniquet: pathophysiological consequences and anaesthetic implications. *Anaesthesia* 2001; 56: 534-45.

Applied pharmacology 2.3: Patient-controlled analgesia

You are called to the ward to assess a patient complaining of severe pain following an abdominal hysterectomy.

What options are available to provide analgesia during the first 24 hours of the postoperative period?

The patient should be receiving regular paracetamol +/- NSAIDs. These can be supplemented with either:

- Patient-controlled analgesia (PCA) - opioid.
- Nurse-controlled IV analgesia.
- IM opioid.
- Regional anaesthesia.

What are the advantages of PCA?

- Associated with a significantly better quality of pain relief than conventional analgesia.
- It is liked by patients.
- No painful IM injections.
- Reduced work load for the nurses.

How would you initiate analgesia with a PCA pump?

Explain the device to the patient and ensure the patient understands the technique and is capable of using the PCA. Make sure that the patient has an IV line and oxygen is available.

For all modes of PCA, there are the following basic variables:

- Choice of drug, e.g. morphine.

- Titration of an initial 'loading' dose to achieve analgesia.
- Setting the demand dose and the lockout interval with or without a background infusion.

What is the principle on which PCA is based?

It is based on the premise that a negative feedback loop exists: when pain is experienced, analgesic medication is demanded; when the pain is reduced, there are no further demands.

For each individual there is a minimum effective analgesic concentration (MEAC): this is the smallest concentration at which pain is relieved. This varies with changes in the level of pain perceived and appears to be largely independent of pharmacokinetic variables. There is marked pharmacodynamic variability in the response to opioids amongst individuals. Once the individual MEAC as been achieved only a small amount of drug needs to be given to ensure effective analgesia and retain the MEAC.

Describe the design of a PCA pump

It is a computerised, programmable, lightweight, battery-operated portable pump with the capability of storage and retrieval of data by a microprocessor. Most PCA devices are microprocessor-controlled pumps triggered by a button. When the pump is triggered, a preset amount of opioid is delivered into the patient's intravenous line. A timer prevents administration of an additional bolus until a specified period (lockout interval) has elapsed. Most pumps can be programmed for two modes of delivery:

- Continuous infusion per hour rate which is pre-programmed combined with a bolus for breakthrough pain; boluses are controlled by the patient.
- Boluses with a set lockout time.

What safety features should be incorporated into a PCA system for adults?

The main aim is to prevent a drug overdose:

- Appropriate concentration: the PCA syringe should ideally be prepared by the pharmacy.

◆ Appropriate lockout time (usually 5 minutes): electronic pumps are programmable. Disposable sets rely on refill of the chamber (this cannot be altered).
◆ Maximum hourly dose: can be adjusted in programmable pumps.
◆ Alarms: these are incorporated in electronic pumps preventing excessive dosing.
◆ Anti-siphoning device: a one-way valve should be incorporated into any system, and the device should not be placed above the level of the patient.
◆ Security: pumps should be lockable so that the patient/others cannot access the syringe.

What are the side effects of an opioid-based IV PCA?

◆ Nausea and vomiting.
◆ Pruritis.
◆ Confusion and sedation.
◆ Respiratory depression.

What safety instructions would you give the ward nurse?

A pre-printed set of standard orders should be used throughout the hospital to facilitate a uniform standard of care, and the following safety instructions should be included:

◆ Sedation scoring and respiratory rate charting - to indicate opioid overdosing.
◆ Reversal of narcosis - prescription for naloxone. Nurses should be allowed to administer according to a set protocol.
◆ Continuous oxygen therapy until the PCA is removed.
◆ Equipment failure - the syringe volume should be checked against cumulative consumption on display.
◆ Medical help - 24-hour access to pain and/or an emergency team for advice and assistance.

What are the other routes by which PCA can be administered?

◆ Epidural PCA.
◆ Peripheral nerve catheter PCA.

◆ Transdermal PCA.
◆ Subcutaneous PCA.

Opioid drugs used as patient-controlled analgesia

Morphine, fentanyl, diamorphine and pethidine are commonly used for intravenous PCA. Epidural PCA usually includes bupivacaine or levobupivacaine +/- fentanyl.

Table 2.4 Dose regimen of commonly used drugs.		
Drug	**Dose**	**Lockout time**
Morphine	0.5-2.0mg	5-10 minutes
Fentanyl	20-50µg	5-10 minutes
Diamorphine	0.5-2.0mg	5-10 minutes
Pethidine	5-20mg	5-15 minutes

Key points

◆ PCA provides a better quality of pain relief than conventional analgesia.
◆ Standard orders should be used throughout the hospital to facilitate a uniform standard of care, and staff should be trained to use PCA safely.
◆ The PCA pump should incorporate safety features to avoid excessive dosing and security features so that others cannot access the programme and syringe.

Further reading

1. Grass JA. Patient-controlled analgesia. *Anaesthesia Analgesia* 2005; 101: S44-61
2. Macintyre PE. Safety and efficacy of patient-controlled analgesia. *British Journal of Anaesthesia* 2001; 87: 36-46.

Equipment, clinical measurement and monitoring 2.4: Defibrillator

How would you treat the following arrhythmia?

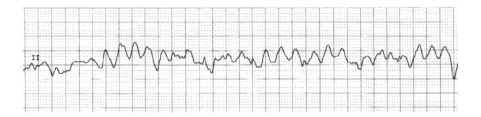

Figure 2.4 ECG.

This ECG shows ventricular fibrillation. This rhythm should be treated with defibrillation.

What is a defibrillator?

It is electrical equipment in which electric charge is stored and released in a carefully controlled fashion. It delivers direct electrical current across the myocardium causing synchronous depolarization of the cardiac muscle. It is used in the treatment of ventricular fibrillation and to convert arrhythmias into normal sinus rhythm.

How does it work? What are the components of a defibrillator circuit?

It has a power source from the mains. A step-up transformer converts 240V to 5000V. A rectifier (diode) is used to convert alternate current (AC) into direct current (DC).

Electric charge is stored in a capacitor, which consists of two plates separated by an insulator. When the defibrillator is activated, it releases the stored charge.

An inductor is included in the output circuit, which lengthens the duration of current pulse. This inductor in the discharge path opposes sudden change in current flow, slows down the rapid discharge from the capacitor, and hence controls the duration shock. It also absorbs some of the electrical charge. Hence, the delivered energy is less than that of stored energy. Energy indicated on the defibrillator is the actual delivered energy, not the stored energy. Maximum energy delivered in the monophasic defibrillator is normally 360J.

Explain the current flow in the circuit during charging and discharging

Whilst charging, the switch (switch A) is activated so that the current flows from the mains to the capacitor. The capacitor charges in an exponential fashion. Initially the voltage at the capacitor plate is low, so more current flows. As the voltage of stored charge on the plate increases, current flow decreases. When the discharge switch (switch B) is activated, current flows from the capacitor to the paddles via the inductor. The current flow across the chest is limited by thoracic impedance; it can be minimised by applying gel pads, and by delivering shock during the expiratory phase.

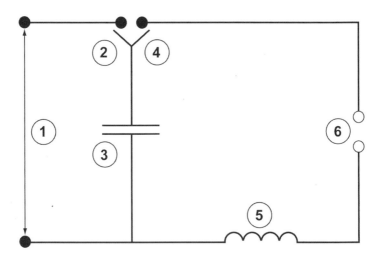

Figure 2.5 The components of a defibrillator circuit
1. Power source; 2. Switch A; 3. Capacitor; 4. Switch B; 5. Inductor; 6. Paddles.

What is capacitance?

This is the ability of the capacitor to hold the electrical charge. It is measured in Farads (F).

What factors determine the capacitance (the quantity of stored charge in the capacitor)?

Surface area of the plate and thickness of the insulating layer.

How would you calculate the stored energy?

Stored energy, $E = \frac{1}{2} QV$, where Q is the charge in millicoulombs and V is the potential (volts).

How does a biphasic differ from a monophasic defibrillator?

A monophasic defibrillator produces a single pulse of current which travels in one direction through the chest. A biphasic defibrillator produces two consecutive pulses, in which the current first travels in one direction and then in the other. In the biphasic type, the defibrillation threshold is lower than the monophasic defibrillator and, hence, is more efficient. It needs a smaller capacitor with less battery power.

Automated implantable cardioverter-defibrillator (AICD)

The AICD is a small defibrillator, the size of an implantable pacemaker. It has its own battery power. It has sensing electrodes that sense the heart rate and rhythm and shocking electrodes to deliver the shock. The energy output varies from 0.1-30J.

The original model was only able to recognise and deliver unsynchronised shock for ventricular fibrillation, but the recent AICDs consist of more complex algorithms to manage ventricular tachycardia and ventricular fibrillation. The AICD can analyse rhythm and perform one of the following actions:

- Synchronised shock.
- Unsynchronised shock.
- Anti-tachycardia pacing.

The AICD also incorporates pacemaker function to provide anti-bradycardia back-up. Similar to pacemaker generic code, a four-letter AICD code has been devised.

The first letter indicates the chamber shocked: atrium (A), ventricle (V) and dual (D).

The second letter indicates the chamber in which anti-tachycardia pacing is administered: atrium (A), ventricle (V) and dual (D).

The third letter indicates the method of detecting rhythm and rate: electrogram (E) and haemodynamic (H).

The fourth letter indicates the chamber in which pacing is delivered: no pacing action (O), atrium (A), ventricle (V) and dual (D).

The effect of electromagnetic interference may include inappropriate inhibition or triggering of pacing activity.

External defibrillation may cause serious damage to the AICD by generating a large amount of electromagnetic interference. The high energy of current induced by the defibrillator can pass through the leads of the AICD and cause myocardial burns.

Key points

♦ The defibrillator stores and releases electrical charge in a controlled fashion.
♦ The capacitor in the defibrillator stores the electrical charge.
♦ The stored energy depends on the potential difference across the plates of the capacitor and the charge.
♦ The AICD senses the heart rhythm and delivers shock when indicated.

Further reading

1. Chaudhari M, Baker PM. Physical principles of the defibrillator. *Anaesthesia and Intensive Care Medicine* 2005; 6: 411-2.
2. Allen M. Pacemakers and implantable cardioverter defibrillators, review article. *Anaesthesia* 2006; 61: 883-90.

Structured oral examination 3

Clinical Anaesthesia

Long case 3

Information for the candidate

History

A 72-year-old female presents on the neurosurgical list for a posterior cervical fusion. She has a history of cervical spondylosis and presented with tingling and numbness of both hands. She also mentions that her husband complains of her snoring at night and that she feels tired all the time.

Her past history includes rheumatoid arthritis, hypertension and glaucoma. She has smoked 15 cigarettes per day for the last 50 years.

Her current medication includes amlodipine 5mg o.d., bendroflumethiazide 5mg o.d., atenolol 50mg o.d., timolol (eye drops), prednisolone 5mg o.d., lansoprazole 20mg o.d., ipratropium bromide inhaler 40μg b.d., salbutamol inhaler 100μg b.d., and diclofenac sodium 50mg t.d.s.

Clinical examination

She is a cheerful 72-year-old lady with rheumatoid changes especially in both hands. Chest and heart examination shows nothing abnormal.

She has very limited neck movement and complains of pins and needles in both hands during attempted neck flexion. She has a full set of dentures.

Table 3.1 Clinical examination.

Weight	65kg
Height	173cm
BMI	22
Heart rate	48 bpm
Respiratory rate	16/minute
Blood pressure	150/80mmHg
Temperature	37.1°C

Investigations

Table 3.2 Biochemistry.

		Normal values
Sodium	136mmol/L	135-145mmol/L
Potassium	3.9mmol/L	3.5-5.0mmol/L
Urea	7.8mmol/L	2.2-8.3mmol/L
Creatinine	92µmol/L	44-80µmol/L

Table 3.3 Haematology.

		Normal values
Hb	12.1g/dL	11-16g/dL
Haematocrit	0.38	0.4-0.5 males, 0.37-0.47 females
RBC	3.75×10^{12}/L	$3.8-4.8 \times 10^{12}$/L
WBC	6.5×10^9/L	$4-11 \times 10^9$/L
Platelets	294×10^9/L	$150-450 \times 10^9$/L
MCV	88.4fL	80-100fL
MCHC	34.2g/dL	31.5-34.5g/dL
Neut	4.54×10^9/L	$2.5-7.5 \times 10^9$/L
Lymp	1.58×10^9/L	$1.5-4.0 \times 10^9$/L
Mono	0.72×10^9/L	$0.2-0.8 \times 10^9$/L
Eos	0.09×10^9/L	$0.04-0.4 \times 10^9$/L
Baso	0.01×10^9/L	$<0.01-0.1 \times 10^9$/L

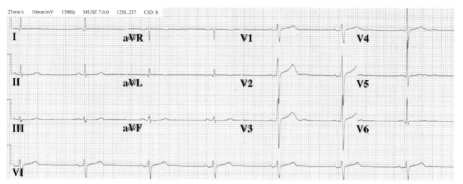

Figure 3.1 ECG.

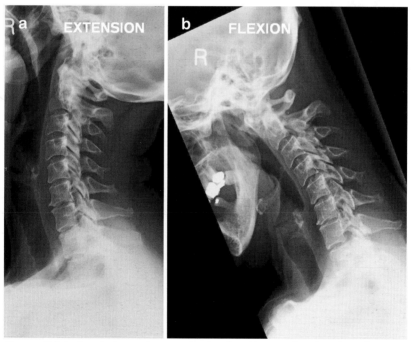

Figure 3.2 Lateral view of a cervical spine X-ray: a) extension view; b) flexion view.

Examiner's questions

Please summarise the case

This is a 72-year-old lady scheduled for a posterior cervical fusion. She has multiple systemic problems which include rheumatoid arthritis, hypertension, sinus bradycardia, glaucoma, possible obstructive airway disease associated with chronic smoking and possible obstructive sleep apnoea. She has a potentially difficult airway due to limited neck movement and an unstable cervical spine. The surgical access will require prone positioning. She needs further investigation to quantify the degree of obstructive sleep apnoea.

What further history and clinical examination are needed?

History

◆ Previous anaesthetic history, noting the management of the airway.
◆ A detailed CVS history to exclude ischaemic heart disease.
◆ A detailed history of the respiratory system in view of her smoking history.
◆ Further history regarding her snoring and somnolence.

Clinical examination

◆ Detailed airway examination.
◆ A neurological examination and documentation of deficits.

Can you interpret the cervical spine X-ray?

This is a lateral X-ray of the cervical spine. Seven cervical vertebrae are visible. The line passing through the anterior aspect of the vertebral canal is disrupted at the C2-C3 level. The posterior spinal line at C2-C3 is also disrupted. The gap between the odontoid process of the axis and anterior arch of the atlas is increased indicating anterior subluxation of the atlas (flexion view). The intervertebral disc space between C6 and C7 is narrowed.

Can you read the ECG in a systematic way?

◆ Confirm the patient's name, age and the date of the ECG.
◆ Rate: 42 per minute.
◆ Rhythm: sinus bradycardia.
◆ Axis: normal axis.
◆ P wave: normal.
◆ P-R interval: 0.16s, within normal limits.
◆ QRS complex: normal duration, <0.12s.
◆ ST segment: normal.
◆ T wave: normal.

This ECG shows sinus bradycardia.

What are the causes of sinus bradycardia?

◆ Physiological:
  - increased vagal tone;
  - athletes.
◆ Intra-cardiac conduction defects:
  - sick sinus syndrome;
  - sino-atrial block;
  - atrioventricular block;
  - myocardial infarction/ischaemia.
◆ Endocrine disorders:
  - hypothyroidism.
◆ CNS:
  - raised intracranial pressure.
◆ Drugs:
  - beta-blockers;
  - calcium channel blockers;
  - anti-arrhythmic drugs.

What is the likely cause of bradycardia in this patient?

Bradycardia in this patient could be due to the beta-blockers she is taking. She is on atenolol 50mg o.d. and also timolol eye drops. Timolol is a topical beta-blocker with systemic side-effects.

What is 'sick sinus syndrome'?

Sick sinus syndrome is the name for a group of arrhythmias in which the sinus node malfunctions. The sinus node beats abnormally causing bradycardia, tachycardia or alternating slow and fast rhythms, or a tachycardia-bradycardia syndrome.

What are the symptoms of sick sinus syndrome?

Most people with sick sinus syndrome have few or no symptoms. Signs and symptoms of sick sinus syndrome may be paroxysmal. They may include:

◆ Fatigue.
◆ Dizziness or light-headedness.
◆ Fainting or near-fainting.
◆ Shortness of breath.
◆ Chest pain.
◆ Trouble with sleeping.
◆ Confusion.
◆ Palpitations.

What are the treatment options for sick sinus syndrome?

◆ Pacemaker - treatment of choice.
◆ AV-node ablation.
◆ Anti-arrhythmia medication.

Do you think the history of snoring in this patient is important?

Yes, the history of snoring in conjunction with the history of somnolence may indicate that the patient has obstructive sleep apnoea.

What is obstructive sleep apnoea?

Obstructive sleep apnoea (OSA) is a syndrome which is characterised by a periodic partial or complete obstruction of the upper airway during sleep. This, in turn, causes repetitive arousal from sleep in order to restore the airway patency, which may result in hypersomnolence during the day. The airway obstruction may also cause episodic sleep-associated oxygen desaturation, episodic hypercarbia and cardiovascular dysfunction.

Apnoea is cessation in airflow. Hypopnoea is reduction in airflow by 50% for more that 10 seconds. In OSA these episodes occur more than five times per hour.

What is the pathophysiology of OSA?

During sleep, the negative pressure created during inspiration leads to collapse of the pharyngeal airway, particularly at the level of the tongue and soft palate. Partial collapse leads to decreased airflow during inspiration (hypopnoea) and complete collapse of the pharynx leads to apnoea. After a period of apnoea or hypopnoea, the increasing $PaCO_2$ and decreasing PaO_2 lead to arousal. The arousal leads to re-opening of the airway and is associated with tachycardia and hypertension. After a brief period of arousal, sleep resumes and airway obstruction develops again. The repeated episodes of hypoxia can lead to pulmonary hypertension and right heart failure. The neurological effects include somnolence, impaired memory, impaired cognition, anxiety, depression, headache and intracranial hypertension.

The severity of OSA is assessed by measuring the frequency of apnoea and hypopnoea episodes, known as the apnoea/hypopnoea index (AHI):

◆ Mild: AHI 5-14 per hour.
◆ Moderate: AHI 15-30 per hour.
◆ Severe: AHI >30 per hour.

What other clinical signs and symptoms may be associated with OSA?

Physical

◆ BMI ≥35.
◆ Neck circumference ≥17 inches (men) or 16 inches (women).
◆ Craniofacial abnormalities affecting the airway.
◆ Anatomical nasal obstruction.
◆ Enlarged tonsils nearly touching in the midline.

History of apparent airway obstruction during sleep

◆ Snoring.
◆ Frequent snoring.
◆ Observed pauses in breathing during sleep.
◆ Awakening from sleep with choking sensation.
◆ Frequent arousals from sleep.

Somnolence (one or more of the following is present)

◆ Frequent somnolence or fatigue despite adequate 'sleep'.
◆ Falls asleep easily in a non-stimulating environment (e.g. whilst watching television, reading, riding in or driving a car) despite adequate 'sleep'.

How would you confirm the diagnosis of OSA?

Polysomnography (PSG) usually involves an overnight sleep study, where numerous bodily functions are monitored and scored (e.g. respiratory pattern, pulse oximetry, electroencephalogram [EEG], electro-oculogram [EOG], and chin electromyogram [EMG]).

Pulse oximetry alone has limited value in diagnosing OSA. The number of desaturation episodes over an hour or total duration of desaturation is counted. When compared to PSG, pulse oximetry has a low specificity and sensitivity.

Would the diagnosis of OSA change your management of this patient?

Yes, during the postoperative period, airway obstruction may be worsened by the effect of residual anaesthetic and sedative drugs. The following are the implications of OSA on anaesthetic management.

Pre-operative

◆ Need to ascertain the severity of the OSA through discussions with the respiratory physician.
◆ Possible institution of pre-operative treatment such as overnight nasal continuous positive airway pressure (nCPAP).

Intra-operative

◆ Possible difficulty in mask ventilation and intubation.
◆ Increased sensitivity to opioids and anaesthetic agents.
◆ Need to ensure complete reversal from muscle relaxants prior to extubation and extubate patients when fully awake and in the semi-upright position.
◆ Need for multimodal analgesia including a local anaesthetic to reduce opioid requirements.

Postoperative

◆ High dependency care.
◆ Supplementary oxygen.
◆ Re-institute nCPAP as soon as possible.

What further investigations would you like to see?

◆ MRI of the cervical spine to assess the severity and location of cord compression.
◆ Clotting screen.
◆ Lung function tests (FEV1, FVC, PEFR).
◆ Blood group and save.

What cervical problems are associated with rheumatoid arthritis?

With rheumatoid arthritis the integration of the vertebral bodies, facet joints, synovial capsules and ligaments can be severely disrupted leading to subluxation. Between 15-85% of patients with rheumatoid arthritis have cervical involvement with a higher incidence in patients who are seropositive for Rheumatoid Factor. This subluxation can be classified as atlanto-axial and sub-axial subluxation.

Atlanto-axial subluxation (AAS)

There are four types:

◆ Anterior (80%). The atlas (C1 vertebra) moves forward on the axis (C2) because of the destruction of the transverse ligament. It is worsened by neck flexion. It exists when the distance between the odontoid peg and the atlas exceeds 4mm.
◆ Posterior (5%). Due to the destruction of the odontoid peg. It is worsened by neck extension.
◆ Vertical (10-20%). The destruction of the lateral mass of C1 vertebrae can lead to the subluxation of the odontoid peg through the foramen magnum.
◆ Lateral due to the destruction of the C1/C2 facet joints.

What clinical signs and symptoms might a patient with rheumatoid arthritis cervical joint disease have?

◆ Occipital headaches (due to entrapment of the C1/C2 nerve roots).
◆ Dysphagia, dysphonia, diplopia (due to cranial nerve compression).
◆ Persistent pain in the neck and arms (due to radicular entrapment).
◆ Involuntary movements of the extremities.
◆ Attacks of dizziness (vertebral artery compression).
◆ Numbness in the upper extremities.

How else can the airway of a patient with rheumatoid arthritis be affected?

◆ Arthritis of the crico-arytenoid joints which can lead to hoarseness, stridor, dyspnoea and possibly a laryngeal mass.

◆ Arthritis of the temporomandibular joints can lead to limited mouth opening.

How would you manage the airway in this patient undergoing posterior cervical fusion?

This patient has a potentially difficult airway due to limited neck extension. Excessive manipulation of the neck may result in damage to the patient's spinal cord and may also lead to vertebral artery insufficiency. During induction, intubation and positioning, care should be taken to minimise the movement of the cervical spine. Manual in-line immobilisation should be applied during laryngoscopy and intubation.

The options for tracheal intubation include:

◆ Awake fibreoptic intubation, which is the preferred option.
◆ Asleep fibreoptic, ensuring that cervical spine movement is kept to a minimum during the procedure.
◆ Intubating LMA and fibreoptic-assisted intubation.

Briefly explain how you would perform an awake fibreoptic intubation

Pre-operative

◆ Discussion and explanation of the procedure with the patient.
◆ Preparation of the equipment and the drugs required for the procedure including sedation and local anaesthetic drugs.

Procedure

◆ IV access and supplementary oxygen.
◆ Monitoring by pulse oximetry, ECG, NIBP and sedation score during the procedure.
◆ Antisialogogue (glycopyrrolate 150-200µg).
◆ Sedation with profopol and fentanyl or remifentanil.
◆ Local anaesthesia with either a topical, nerve block or 'spray-as-you-go' technique.

(For further details refer to SOE 7, Applied anatomy 7.1.)

What position would this patient be in for the posterior cervical fusion?

Prone position.

Describe how you would turn this patient into the prone position

The patient is first anaesthetised on the trolley and then moved to the operating table. The appropriate equipment and padding to support the pressure points should be checked and ready to use. Positioning the patient into the prone position requires at least six people.

Airway management

This patient requires a well-secured, armoured endotracheal tube.

C-spine

The c-spine needs to be immobilised during the moving of the patient after she has been anaesthetised.

Eyes

Adequate eye protection is important to avoid corneal abrasion and padding to avoid pressure on the eye, which can cause retinal artery occlusion and optic neuropathy. This is of particular importance as this patient has glaucoma.

Intravenous and arterial lines

Intravenous and arterial lines should be carefully secured before turning the patient - it may be easier to disconnect them beforehand.

Positioning into the prone position

An adequate number of persons are required to turn the patient prone safely; the larger the patient the greater the number of assistants required. The neurosurgeon should be present to direct the correct surgical positioning.

The head is positioned face down on a piece of hollow foam or headrest. The pressure should be limited to the forehead. In this patient, as surgical access is required in the upper cervical region, the surgeon may prefer to position the head using head pins and a Mayfield skull clamp. Avoid any pressure on the eyes. Ensure that the endotracheal tube is secured, not kinked and has not migrated into the right main bronchus. The neck should be minimally flexed and the chin should be free from the chest.

The arms are positioned fully adducted so they lie by the patient's side. Undue pressure in the axillae should be avoided as axillary nerve or brachial plexus neuropraxia may occur from overstretching. Finally, check that the patient is not lying on any cables, leads or tubing.

What are the main pressure points to be checked and which nerves are at risk?

- Face (eyes in particular); this patient may have increased intra-ocular pressure due to glaucoma.
- Chest and breast tissue.
- Anterior superior iliac spines.
- Knees and feet.
- Genitalia.
- Nerves at risk are the supra-orbital, infra-orbital, optic, facial, brachial plexus, ulnar nerve at the elbow, radial and median nerve at the wrist, femoral nerve under the inguinal ligament and the lateral cutaneous nerve of the thigh at the level of the anterior superior iliac spine.

What are the main physiological changes that may occur in the prone position?

Respiratory system

Lung compliance is reduced due to decreased chest wall and diaphragmatic excursion. To aid compliance, a 'Montreal' mattress (a rectangular mattress with a hole in its centre) may be used to prevent the abdominal contents forcing the diaphragm upwards. Alternatively, pillows should be placed under the iliac crests and chest, leaving the abdomen unhindered.

Cardiovascular system

Increased intra-abdominal pressure may lead to a decreased venous return and a reduction in cardiac output.

Gatrointestinal system

There may be an increased risk of regurgitation.

Neurological system

Increased intra-abdominal pressure will impair drainage from epidural veins; this can lead to increased venous ooze at the surgical site.

How would you manage this patient during recovery and in the postoperative period?

Care needs to be taken to turn the patient into the supine position again with c-spine immobilisation. Ensure that the neuromuscular blocking agents are adequately reversed and the patient is awake before extubation, as emergency re-intubation may be difficult.

Check neurological function to rule out surgical complications.

The patient will require monitoring in a high dependency unit

Rheumatoid arthritis

Rheumatoid arthritis is a typically persistent, symmetrical, deforming peripheral arthropathy. Its peak onset is in the 5th decade and it is three times more common in women than men. Seventy percent of cases are associated with the HLA-DR4 subtype.

Clinical features

The common articular signs include swollen, warm, painful and stiff joints, deformities and nodules. These symptoms tend to be episodic lasting for weeks to months followed by asymptomatic periods. Repeated episodes can lead to progressive joint damage and deformity.

Extra-articular manifestations are common and occur in more than 50% of cases.

Cardiovascular system
- Pericarditis, pericardial effusions and tamponade.
- Myocarditis.
- Endocarditis.
- Cardiac failure.
- Peripheral vasculitis.
- Atherosclerosis and ischaemic heart disease.

Respiratory system
- Fibrosing alveolitis - restrictive defect.
- Rheumatoid nodules.
- Costochondral rheumatoid arthritis leading to reduced chest wall compliance.
- Pleural effusions.

Haematological system
- Anaemia - iron deficiency and a normocytic, normochromic picture.

Other
- Hepatomegaly.
- Splenomegaly.
- Decreased albumin.
- Autonomic dysfunction.
- Peripheral neuropathy.

Drug therapy and side effects

- Symptomatic relief: paracetamol, NSAIDs and corticosteroids.
- Anti-cytokine agents: anti-TNF (tumour necrosis factor).
- Disease-modifying drugs.

Table 3.4 Drug therapy and side effects.

Drug	Side effects
Sulphasalazine	Bone-marrow suppression, aplastic anaemia and fibrosing alveolitis
Methotrexate	Pneumonitis and cirrhosis
Cyclosporine	Hypertension and renal impairment
Gold	Bone-marrow suppression, hepatitis, pulmonary fibrosis, nephritic syndrome
Azathioprine	Bone-marrow suppression, cholestatic hepatitis
Penicillamine	Bone-marrow suppression, proteinuria, myasthenic syndrome, haemolytic anaemia
Hydroxychloroquine	Renal impairment and hypertension

Key points

- Polysomnography is the investigation of choice for diagnosing obstructive sleep apnoea.
- The residual effect of general anaesthetics and sedative drugs may worsen the hypoxic episodes in patient with obstructive sleep apnoea.
- In patients with rheumatoid arthritis involving the cervical spine, great care should be taken to immobilise the cervical spine during induction, intubation and positioning.

Further reading

1. Macarthur A. Kleiman S. Rheumatoid cervical joint disease - a challenge to the anaesthetist. *Canadian Journal of Anesthesia* 1993; 40: 154-9.

2. Practical guidelines for the peri-operative management of patients with obstructive sleep apnoea. *Anaesthesiology* 2006; 104: 1081-93.
3. Management of obstructive sleep apnoea/hypopnoea syndrome in adults: a national clinical guideline. www.sign.ac.uk/pdf/sign73.pdf.
4. Edgcombe H, Carter K, Yarrow S. Anaesthesia in the prone position. *British Journal of Anaesthesia* 2008; 100: 165-83.

Short case 3.1: Down's syndrome

A 28-year-old male patient with Down's syndrome presents for a dental procedure as a day case.

What are the problems associated with Down's syndrome?

There are many clinically significant problems that anaesthetists may encounter when providing anaesthesia to patients with Down's syndrome. Safe anaesthetic management depends on an awareness of the multi-systemic nature of this condition.

Central nervous system

Mental retardation is very common with an incidence of 95%-99%. Epilepsy occurs in up to 10% of individuals.

Musculoskeletal system

Atlanto-axial instability (AAI) has an incidence which varies between 12%-30%. The main cause of AAI is the laxity of the transverse ligament. Other causes, e.g. hypoplasia, malformation or absence of the odontoid process, also predispose to C1-C2 instability. Subluxation at C1-C2 may cause spinal cord compression.

The normal atlanto-axial gap (distance between the odontoid process and anterior arch of the atlas) on lateral cervical spine X-ray is <4.0mm. Most patients have neurological symptoms if the gap is >7mm.

The signs and symptoms of AAI include:

◆ Positive Babinski test.
◆ Hyperactive deep tendon reflexes including ankle clonus.
◆ Muscle weakness.
◆ Increased muscle tone.
◆ Abnormal gait and walking difficulty.
◆ Neurogenic bladder.

Airway

Airway management can be potentially difficult due to a relatively large tongue, crowding of mid-facial structures, a high arched plate, a short broad neck and micrognathia. There is also a high incidence of tonsillar and adenoidal hypertrophy.

Respiratory system

Upper and lower respiratory tract infection are frequent. In children with Down's syndrome, congenital anomalies of the lower airways are common and include stenotic anomalies, tracheo-oesophageal fistulae and branching anomalies. Airway obstruction and obstructive sleep apnoea are common.

Cardiovascular system

Congenital cardiac anomalies are common with an overall incidence of approximately 40%:

◆ The majority of congenital cardiac defects involve a left to right shunt, thus leading to possible pulmonary hypertension.
◆ A ventricular septal defect and complete atrioventricular defect occur in 30%-60% of all patients with Down's syndrome.
◆ A patent ductus arteriosus (12%) and Tetralogy of Fallot (8%) occur less frequently.
◆ There is an increased incidence of mitral valve prolapse and aortic regurgitation in adults.

Gastrointestinal system

There is increased risk for gastro-oesophageal reflux.

Haematological system

Neonates with Down's syndrome are prone to polycythaemia. There is also a risk of leukaemia in children.

Endocrine system

Congenital hypothyroidism is more common. Insulin-dependent diabetes is also more likely to occur.

Immunological system

There is an increased susceptibility to all infections because of immune deficiency.

How would these factors affect your anaesthetic management of this patient?

Pre-operative assessment

It may be difficult or impractical to obtain a proper history from the patient. They may not co-operate for the pre-operative investigations. Any previous surgical correction or other invasive procedure that has been performed for previous or currently existing cardiac abnormalities should be noted.

A thorough clinical examination of the respiratory and cardiovascular systems is essential. If clinical symptoms and signs are suggestive of atlanto-axial subluxation, c-spine X-rays should be reviewed prior to induction of anaesthesia.

Pre-operative prophylaxis for gastro-oesophageal reflux is advisable.

Induction of anaesthesia and airway management

Induction may be difficult due to a lack of co-operation. The presence of a guardian or carer at induction may improve co-operation. Topical ametop or EMLA should be considered to facilitate intravenous induction. Hypotonia may make it difficult to maintain an adequate airway during induction. Excessive neck movement should be avoided to minimise damage to the spinal cord. A smaller endotracheal tube than normal may be necessary.

Maintenance of anaesthesia

Hypoventilation frequently occurs during spontaneous ventilation, so a method using IPPV should be considered.

Recovery and emergence from anaesthesia

There is a higher incidence of postoperative agitation which may require sedation.

Is this patient suitable for day-case anaesthesia?

Provided there are no significant cardiovascular problems with this patient, this procedure can be done as a day case.

What are the criteria for day-case anaesthesia?

Surgical

Surgical procedures of moderate duration associated with mild to moderate postoperative pain can be performed as a day-case procedure. Surgical procedures with significant postoperative pain, haemorrhage and prolonged immobility should not be performed as day-case procedures.

Medical

Day-case surgery is usually restricted to patients with ASA grades 1 and 2. Patients with angina, a significant arrhythmia and overt cardiac failure are not suitable. Age alone is not a strict criterion; physiological fitness should be considered rather than age alone.

Social

Patients should have appropriate care and facilities at home; they should have easy access to a telephone and transport. All patients should be escorted home by a responsible adult and should be adequately supervised by a responsible adult for the first 24 hours. They should be living within a reasonable distance so that they are able to get back to the hospital if necessary (about 60 minutes travel time).

Down's syndrome

Down's syndrome is one of the commonest congenital abnormalities. In Down's syndrome the cell contains 47 chromosomes with an extra chromosome linked to chromosome 21, known as Trisomy 21.

Although moderate to severe mental retardation is seen in Down's patients, the majority of patients are cheerful and calm. A few patients exhibit anxiety and stubbornness. Short stature and obesity is seen at adolescence. The characteristic facial features include microcephaly or brachycephaly, a sloping forehead, a flat occiput, a flat nasal bridge and upslanting palpebral fissures with bilateral epicanthic folds. They have a tendency to keep the mouth open with a protruding tongue. Chronic otitis media with hearing loss is common.

Key points

- In addition to dysmorphic features and mental retardation, Down's syndrome may involve other systems.
- Airway management can be potentially difficult due to a large tongue, high arched plate, micrognathia and short neck.
- Congenital heart disease is more common in Down's syndrome.

Further reading

1. Mitchell V, Howard R, Facer E. Down's syndrome and anaesthesia. *Paediatric Anaesthesia* 1995; 5: 379-84.
2. Meitzner MC, Skurnowicz JA. Anaesthetic considerations for patients with Down syndrome. *AANA Journal* 2005; 73: 103-7.
3. Allt JE, Howell CJ. Down's syndrome. *British Journal of Anaesthesia CEPD Review* 2003; 3: 83-6.

Short case 3.2: Transurethral resection of the prostate (TURP)

A 70-year-old male patient presents for TURP. What problems would you anticipate in this patient pre-operatively?

Elderly patients presenting for TURP have reduced physiological reserve and are likely to have multiple co-existing diseases.

Cardiovascular system

Elderly patients have reduced ventricular compliance and myocardial contractility. Similarly, vascular compliance is reduced predisposing them to swings in blood pressure. Atherosclerosis, hypertension, ischaemic heart disease (IHD) and arrhythmias (particularly atrial fibrillation) are common.

Respiratory system

The closing capacity approaches functional residual capacity even in the sitting position. There is more likelihood of airway collapse, increasing ventilation perfusion mismatching and the resultant increase in alveolar-arterial oxygen difference. The response to hypoxia and hypercarbia is blunted. Smoking and COAD may lead to a marked decrease in respiratory reserve.

Musculoskeletal system

Degenerative changes in the vertebral column may make subarachnoid block (SAB) technically difficult. Arthritic joints or joint replacements are susceptible to damage or dislocation when the patient's legs are placed in the lithotomy position for the procedure.

Nervous system

Decreasing density of neurons and reduction in neurotransmitter levels are seen with advancing age. Dementia, confusion and cerebrovascular accidents are more common.

Other systems

Hypothyroidism and diabetes mellitus are more likely. Marked hypothermia may occur during the peri-operative period. Renal impairment may occur due to obstructive uropathy.

Pharmacology

Both pharmacokinetics and pharmacodynamics are altered in elderly patients. They are often on multiple drugs with potential drug interaction. A high proportion of elderly patients take cardiovascular medications (diuretics, beta-blockers, ACE inhibitors, digoxin and aspirin). The first-line medical treatments for benign prostatic hypertrophy are alpha-blockers, and the combined effect of these drugs, cardiovascular drugs and anaesthesia may result in severe hypotension during the intra-operative period.

What anaesthetic options are available for TURP?

♦ Spinal anaesthesia with or without sedation.
♦ General anaesthesia: spontaneous breathing technique with laryngeal mask airway.
♦ General anaesthesia: positive pressure ventilation with endotracheal intubation.

What are the benefits of spinal anaesthesia for TURP?

The advantages of a regional technique include:

♦ Early detection of complications such as TUR syndrome and bladder perforation.
♦ Possible reduction in blood loss thus reducing the transfusion requirement.
♦ Avoidance of the effects of general anaesthesia on the cardiorespiratory system.
♦ Provision of postoperative analgesia during the early postoperative period.
♦ Reduced incidence of postoperative DVT and PE.

♦ Reduced incidence of postoperative nausea and vomiting (PONV).
♦ Rapid return to normal oral intake (particularly important for patients with diabetes).

What problems might you encounter intra-operatively?

Hypotension

This may be due to sympathetic blockade associated with spinal anaesthesia in combination with any pre-operative hypotensive medications (ACE inhibitors) or due to hypovolaemia related to blood loss.

Bleeding

Blood loss during TURP is difficult to assess due to dilution with irrigating fluid. Monitoring serial haemoglobin can be useful in assessing blood loss. The amount depends on the duration and extent of resection. A rough estimate is 2-5ml per minute of resection time or 20-50ml per gram of prostate tissue resected.

Hypothermia

Large volumes of cold irrigating fluid may contribute to peri-operative hypothermia.

TUR syndrome

This is due to the absorption of large volumes of irrigating fluid through the venous sinuses, resulting in fluid overload, dilutional hyponatraemia and pulmonary oedema.

Bladder perforation

Extraperitoneal bladder rupture may cause peri-umbilical or suprapubic pain in the awake patient under regional anaesthesia. Intraperitoneal bladder perforation leads to generalised abdominal pain, which may be referred from the diaphragm to the chest or shoulder. It may also be associated with pallor, sweating, hypotension, and nausea and vomiting.

Bacteraemia and sepsis may rarely occur following TURP. Septic shock following TURP has a high mortality rate. Antibiotic prophylaxis with a single dose of gentamicin 3-4mg/kg on induction should be considered.

What are the clinical features of TUR syndrome?

Intravascular absorption of irrigating fluid results in symptoms and signs related to the cardiovascular and central nervous system.

Cardiovascular system

◆ Increase in systolic BP and a wide pulse pressure (fluid overload), then hypotension (cardiac failure).
◆ Bradycardia.
◆ Chest pain.
◆ Shortness of breath due to pulmonary oedema.
◆ Arrhythmias.
◆ Cardiovascular collapse.

Central nervous system

◆ Nausea and vomiting, caused by hyponatraemia and cerebral oedema.
◆ Altered level of consciousness, confusion and disorientation, also caused by hyponatraemia and cerebral oedema.
◆ Visual disturbance and transient blindness caused by glycine toxicity.
◆ Convulsions.
◆ Coma when the serum sodium concentration falls to less than 100mmol/L.

What is the pathophysiology of TUR syndrome?

The resection of prostate tissue opens an extensive network of venous sinuses, which allows the electrolyte-free irrigation fluid to be absorbed into the systemic circulation, causing an increase in intravascular volume. The glycine-containing irrigation solution is hypo-osmotic (188mosm/L) and results in:

◆ Dilutional hyponatraemia. Encephalopathy with seizures occurs when the sodium concentration falls below 120mmol/L.

- Fluid overload may cause pulmonary oedema and cardiac failure.
- Glycine toxicity may contribute to a reduced level of consciousness and visual impairment.

What are the factors that may affect the absorption of fluid?

- Number and size of the venous sinuses opened. This depends on the size of the gland; a prostate size larger than 60-100g increases the risk of TUR syndrome.
- Experience of the surgeon.
- Duration of the procedure; if longer than 1 hour the risk is increased.
- Hydrostatic pressure >60cm H_2O (height of bag above patient).
- Volume and type of irrigation fluid: use of large volumes of hypotonic intravenous fluids such as 5% dextrose.
- Reduced peripheral venous pressure (dehydration).
- Pre-existing hyponatraemia or pulmonary oedema.

How would you confirm the diagnosis of TUR syndrome?

- Low serum sodium. Levels ≤120mmol/L are invariably symptomatic but a rapid fall is more likely to produce symptoms.
- Low serum osmolality and a high anion gap caused by the presence of glycine.
- ECG manifestations of hyponatraemia such as QRS widening, ST segment elevation and T-wave inversion usually only occur below 115mmol/L.
- Hyper-ammonaemia is a common finding; it is a by-product of glycine metabolism.

What is meant by the term 'anion gap'?

The anion gap is the difference between the measured cations and anions. It represents the unmeasured anions in serum (proteins, phosphates, sulphates and organic acids). The 'measured' cations are sodium (Na^+), potassium (K^+), calcium (Ca^{2+}) and magnesium (Mg^{2+}). The 'measured' anions are chloride (Cl^-), bicarbonate (HCO_3^-) and phosphate (PO_3^-).

The anion gap is calculated as follows:

$$\text{Anion gap} = Na^+ + K^+ - (Cl^- + HCO_3^-)$$

The normal range is 4-12. In normal health there are more unmeasured anions in the serum, therefore, the anion gap is usually positive. But any increase in unmeasured anions (such as glycine) will cause a raised anion gap.

What are the causes of a raised anion gap?

A high anion gap indicates that there is loss of HCO_3^- without a concurrent increase in Cl^- (measured anion). HCO_3^- is replaced by the unmeasured anion resulting in a high anion gap.

The other causes of an increased anion gap include:

◆ Ketoacidosis.
◆ Uraemic acidosis.
◆ Salicylate poisoning.
◆ Methanol and ethanol.
◆ Lactic acidosis.

Which type of acidosis has a normal anion gap?

In patients with a normal anion gap the drop in HCO_3^- is compensated for almost completely by an increase in Cl^-. Causes are hyperchloraemic acidosis, e.g. gastrointestinal loss of HCO_3^- in diarrhoea, renal dysfunction and renal tubular acidosis.

How would you monitor fluid absorption?

Repeated measurements of serum sodium

This is not practicable in routine clinical practice.

Volumetric fluid balance

Measuring input and output of irrigating fluid. The difference is a guide to the amount absorbed or extravasated. It is difficult to do in practice as it is not possible to collect and measure all the output irrigating fluid. Spillage, urine output and blood loss hamper the accuracy of measurement.

Gravimetry

Checking the weight of the patient during the intra-operative period using an operating table with a facility to weigh the patient. The weight gain accounts for the amount of fluid absorbed. The blood loss and intravenous fluid administration should also be taken into account.

CVP

Increases transiently. More than 500ml of fluid absorption within 10 minutes is needed to demonstrate a change in CVP. The CVP value is altered by blood loss, IV fluid administration, patient position and positive pressure ventilation.

Ethanol

The irrigating fluid should contain 1% ethanol. Detection of ethanol in the expired breath gives an indication of the amount of fluid absorbed.

TUR syndrome

TUR syndrome is a recognised complication of transurethral resection of the prostate. Mild TUR syndrome may occur in about 5-10% of patients undergoing TURP. A large amount of fluid absorption can lead to signs and symptoms which can be severe enough to warrant an intensive care admission. The irrigating fluid is directly absorbed into the systemic circulation when the pressure of the irrigating fluid is greater than venous pressure (15cm H_2O).

The ideal irrigating fluid should be isotonic, non-haemolytic, non-toxic, should allow clear visibility, be rapidly excreted and should not influence the plasma osmolality. Glycine 1.5% is used as irrigating fluid as it is cheap and has a low incidence of allergic reactions. The distribution half-life of glycine is 6 minutes; the terminal half-life varies between 40 minutes to several hours. It is metabolised to ammonia in the liver.

Normal saline has been used, but it causes greater volume expansion, and due to excessive chloride content it causes hyperchloraemic acidosis. Sterile water provides clear visibility, but causes cerebral oedema more rapidly than other electrolyte-free irrigation fluids.

Table 3.5 Plasma concentration of glycine and symptoms.

Plasma concentration	Symptoms
5-8mmol/L	Visual disturbance
>10mmol/L	Nausea and vomiting
>21-80mmol/L	Fatal TUR syndrome

Table 3.6 Plasma concentration of sodium and ECG changes.

Plasma concentration	ECG changes
120mmol/L	Possibly wide QRS
115mmol/L	Wide QRS, ST elevation
100mmol/L	VT/VF

Management of TUR syndrome

Initial management should follow the airway, breathing and circulation (ABC) approach. Awake patients may need to be sedated and ventilated, whilst anaesthetised patients breathing spontaneously may need to be intubated and ventilated. The surgeon needs to be informed and the surgery should be completed or terminated as soon as possible. The patient should be managed in an intensive or high dependency care unit and the main aspect of the treatment is supportive.

The principles of managing TUR syndrome involve:

◆ Ensuring adequate oxygen delivery.
◆ Maintaining an adequate circulation.
◆ Correcting hyponatraemia and acid-base imbalance.
◆ Reducing intracranial pressure.
◆ Controlling convulsions.

The management of fluid overload and hyponatraemia involves restricting IV fluids and giving IV frusemide to promote diuresis. Hypertonic saline solutions (1.8%, 3% or 5%) can be used if the serum sodium is lower than 120mmol/L. The rate of increase in the serum sodium level should not be more than 1mmol/L/hour. The rate of correction should not exceed 20mmol/L in the first 48 hours of therapy. Hypertonic saline should be stopped when symptoms cease or the sodium level reaches ≥125mmol/L. The sodium levels should be checked regularly as the rapid correction of sodium may cause central pontine myelinolysis, which causes irreversible brain damage.

Convulsions should be treated initially with a benzodiazepine or small doses of thiopentone. If the seizures are intractable, the sodium level may be corrected more rapidly.

Preventative measures include limiting the height of the bag of irrigating fluid to 60cm above the patient (limiting the infusion pressure to 60cm H_2O), limiting the volume of irrigant used and limiting the resection time to 1 hour.

Key points

◆ Patients undergoing TURP often have many comorbidities.
◆ Spinal anaesthesia allows early detection of mental changes associated with TUR syndrome.
◆ TUR syndrome requires prompt recognition and treatment.

Further reading

1. Porter M, McCormick C. Anaesthesia for transurethral resection of the prostate. *Update in Anaesthesia* 2003; 16(8). Available at: http://www.nda.ox.ac.uk/wfsa/html/u16/u1608_01.htm.
2. Hahn RG. Fluid absorption in endoscopic surgery. *British Journal of Anaesthesia* 2006; 96: 8-20.
3. Jensen V. The TURP syndrome. *Canadian Journal of Anesthesia* 1991; 38: 90-7.

Short case 3.3: Head injury

You have been alerted to attend a trauma case in the emergency department. A 25-year-old male patient and driver of a car involved in a road traffic accident is due to arrive in 10 minutes.

How would you manage this clinical scenario?

◆ Attend the trauma resuscitation room in the emergency department, ensuring that resuscitation equipment and anaesthetic drugs are available.
◆ Formulate a plan with other members of the team (team leader delegating the task to other members).
◆ Follow the ATLS® protocol of primary survey which includes finding any life-threatening problems and managing them before proceeding to the next step:
  - Airway with C spine control: the airway is assessed for patency and signs of airway obstruction if any. Only a jaw thrust should be applied to open the airway;
  - Breathing and ventilation: expose the patient's chest and observe for chest movement, respiratory rate, pattern of respiration, and auscultate the chest for bilateral air entry;
  - Circulation: assessed by skin colour, pulse, capillary refill, and an attempt is made to control any obvious bleeding;
  - Disability: neurological assessment is conducted by using the AVPU scale or the Glasgow Coma Scale and examining the size and reactivity of the pupils. (AVPU = alert, vocalising, responding to pain, unconscious);

- Exposure: the patient should be completely exposed and examined for any obvious injuries. Care should be taken to prevent hypothermia.

What are the indications for intubation and ventilation of a head-injured patient?

Intubation and ventilation is indicated immediately in the following circumstances:

- ◆ Coma or GCS of ≤8.
- ◆ Loss of protective laryngeal reflexes.
- ◆ Ventilatory insufficiency as judged by arterial blood gases: hypoxaemia (PaO_2 <13kPa on oxygen) or hypercapnia ($PaCO_2$ >6kPa).
- ◆ Spontaneous hyperventilation causing a $PaCO_2$ of <4kPa.
- ◆ Irregular respiration.

The patient should be intubated and ventilated before the start of the transfer in the following circumstances:

- ◆ Significantly deteriorating conscious level.
- ◆ Unstable fractures of the facial skeleton.
- ◆ Copious bleeding into the mouth.
- ◆ Seizures.

What are the indications for an immediate CT scan after a head injury?

These are the criteria in adults:

- ◆ A GCS of less than 13 on initial assessment in the emergency department.
- ◆ A GCS of less than 15 at 2 hours after the injury on assessment in the emergency department.
- ◆ Suspected open or depressed skull fracture.
- ◆ Any sign of basal skull fracture such as haemotympanum, bruising around the eyes, cerebrospinal fluid leakage from the ear or nose, and bruising behind the ears (Battle's sign).
- ◆ Post-traumatic seizure.

- Focal neurological deficit.
- More than one episode of vomiting.
- Amnesia for events more than 30 minutes before impact.
- Loss of consciousness or amnesia in a patient with a history of coagulopathy.
- The mechanism of injury suggests a possible intracranial bleed (e.g. a pedestrian or cyclist struck by a motor vehicle, or an occupant ejected from a motor vehicle or a fall from a height of greater than 1m or five stairs).

This patient has a GCS of 12 and the CT scan shows a left-sided extradural haematoma. How would you prepare for a transfer to a specialist neurosurgical unit?

Prior to transfer to the neurosurgical unit, this patient will require tracheal intubation and ventilation. He will then require intravenous sedation (propofol infusion), analgesia (intermittent fentanyl or alfentanil infusion) and muscle paralysis with an appropriate neuromuscular blocking drug. The trauma team leader or a consultant surgeon should discuss the transfer with a neurosurgeon in the specialist unit. The fundamental requirement during transfer is to ensure satisfactory cerebral perfusion and oxygen delivery. MAP should be maintained above 80mmHg using a vasopressor infusion and IV fluids. PaO_2 should be maintained above 13kPa and $PaCO_2$ should be maintained between 4.5 and 5.0kPa.

Availability of oxygen cylinders, infusion pumps with an adequate battery charge, and a transfer pack containing resuscitation drugs and equipment should be checked. If the patient has suffered convulsions a loading dose of phenytoin 15mg/kg should be considered prior to transfer.

As IV fluids, a warm crystalloid solution should be used for resuscitation of hypovolaemia. 5% dextrose should be avoided. Blood should be cross-matched and sent in the transferring ambulance.

A large-bore orogastric tube should be passed and left to drain freely. In the presence of associated chest injury (rib fractures) the possibility of pneumothorax should be considered before transferring. If in doubt a chest drain should be inserted.

What parameters would you monitor during transfer?

The following parameters should be monitored during transfer:

- Pupil size and reaction to light.
- Continuous ECG.
- Pulse oximetry.
- $EtCO_2$.
- Invasive blood pressure.
- Urine output.
- Central venous pressure monitoring (if hypovolaemia is suspected).
- Temperature.

What investigations would you undertake prior to transfer?

- Measurement of arterial blood gases (PaO_2, $PaCO_2$ and pH).
- X-rays: chest, cervical spine and pelvis.
- Haematology: FBC and coagulation screen.
- Biochemistry: blood sugar levels.
- Other investigations as appropriate: CT scan of the head, cervical spine, etc.

Anaesthetic management for craniotomy

Once the patient has been reviewed by the neurosurgical team, he will be transferred to the operating theatre. ECG, invasive BP, CVP, $ETCO_2$, urine output, and temperature monitoring should be continued during the peri-operative period.

A slight head-up tilt (10-15°) position facilitates venous drainage; care should be taken to avoid kinking and obstruction of major veins of the neck. Anaesthesia can be maintained either with a total intravenous anaesthesia (TIVA) technique or with oxygen, air and a volatile anaesthetic.

Blood loss and hourly urine output should be monitored during the intra-operative period. MAP should be maintained above 80mmHg and $PaCO_2$ between 4.5 to 5kPa. Mannitol (0.5-1g/kg) and dexamethasone (8-10mg) may be required intra-operatively to reduce cerebral oedema.

Dexamethasone can cause hyperglycaemia; glucose should be checked and hyperglycaemia should be controlled with insulin infusion.

Postoperatively this patient needs to be transferred to the intensive care unit.

Intensive care management

The main goal is to minimise the secondary brain insult from systemic and intracranial causes. Maintaining adequate perfusion pressure and reducing intracranial pressure are important aspects of intensive care management. The intensive care management of head injury patients includes the following measures:

◆ Sedation, analgesia, paralysis and ventilatory support should be continued to maintain PaO_2 above 11kPa and $PaCO_2$ between 4.5 to 5kPa. Hyperventilation to a target $PaCO_2$ of 4.0 to 4.5 kPa is reserved for those with intractable intracranial hypertension. Adequate sedation minimises anxiety, agitation and reduces the cerebral metabolic rate.

◆ Maintaining perfusion pressure: ICP is defined as the pressure exerted by the contents (blood, CSF and brain) within the rigid skull. Since cerebral perfusion pressure (CPP) = MAP-ICP, any increase in ICP reduces CPP. To maintain the CPP, the MAP should be increased. Hypotension should be avoided, as it causes reduced cerebral perfusion and cerebral ischaemia. Hypotension should be initially treated with volume resuscitation (colloid or crystalloid) to maintain CVP between 5-10mmHg. If required vasopressor or inotropic support should be initiated to maintain MAP.

◆ Nutrition. Early enteral feeding should be considered if there is no associated abdominal injury, in which case parenteral nutrition should be initiated.

◆ Hyperglycaemia is associated with cerebral oedema and an increased ICP. Maintaining glucose at normal levels using insulin therapy has shown to reduce the mortality in patients with severe head injury.

◆ Hyperthermia has adverse effects on the ischaemic brain. Temperature should be regularly monitored and temperature should be carefully controlled.

◆ DVT prophylaxis should be considered using TED (thromboembolic deterrent) stockings and low-molecular-weight heparin.

Table 3.7 Causes of secondary brain insult.

Systemic causes	Intracranial
Hypotension	Cerebral oedema
Hypoxia	Cerebral vasospasm
Hypo / hyperglycaemia	Seizures
Hyperthermia	Infection
Acidosis	
Anaemia	

Role of $PaCO_2$ in cerebral protection

Hyperventilation reduces $PaCO_2$. Cerebral blood flow and $PaCO_2$ are linearly related; a reduction in $PaCO_2$ reduces cerebral blood volume offsetting the increased intracranial pressure. Hyperventilation-induced vasoconstriction, however, reduces blood flow to the injured brain tissue. There is limited evidence for the therapeutic benefit of hyperventilation. However, hypoventilation and hypercapnia must be avoided in patients with a head injury because of the increase in intracranial pressure.

Key points

♦ Initial management of a trauma patient should follow the ATLS® protocol of the ABCDE approach.
♦ The main goal in managing head injury is minimising secondary brain insult.
♦ Adequate perfusion of the injured brain is achieved by maintaining an adequate MAP.
♦ Prior to transfer to another centre the patient should be appropriately resuscitated and stabilised.

Further reading

1. Recommendations for safe transfer of patients with brain injury. http://www.aagbi.org/publications/guidelines/docs/braininjury.pdf.

2. Triage, assessment, investigation and early management of head injury in infants, children and adults. London: NICE guidelines CG 56, September 2007. http://www.nice.org.uk/CG56.
3. Fukuda S, Warner DS. Cerebral protection. *British Journal of Anaesthesia* 2007; 99: 10-7.
4. Helmy A, Vizcaychipi M and Gupta AK. Traumatic brain injury: intensive care management. *British Journal of Anaesthesia* 2007; 99: 32-42.

Applied anatomy 3.1: Pain pathways

You are called to the recovery area to assess a patient who is complaining of pain following an orthopaedic procedure on the foot.

What are the goals of pain assessment?

The goals of pain assessment are to:

◆ Define the severity of pain.
◆ Assist in the selection of appropriate analgesia.
◆ Evaluate the response to treatment.

How would you assess the severity of the pain?

Several pain scales are used to assess its severity and evaluate the response to treatment:

◆ Numerical pain scales, e.g. Visual Analogue Score (VAS). This quantifies the intensity of pain and discomfort using numbers ranging from 0 to 10.
◆ Verbal Pain Scale/Category Rating Scale. Includes frequently used words such as 'low', 'mild' or 'excruciating' to describe the intensity or severity of discomfort. These verbal scales are useful because the expressions are relative, so one focuses on the quality of the pain.
◆ Visual Pain Scale. The Wong-Baker faces rating scale is useful for children who may not have the required vocabulary. Their facial appearance gives an estimate of the severity of pain.

What is the anatomy of the basic pain pathway?

Nociceptors are specific nerve terminals which are activated by mechanical, chemical or thermal stimuli. Nociceptors are served by two types of afferent nerve fibres, A-delta and C fibres.

A-delta fibres are myelinated, and are stimulated by mechanical and thermal stimuli of low or high threshold and transmit immediate sharp pain. C fibres are unmyelinated and are stimulated by high-threshold chemical, thermal and mechanical stimuli. All nociceptors are free nerve endings that have their cell bodies outside the spinal column in the dorsal root ganglia. The afferent fibres synapse in the dorsal horn of the spinal cord (laminae I-II).

The fibres cross over and ascend in the spinothalamic tract to the thalamus. They then project to the somatosensory cortex and limbic system.

Describe the visceral pain pathway

The viscera are innervated mainly by C fibres or unmyelinated fibres which are activated by the distension of hollow viscera, ischaemia, inflammation, traction and muscle spasm. The visceral afferent neurons travel in autonomic nerves, from both the sympathetic and parasympathetic system. The afferent neurons terminate in the dorsal horn laminae where they form synapses with somatic pain afferents and ascend in spino-thalamic tracts to the cerebral cortex.

Which neurotransmitters are involved with pain transmission?

The cell bodies of afferent neurons in the dorsal horn of the spinal cord release two types of excitatory neurotransmitters:

◆ Neuropeptides: substance P, neurokinins, calcitonin gene-related peptide (CGRP), cholecystokinin (CCK), vasoactive intestinal polypeptide and somatostatin.
◆ Amino acids: glutamate, N-methyl D-aspartate (NMDA) and α-amino-3-hydroxyl-5-methyl-4-isoxazole-propionate (AMPA).

What do you understand by the gate control theory of pain?

The gate control theory asserts that activation of nerves which do not transmit pain signals, called non-nociceptive fibres, can interfere with signals from pain fibres, thereby inhibiting pain. Large-diameter Aß fibres are non-nociceptive and inhibit the effects of firing by Aδ and C fibres. If the relative amount of activity is greater in the Aß fibres, there should be little or no pain. If there is more activity in small nerve fibres, then there will be pain.

Are you aware of any clinical applications of the gate control theory of pain?

In transcutaneous electrical nerve stimulation (TENS), non-nociceptive fibres are selectively stimulated with electrodes in order to produce this effect and thereby reduce pain.

Which analgesia would you select for this patient?

The analgesia that the patient has already received should be checked.

The analgesia should be tailored to the severity of pain, but a combination of simple analgesia, e.g. paracetamol, non-steroidal analgesia and opiates, should be considered. The route of administration depends on the severity and intensity of the pain. When giving opioid drugs the intravenous route is preferred to achieve rapid onset pain relief.

What is the mechanism of action of paracetamol?

The mechanism of the analgesic and antipyretic effects of paracetamol is still debated. The probable mechanisms of action are as follows:

- Inhibition of the cyclo-oxygenase-isoenzymes.
- Modulation of the endogenous cannabinoid system.

What is the mechanism of development of liver toxicity with paracetamol overdose?

Paracetamol is metabolised in the liver, primarily by sulphation and glucuronidation to inactive sulphate and glucuronide conjugates, which are then excreted by the kidneys. A small amount is metabolised by the hepatic cytochrome P450 system producing an alkylating metabolite (N-acetyl-p-benzo-quinone imine) which is conjugated with glutathione (the sulfhydryl group) and renally excreted.

In paracetamol toxicity, the sulphate and glucuronide pathways become saturated and more paracetamol is metabolised by cytochrome P450; the hepatocellular glutathione stores become depleted and the alkylating metabolite causes hepatocellular damage.

What is the definitive treatment of paracetamol toxicity and what is its mechanism of action?

N-acetylcysteine can be given. This supplies sulfhydryl groups which react with the metabolite so that it can be safely excreted without causing hepatocellular damage. The dose of N-acetylcysteine is given according to a nomogram. It should be given if the serum paracetamol level is more than 200mg/L at 4 hours, 100mg/L at 8 hours or 50mg/L at 12 hours of ingestion. Liver function, creatinine, INR and blood gas analysis should be performed if the presentation is delayed. The patient should be transferred to a specialist unit if there are signs of cerebral encephalopathy, an INR >2.0, presence of acidosis or renal impairment.

What is the mechanism of action of morphine?

Morphine acts at the opioid receptors, activation of which leads to the reduction of neuronal cell excitability. This then leads to a reduction in nerve impulse transmission and the inhibition of neurotransmitter release. The opioid receptors are G-protein-coupled receptors and activation of these leads to the closing of voltage-sensitive calcium channels, potassium efflux and subsequent hyperpolarisation and reduction of c-AMP

Role of gabapentin in acute pain

There has been recent evidence demonstrating the usefulness of gabapentin and pregabalin in the treatment of acute pain, leading to a reduction in morphine requirements.

The mechanism of action has an overlap in the pathophysiology of acute and chronic pain. Sensitisation of the dorsal horn neurons has been demonstrated in acute pain, for instance, postoperatively and following trauma, leading to allodynia and hyperalgesia.

Gabapentin has a high affinity for the $\alpha2\delta$ subunit of the pre-synaptic voltage-gated calcium channels. These receptors are up-regulated in the dorsal root ganglia and spinal cord following peripheral nerve damage. When it binds with these receptors gabapentin inhibits calcium influx and the subsequent release of excitatory neurotransmitters such as glutamate in the pain pathways. Gabapentin may also reduce or reverse opioid tolerance and there seems to be a synergistic effect with morphine.

Key points

◆ The severity of acute pain can be assessed using numerical, verbal or visual analogue scales.
◆ Pain sensation from nociceptors is carried by the spinothalamic tract to the cerebral cortex.
◆ Gabapentin has been found to be useful in managing acute pain.

Further reading

1. Rowbotham DJ. Gabapentin: a new drug for postoperative pain? *British Journal of Anaesthesia* 2006; 96: 152-5.
2. Seib RK, Paul JE. Preoperative gabapentin for postoperative analgesia: a meta-analysis. *Canadian Journal of Anesthesia* 2006; 53: 461-9.

Applied physiology 3.2: Oxygen delivery

You have been asked to review a 68-year-old female patient in the critical care unit who underwent an emergency laparotomy for a perforated bowel 24 hours ago. She is breathing spontaneously, and her respiratory rate is 18 per minute. Her systolic blood pressure has been between 70 to 100mm Hg for the past 2 hours and her heart rate is 94 per minute. Her blood gas analysis shows a lactate level of 5.4mmol/L.

Can you comment on the lactate level?

The normal lactate concentration in the arterial blood is less than 1.5mmol/L. This patient has an increased lactate level in the blood indicating lactic acidosis.

What is the cause of lactic acidosis?

The cause of lactic acidosis is excessive production of lactic acid as a result of anaerobic metabolism. Blood lactate is mainly metabolised to glucose in the liver.

There are two types of lactic acidosis: type A and type B. Type A is due to excessive production of lactate due to tissue hypoxia and type B occurs in the absence of tissue hypoxia. Accelerated aerobic glycolysis and pyruvate production in excess of mitochondrial needs may produce lactic acidosis. In sepsis increased muscle Na^+/K^+ ATPase activity produces lactic acidosis. Type B occurs in association with diabetes, renal failure and hepatic failure. Certain drugs such as biguanides, salicylates and isoniazid can result in lactic acidosis.

What is the most likely cause of lactic acidosis in this patient?

She is most likely suffering from type A lactic acidosis. This could be due to excessive production of lactic acid resulting from hypoperfusion of the tissues, which will cause hypoxia resulting in anaerobic metabolism.

How is oxygen delivery determined?

Oxygen delivery is dependent on blood flow (cardiac output) and the oxygen content of the arterial blood (haemoglobin and dissolved oxygen). The oxygen delivery can be calculated as follows:

Oxygen delivery = CO [(Hb × 1.34) x SaO_2 x 0.01 + (PaO_2 × 0.023)]

where CO = cardiac output in dL, Hb = haemoglobin/dL, SaO_2 = arterial oxygen saturation, PaO_2 = partial pressure of oxygen in the arterial blood in kPa.

Oxygen delivery can be improved by optimising the factors involved in the above formula.

How would you optimise her cardiac output?

Cardiac output depends on heart rate and stroke volume. The heart rate should be maintained within the normal range. The stroke volume is determined by the preload, myocardial contractility and afterload.

The Frank-Starling law states that the force of contraction of a muscle fibre is proportional to its initial length. In the heart, within physiological limits, an increase in end-diastolic volume (EDV) produces a more forceful contraction and an increase in stroke volume.

Maintaining an optimum preload ensures good contraction of the myocardium and a good stroke volume. The ventricle with normal compliance follows the Frank-Starling relationship whereby increasing the preload increases the stroke volume. The preload is mainly dependent on the return of venous blood from the body. Venous return is influenced by changes in position, intrathoracic pressure, blood volume and the balance of constriction and dilatation in the venous system.

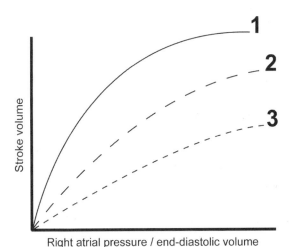

Figure 3.3 Frank-Starling curve and effect of inotropic drugs.
1. Positive inotropic effect; 2. Normal curve; 3. Negative inotropic effect.

What factors may adversely affect the Frank-Starling curve?

The curve is shifted rightward and downward in cardiac failure. Drugs that reduce the contractility such as beta-blockers, hypoxia and acidosis also cause a right and downward shift of the curve. In these circumstances the stroke volume fails to improve despite adequate preload.

Sympathetic stimulation and inotropes can shift the curve upwards and to the left, increasing the stroke volume.

How does afterload affect the stroke volume?

Afterload is the resistance to ventricular ejection. This is reflected as systemic vascular resistance which is determined by the diameter of the arterioles and pre-capillary sphincters. The level of systemic vascular resistance is controlled by the sympathetic system. Increasing afterload decreases the stroke volume.

What other factors can improve oxygen delivery?

Haemoglobin content

If the haemoglobin is lower than the transfusion threshold (7g/dL), red blood cell transfusion should be given to increase the level.

Arterial oxygen saturation

If the SaO_2 is low, oxygen delivery to the lungs should be maximised. This can be accomplished by increasing the concentration of inspired oxygen (FiO_2), increasing the level of PEEP, and by other manoeuvres that will improve ventilation and perfusion (V/Q) matching and decrease intrapulmonary shunting (e.g. chest physiotherapy, prone position, bronchodilators and diuresis).

Partial pressure of oxygen in the arterial blood (PaO_2)

The amount of dissolved oxygen in the arterial blood is directly proportional to PaO_2 (Henry's law).

Dissolved oxygen in 100ml of blood $= 0.023\text{mL}/PaO_2$ in kPa
$$= 0.2\text{ml}/100\text{ml when } PaO_2 \text{ is } 10\text{kPa}$$
$$= 2\text{ml}/100\text{ml when } PaO_2 \text{ is } 100\text{kPa}$$

The average metabolic consumption of oxygen by the human body at sea level is 6.6ml/100ml of blood.

At a PaO_2 of 300kPa, the amount of dissolved oxygen is (6ml/100ml) approximately equal to the metabolic requirement.

Hyperbaric oxygen therapy increases the partial pressure of inspired oxygen and increases the amount of dissolved oxygen.

What are the indications for hyperbaric oxygen therapy (HBO)?

HBO is useful in treating moderate to severe carbon monoxide (CO) poisoning. The indications for HBO in CO poisoning include neurological impairment, loss of consciousness, pregnancy, myocardial dysfunction (chest pain, elevated cardiac enzymes), acidosis, severe hypoxia, and asymptomatic poisoning with a carboxyhaemoglobin level of greater than 15%.

Table 3.8 Indications for hyperbaric oxygen therapy.

Main therapy	Adjunctive therapy
Carbon monoxide poisoning	Radiation tissue damage
Air or gas embolism	Prevention of osteo-radio-necrosis
Decompression sickness	Acute ischaemia and/or crush injuries
Clostridial gas gangrene	Necrotising infections Acute exceptional blood loss Acute thermal burns Compromised skin grafts or flaps Refractory osteomyelitis

What are the physiological effects of hyperbaric oxygen?

Oxygen-carrying capacity

It increases the amount of dissolved oxygen in the arterial blood. As the oxygen diffusion across the tissue depends on the partial pressure gradient it will increase oxygen diffusion.

Decreased size of gas bubble

According to Boyle's law, at constant temperature, the volume of a gas is inversely proportional to pressure exerted on it. During HBO gas bubbles causing vascular obstruction will move to smaller vessels. Due to increased PaO_2, dissolution of bubbles is enhanced by replacing the inert gas within the bubbles by oxygen. These physiological effects are useful in treating gas emboli.

Cardiovascular system

HBO causes vasoconstriction and decreases oedema. It promotes new vessel formation and wound healing. Systemic vascular resistance is increased due to vasoconstriction. Blood pressure increases and a reflex fall in heart rate and cardiac output may be observed.

Effect on bacterial growth

A high PaO_2 prevents the growth of anaerobic bacteria. It decreases the production of clostridial alpha toxins.

Effect on reperfusion injury

HBO therapy modifies the reperfusion injury by inhibiting lipid peroxidation and reducing oxygen-free radicals.

What are the side effects of hyperbaric oxygen therapy?

The side effects related to hyperbaric oxygen therapy can be classified as:

- Those due to high ambient pressure.
- Those due to high PaO_2.

Effects due to high ambient pressure

♦ Increased middle ear pressure may lead to tympanic membrane perforation.
♦ Decompression sickness. With increasing barometric pressure, increasing amounts of nitrogen dissolve and accumulate in the lipid component of tissues. Decreasing barometric pressure too quickly causes the dissolved nitrogen to return to gas while still in the blood or tissues, causing bubbles to form. This can be prevented by slow decompression. The risk of decompression sickness is minimal during HBO because the patient is breathing 100% oxygen, with very minimal nitrogen in the blood.

Effects due to high PaO_2

The adverse effects due to high PaO_2 (oxygen toxicity) depends on the duration of exposure and the partial pressure of oxygen. The mechanism can be explained by the free radical theory. Various highly reactive and potentially cytotoxic free radicals are produced in the mitochondria during the metabolism of oxygen. The short lived O_2 metabolites include:

♦ Superoxide anion (O_2^-).
♦ Hydroxyl radical (OH^-).
♦ Hydrogen peroxide (H_2O_2).
♦ Singlet oxygen.

These metabolites of oxygen can cause inactivation of sulfhydryl enzymes, disruption of DNA and peroxidation of unsaturated membrane lipids with resultant loss of membrane integrity. The cell is also equipped with an array of antioxidant defences, including the enzymes, superoxide dismutase (SOD), catalase, glutathione peroxidase, vitamin E and ascorbate. During hyperoxia, the intracellular generation and influx of free radicals is believed to increase markedly and may overwhelm the detoxifying capacity of the normal complement of antioxidant defences, with resultant cytotoxicity.

Pulmonary toxicity

Pulmonary toxicity can develop after prolonged exposure to oxygen at concentrations between 0.5-1.0 atmospheres. The pathological changes consist of atelectasis, oedema, alveolar haemorrhage, inflammation, fibrin deposition and thickening of alveolar membranes.

Exposure to 100% O_2 for 12-24 hours causes irritation and substernal discomfort.

Exposure to 100% O_2 for 24-26 hours causes reduced vital capacity, compliance and diffusing capacity, decreased surfactant production, increased ventilation/perfusion mismatch and increased capillary permeability.

Neurological toxicity
Symptoms include muscle twitching, nausea, tinnitus, vertigo, visual field defects, hallucinations and dysphoria. Convulsions may occur at an inspired oxygen pressure of about 2-3 atmospheres.

Systemic oxygen toxicity
Systemic oxygen toxicity is related to arterial O_2 tension, whereas pulmonary oxygen toxicity depends on alveolar O_2 tension. Retrolental fibroplasia has been reported in the premature neonate after exposure to PaO_2 at more than 10-20kPa for a few hours. Reversible myopia due to the effect on the lens is one of the common side effects. Oxygen toxicity can be prevented by using air in the chamber for 5 minutes for every 30 minutes (air breaks).

Carbon monoxide poisoning

Carbon monoxide (CO) affects oxygen transport and utilization. It binds to haemoglobin with an affinity 200 times that of oxygen. CO poisoning causes hypoxia by the following mechanisms:

- Reduces the amount of haemoglobin available for O_2 transport.
- Shifts the oxygen dissociation curve to the left, so impairing oxygen delivery to the tissues.
- Binds to cytochrome oxidase and impairs tissue oxygen utilization.

CO also binds to the large pool of myoglobin, increasing tissue hypoxia.

Clinical features of carbon monoxide poisoning

Central nervous system
Drowsiness, headache, dizziness, stupor, seizures and loss of consciousness.

Cardiovascular system
Tachycardia, myocardial ischaemia, arrhythmias, hypotension or hypertension.

Respiratory system
Tachypnoea, dyspnoea and pulmonary oedema.

Metabolic system
Metabolic acidosis.

Pulse oximetry

Oxygen saturation may remain in the normal range despite cyanosis and tissue hypoxia (false high reading). CO poisoning typically produces a pulse oximetry gap (the difference between the pulse oximeter reading and the spectrophotometrically measured oxyhaemoglobin saturation). The clinical features and severity of CO poisoning do not correlate well with the carboxyhaemoglobin concentration.

Management of CO poisoning

Initial management involves an airway, breathing and circulation approach. 100% oxygen decreases the half-life of carboxyhaemoglobin from about 5 hours to 1 hour. Hyperbaric oxygen can reduce the half-life to about 20 minutes. Hyperbaric oxygen also provides an alternate source of tissue oxygenation through oxygen dissolved in plasma. In addition, hyperbaric oxygen dissociates CO from cytochrome oxidase improving electron transport and cellular energy state.

Key points

◆ Oxygen delivery is determined by arterial oxygen content and cardiac output.

◆ Cellular hypoxia due to hypoperfusion leads to anaerobic metabolism and lactic acidosis.

◆ Hyperbaric oxygen therapy increases the amount of dissolved oxygen in the plasma thereby increasing the oxygen-carrying capacity of the blood.

◆ Carbon monoxide poisoning is one of the main indications for hyperbaric oxygen therapy.

Further reading

1. Phypers B, Pierce TJM. Lactate physiology in health and disease. *British Journal of Anaesthesia CEACCP* 2006; 6: 128-32.
2. Pitkin AD. Hyperbaric oxygen therapy. *British Journal of Anaesthesia CEPD review* 2001; 1: 150-6.
3. Taneja R, Vaughan RS. Oxygen. *British Journal of Anaesthesia CEPD review* 2001; 4: 104-7.

Applied pharmacology 3.3: Neuromuscular blocking drugs

A 35-year-old male patient with end-stage renal failure on haemodialysis is scheduled on the emergency list for a renal transplant using a cadaveric kidney.

Would you use succinylcholine in this patient?

Post-dialysis serum potassium (K^+) levels should be checked. If K^+ is within the normal range (3.5-5.0mmol/L), a normal dose of succinylcholine can be used. Succinylcholine causes an increase in serum K^+ by 0.5mmol/L. If the serum K^+ level is greater than 5.5mmol/L, succinylcholine should be avoided.

What are the other side effects of succinylcholine?

◆ Myalgia: more common in young females and ambulatory patients following minor surgery.
◆ Sinus bradycardia: more commonly seen in children and after repeated doses.
◆ Succinylcholine apnoea: a prolonged neuromuscular block after succinylcholine is due to a deficiency in the cholinesterase enzyme.
◆ Increased intra-ocular pressure (IOP): occurs within 1 minute of injection and lasts for about 6 minutes.
◆ Increased intragastric pressure: as the lower oesophageal sphincter tone also increases, normally there is no increased risk of regurgitation.
◆ Malignant hyperpyrexia: succinylcholine is one of the triggering agents for malignant hyperthermia.
◆ Tachyphylaxis and Phase II block (dual block): a decreased response may be observed with repeated doses and this may precede the gradual development of Phase II block (change of characteristics of block to a non-depolarising block). This is most commonly seen when large doses or prolonged infusions are used.

Which muscle relaxants would you choose in a patient with renal failure?

Non-depolarising neuromuscular blockers (NDNMBs) such as atracurium and cisatracurium (benzylisoquinolinium esters) are preferred in patients with renal failure. They are broken down by enzymatic ester hydrolysis and non-enzymatic alkaline hydrolysis (Hoffmann elimination) to inactive products with minimal renal excretion of the parent compound. They are not dependent on renal or hepatic excretion for termination of action. Therefore, the elimination half-lives of atracurium and cisatracurium are not affected by renal failure.

What are the differences between depolarising and non-depolarising blockade?

Depolarising muscle relaxants produce a faster onset of block characterised by muscle fasciculation. Neuromuscular stimulation shows reduced single twitch height and reduced train of four twitches; all are of equal amplitude. Tetanic stimulation does not elicit any fade. Post-tetanic potentiation which is seen with non-depolarising blockade is not observed with a depolarising relaxant. The block cannot be antagonised by increasing the acetyl choline levels.

Non-depolarising blockade is of relatively slower onset and does not produce muscle fasciculation. Neuromuscular simulation shows reduced single twitch height, a decreasing height of train of four twitches, tetanic fade and post-tetanic facilitation. This is a competitive block and can be antagonised by increasing the cholinesterase levels at the neuromuscular junction.

Discuss the excretion of other NDNMBs

NDNMBs used in clinical practice include mivacurium, vecuronium and rocuronium.

Mivacurium is a benzylisoquinolinium ester. It is hydrolysed by plasma cholinesterase at a rate of 70% of that of succinylcholine. It is partly metabolised by the liver and less than 5% of mivacurium is eliminated by the kidneys. Elimination half-life remains largely unchanged in renal failure.

Vecuronium and rocuronium are amino-steroids which are excreted mostly by the liver, with about 40% excreted by the kidneys. The duration of neuromuscular blockade by vecuronium and rocuronium is therefore prolonged in patients with renal disease. An intubating dose would be expected to last about 50% longer in patients with end-stage renal disease.

Other NDNMBs such as doxacurium, pipecuronium and pancuronium are dependent mainly on renal excretion. Pancuronium is largely excreted in the urine, after biotransformation to less active 3-hydroxy and 3, 17 dihydroxypancuronium. The elimination half-life of pancuronium is prolonged by more than 95% in patients with end-stage renal failure.

What other conditions can prolong the neuromuscular block?

Electrolyte imbalance

♦ Hypokalaemia and hypernatraemia can increase the trans-membrane potential and post-junctional membrane threshold for depolarization and thus increases the action of NDNMBs.

◆ Hypermagnesaemia enhances the action of non-depolarising muscle relaxants by decreasing the release of acetylcholine from the nerve terminal and reducing the sensitivity of the post-junctional membrane to acetylcholine.

◆ Calcium appears to be effective in antagonising neuromuscular blockade associated with muscle relaxants, magnesium and antibiotics.

Acid-base imbalance

◆ Metabolic and respiratory acidosis may potentiate non-depolarising relaxants.

Drug interactions

◆ Antibiotics such as aminoglycosides and tetracycline decrease acetylcholine release by blocking the influx of calcium ions necessary for transmitter release.

◆ Antiarrhythmic drugs suich as lidocaine, procainamide and quinidine enhance the effects of NDNMBs.

◆ Calcium channel blockers, e.g. verapamil, enhance NDNMBs.

◆ Hypothermia reduces serum clearance, renal and biliary excretion of NDNMBs.

How would you reverse the non-depolarising neuromuscular block?

The NDNMB (competitive block) is reversed using neostigmine, an anticholinesterase. It is a quaternary amine compound that antagonises the acetylcholinesterase enzyme. Normally each acetylcholine molecule comes in contact with one or two post-junctional receptors before being destroyed by the acetylcholinesterase. However, if the acetylcholinesterase is antagonised, each acetylcholine molecule will stay for a longer duration at the junctional cleft and be able to make contact with several receptors.

The carbamyl group of neostigmine binds to the anionic site of the acetylcholinesterase enzyme and forms a carbamylated enzyme complex; it reversibly prevents the binding of acetylcholine to the enzyme. It also acts on the pre-synaptic receptors to increase the release of acetylcholine.

Excessive doses of neostigmine cause a depolarizing type block due to predominance of acetylcholine activity.

The cholinergic effects are not limited to the neuromuscular junction alone, but increased muscarinic activity results in bradycardia, hypotension and reduced vasomotor tone, hence an anticholinergic agent such as glycopyrrolate or atropine should be given along with neostigmine. Glycopyrrolate is better matched to the onset and duration of neostigmine.

Pharmacokinetics

Neostigmine has very low bioavailablity after oral administration (<1%). It is metabolised by plasma esterase to a quaternary alcohol, and most of the drug is excreted in the urine.

The dose is 0.05-0.08mg/kg as an IV bolus used for reversing the effect of non-depolarising agents.

Pharmacodynamics

The onset of action is within 1 minute, with a peak effect at 10 minutes. The duration of action is 20-30 minutes. The following are systemic effects due to muscarinic activity.

Cardiovascular system
* Bradycardia.
* Hypotension.

Respiratory system
* Bronchoconstriction.
* Bronchospasm.

Central nervous system
* In high doses can cause miosis.

Gastrointestinal tract
* Increased gastrointestinal peristalsis.
* Increased salivation.
* Increased lower oesophageal sphincter pressure.

Sugammadex

Sugammadex is a new compound which is a modified gamma-cyclodextrin. Su refers to sugar and gammadex refers to the structural molecule, gammadextrin.

Sugammadex exerts its effect by forming very tight complexes at a 1:1 ratio with steroidal neuromuscular blocking drugs.

During rocuronium-induced neuromuscular blockade, sugammadex rapidly removes free rocuronium molecules from the plasma. This creates a concentration gradient favouring the movement of the remaining rocuronium molecules from the neuromuscular junction back into the plasma, where they are encapsulated by free sugammadex molecules. The sugammadex molecules also enter the tissues and form a complex with rocuronium. The neuromuscular blockade of rocuronium is therefore terminated rapidly by the diffusion of rocuronium away from the neuromuscular junction back into the plasma. Most sugammadex is excreted unchanged in the urine in the first 8 hours.

Table 3.9 Dose of sugammadex.

Dose	2mg/kg	4mg/kg	16mg/kg
Depth of blockade	Moderate T_2 present	Deep PTC: 1 to 2	Immediate reversal of rocuronium

T_2 = second twitch of TOF
PTC = post-tetanic count

Key points

◆ Succinylcholine should be avoided in the presence of hyperkalaemia.
◆ Atracurium and cisatracurium are the neuromuscular blocking drugs of choice in renal failure.

- An anticholinergic agent such as glycopyrrolate should be administered along with neostigmine.
- Sugammadex can immediately reverse rocuronium-induced neuromuscular block.

Further reading

1. Naguib M. Sugammadex. Another milestone in clinical neuromuscular pharmacology. *Anesthesia and analgesia* 2007; 104: 575-81.
2. Peck TE, Williams M, Hill SA. Muscle relaxants and anti-cholinesterases. In: *Pharmacology for anaesthesia and intensive care*, 2nd ed. Cambridge: Cambridge University Press, 2003: 161-87.
3. Appiah-Ankam J, Hunter JM. Pharmacology of neuromuscular blocking drugs. *British Journal of Anaesthesia CEACCP* 2004; 4: 1-7.
4. Nair VP, Hunter JM. Anticholinestarases and anticholinergic drugs. *British Journal of Anaesthesia CEACCP 2004;* 4: 164-8.
5. Mirakhur RK. Sugammadex in clinical practice. *Anaesthesia* 2009; 64 (Suppl 1): 45-54.

Equipment, clinical measurement and monitoring 3.4: Capnometry

How would you confirm successful tracheal intubation?

There are a number of methods described to confirm the successful placement of a tracheal tube. Clinical signs of tracheal intubation are:

- Direct visualisation of passage of the tracheal tube through the vocal cords.
- Bilateral chest movements.
- Bilateral air entry on auscultation over the chest.
- Water condensation on the tracheal tube.
- Compliance of the reservoir bag.
- Palpation of the tube passing through the larynx.

The above clinical signs are not always reliable. The correct placement of a tracheal tube should be confirmed using the following devices:

- Capnography.
- Fenum CO_2 analyser.
- Fibreoptic bronchoscopy.
- Wee's oesophageal detector device.

Direct visualisation and presence of $ETCO_2$ consecutively for six breaths is the gold standard for confirming tracheal intubation. Presence of carbonated drinks and alveolar gas from air in the stomach may give rise to some false positive readings during the initial few breaths following oesophageal intubation.

The Fenum CO_2 analyser contains a chemical that changes colour on exposure to CO_2.

Wee's oesophageal detector works on the principle that application of negative pressure causes collapse of the oesophagus, preventing further aspiration. The negative pressure applied will aspirate gas from the trachea, as the trachea with rigid walls fails to collapse.

Describe the principles of measuring $ETCO_2$

CO_2 concentration in a gas mixture can be measured using the following four methods:

- Mass spectrometry.
- Infrared spectrometry.
- Raman spectrometry.
- Photo-acoustic spectroscopy.

Infrared (IR) spectrometry uses a compact device and is less expensive than other methods of measurement. It is the most popular method currently used to monitor $ETCO_2$. The wave length of IR rays is $>1.0\mu m$ while that of visible light lies between 0.4 and $0.8\mu m$. Gases with molecules containing two or more different atoms absorb radiation in the infrared region of the spectrum. CO_2 has a strong absorption band at a wavelength of $4.26\mu m$.

What types of infrared analysers are there?

There are two types of capnometers used in clinical practice: mainstream and sidestream analysers.

Mainstream analyser

A cuvette with a quartz window is placed between the breathing system and the tracheal tube connector. As expired and inspired gases flow past the window in the cuvette, a beam of infrared radiation (wavelength 4.3µm) is directed through the window. There is no need for gas sampling. Water vapour can condense on the sensor which can result in a false high reading. To overcome this, the sensor is heated to 39°C. It is heavy and cumbersome.

Sidestream analyser

The sensor is located in the main unit; gas is aspirated using a small pump via a sampling tube at a rate of 50-150ml/minute. As this gas also contains anaesthetic agent, it should be scavenged or returned to the patient's breathing system.

Describe the principle of mass spectrometry and Raman spectrometry

The mass spectrograph separates gases and vapours of differing molecular weights. The gas sample is aspirated into a high vacuum chamber where an electronic beam ionizes and fragments the components of the gas sample. The ions are accelerated by an electric field into a final chamber, which has a magnetic field, perpendicular to the path of the ionized gas stream. In the magnetic field the charged ions are deflected. The radius (arc) of deflection depends on the charge: mass ratio. Lighter ions are deflected most. Detector plates placed at various distances will detect and measure the molecules. It has a rapid response time enabling breath by breath analysis of gas. This system is very expensive and too bulky to use in the operating theatre.

Raman spectrometry uses the principle of 'Raman scattering' for CO_2 measurement. The gas sample is aspirated into an analyzing chamber, where the molecules interact with a monochromatic beam of an argon laser. During this stage the rotational energy and vibrational energy of the gas molecules are changed (Raman scattering). Transfer of energy between gas molecules and light results in the change of wavelength which depends on the characteristics of the gas molecule.

What is the principle of photo-acoustic spectroscopy?

Photo-acoustic gas measurement is where a sample of gas is passed through a source of pulsatile infrared radiation. The gas molecules absorb IR energy and expand. This occurs in pulses. The acoustic signal generated due to the increase in pressure in pulses is detected by a microphone.

What do you understand by the term 'end-tidal CO_2 (ETCO$_2$) concentration'?

ETCO$_2$ is the tension of CO_2 in the exhaled gas at the end of expiration. Because the gas originates from the alveoli, it is considered to represent the CO_2 tension in the alveolar gas (PACO$_2$). The PACO$_2$ results from the combination of gases: gases from ideal alveoli and gases from the alveolar dead space region. In ideal alveoli the ventilation and perfusion are perfectly matched and the CO_2 concentration is the same as arterial (PaCO$_2$). The alveoli that are ventilated but not perfused contribute to alveolar dead space where CO_2 concentration is the same as the inspired CO_2 (PICO$_2$) and is normally zero.

What are the factors that influence the ETCO$_2$ concentration?

The ETCO$_2$ concentration depends on the partial pressure of alveolar CO_2 (PACO$_2$) and volume of dead space.

The PACO$_2$ depends on the following factors:

- Production of CO_2 in the tissues.
- Cardiac output and pulmonary blood flow to carry CO_2 to the lungs.
- Alveolar ventilation.

Table 3.10 Causes for increased $ETCO_2$.

Increased production of CO_2	Alveolar perfusion	Alveolar ventilation	Technical factors
Fever	Increased cardiac output	Hypoventilation	Exhausted CO_2 absorber
Thyrotoxicosis		Endobronchial intubation	Breathing system leak
Malignant hyperthermia			Malfunction unidirectional valves
Tourniquet release			Ventilator malfunction
Administration sodium bicarbonate			

Table 3.11 Causes for decreased $ETCO_2$.

Decreased production of CO_2	Alveolar perfusion	Alveolar ventilation	Technical factors
Hypothermia	Reduced cardiac output	Hyperventilation	Breathing system disconnection
	Hypotension	Total airway obstruction	Leak in the sampling tube
	Hypovolaemia	Accidental tracheal extubation	
	Pulmonary embolism		
	Cardiac arrest		

What factors affect the accuracy of IR capnography?

♦ Atmospheric pressure. An increase in the atmospheric pressure increases the density of IR absorbing molecules within the sample chamber. This results in a small increase in the IR energy being absorbed giving rise to a small error in the reading.
♦ Presence of nitrous oxide. Nitrous oxide absorbs IR energy at 4.5μm close to CO_2 absorption frequency. The presence of nitrous oxide causes a 'collision broadening effect'. Because of collision with nitrous oxide molecules, more energy from the infrared beam is absorbed, leading to a false high reading.
♦ Presence of water vapour. Water vapour may absorb IR energy giving rise to false high readings.
♦ Response time. The accuracy also depends on the response time of the monitor. A faster response leads to a more accurate reading. The response time depends on the transit time and rise time. The transit time is the time taken for the sample to travel from the catheter mount at the ETT end to the detector cell in the monitor. With a sidestream analyser, this depends on the sampling flow rate and the length of the sampling tube. The rise time is the time taken to change the output of the capnometer in response to a step change in PCO_2.

Capnography

Capnography is the graphic display of measured CO_2 concentration versus time. Capnometry is the measurement and display of CO_2 concentration in the expired gas.

A normal capnograph trace has four phases:

♦ Inspiratory baseline. This should be at 0, since any elevation of the baseline indicates re-breathing of CO_2.
♦ Expiratory upslope phase (onset of expiration). This is usually a steep upstroke; if shallow, this indicates airway obstruction. The maximum expired CO_2 is usually considered to be the end-tidal CO_2.
♦ Alveolar plateau. This represents mixing of alveolar gas; if sloped rather than flat, this indicates uneven mixing, as in chronic obstructive airway disease.
♦ Inspiratory down-stroke. During commencement of inspiration, fresh gas is inhaled past the sensor and the capnogram falls sharply to the baseline ($PCO_2=0$).

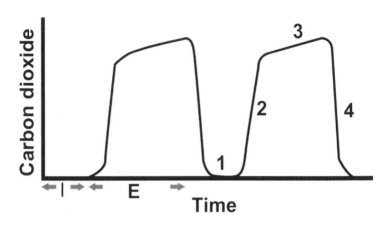

Figure 3.4 Normal capnograph.

Key points

- Clinical signs of tracheal intubation are not always reliable.
- Direct visualisation and presence of $ETCO_2$ consecutively for six breaths confirm tracheal intubation.
- There are two types of IR CO_2 analysers: sidestream and mainstream analysers.
- Sidestream analysers are more convenient but there may be a delay in the response, which depends on transit time and rise time.

Further reading

1. Bhavani-Shnakar K, Moseley H. Capnometry and anaesthesia. *Canadian Journal of Anesthesia* 1992; 39: 617-32.
2. Anderson CT, Breen H. Carbon dioxide kinetics and capnography during critical care. *Critical Care* 2000; 4: 207-5.

Structured oral examination 4

Long case 4

Information for the candidate

History

A 38-year-old Afro-Caribbean female patient is scheduled for an elective subtotal thyroidectomy. She gives a history of intolerance to heat, palpitations, lethargy and weight loss. She had failed radio-iodine therapy 3 years ago. She has a sickle cell trait. She had an uneventful pregnancy 5 years ago. Her current medications are carbimazole 20mg o.d., the oral contraceptive pill and methylcellulose eye drops.

Clinical examination

She is breathless, sweaty and clammy. She has a large diffuse goitre.

Table 4.1 Clinical examination.	
Weight	56kg
Height	170cm
Heart rate	120 bpm
Blood pressure	110/75mmHg
Temperature	36.7°C

Investigations

Table 4.2 Biochemistry.

		Normal values
Sodium	142mmol/L	135-145mmol/L
Potassium	4.1mmol/L	3.5-5.0mmol/L
Urea	3.5mmol/L	2.2-8.3mmol/L
Creatinine	63µmol/L	44-80µmol/L
Blood glucose	5.5mmol/L	3.0-6.0mmol/L

Table 4.3 Haematology.

		Normal values
Hb	10.2g/dL	11-16g/dL
Haematocrit	0.34	0.4-0.5 males, 0.37-0.47 females
RBC	3.7×10^{12}/L	$3.8-4.8 \times 10^{12}$/L
WBC	3.2×10^9/L	$4-11 \times 10^9$/L
Platelets	95×10^9/L	$150-450 \times 10^9$/L
INR	1.0	0.9-1.2
PT	12.5 seconds	11-15 seconds
APTT ratio	1	0.8-1.2

Table 4.4 Thyroid function tests.

T4	30.7pmol/L	10-22pmol/L
Free T3	10.5pmol/L	2.8-7.1pmol/L
TSH	0.1mU/L	0.3-4.6mU/L

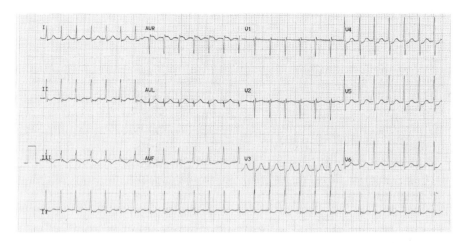

Figure 4.1 ECG.

Examiner's questions

Please summarise the case

This is a 38-year-old lady with thyrotoxicosis and anaemia who is known to have a sickle cell trait. She is listed for an elective thyroid operation. She is clearly hyperthyroid despite her antithyroid medications.

Prior to surgery, thyrotoxicosis should be controlled by optimising drug therapy. She needs further airway assessment and further investigations such as nasoendoscopy, a thoracic inlet X-ray and a CT scan as indicated from clinical history and examination. The full blood count shows pancytopenia which may be related to carbimazole.

What could be the cause for this patient's hyperthyroid state?

Since this lady is on methylcellulose eye drops (artificial tear drops), she most probably has eye signs. Therefore, this is most likely to be Graves' disease.

What are the causes of hyperthyroidism?

The causes of hyperthyroidism can be classified as follows.

Common causes

- Graves' disease (autoimmune).
- Toxic multinodular goitre.
- Solitary toxic nodule/adenoma.

Uncommon causes

- Acute thyroiditis: viral, autoimmune and post-irradiation.
- Neonatal thyrotoxicosis (maternal thyroid antibodies).
- Exogenous iodine.
- Drugs (e.g. amiodarone).

What are the abnormal findings in the investigations provided?

The full blood count shows a low haemoglobin, a low white cell count and low platelets suggesting pancytopenia. Carbimazole can cause bone marrow suppression and pancytopenia.

A low haemoglobin level can also be caused by bone marrow suppression as a result of aplastic crises which usually follow infection with parvovirus B19 and may also cause pancytopenia. A haemoglobin concentration above 8g/dL is an adequate level during the pre-operative period, so this patient does not require pre-operative transfusion.

A marked increase in haemoglobin may increase blood viscosity and precipitate a vaso-occlusive crisis. If the patient has received multiple blood transfusions in the past, there is a possibility of developing red cell antibodies.

Her thyroid function tests show a very low thyroid stimulating hormone (TSH) and elevated free T3 and T4 suggesting that her thyrotoxicosis is not controlled.

The ECG shows narrow complex regular tachycardia with a rate of 150 bpm, most likely to be atrial flutter. There is ST segment depression in V4-V6 and T-wave inversion in leads II, II and aVF.

Can you explain the synthesis of thyroid hormones?

The thyroid hormones, thyroxine (T4) and tri-iodothyronine (T3), are synthesized in the follicular cells. The synthesis of thyroid hormones involves the following steps:

- Iodide trapping. Iodide from dietary sources is actively absorbed from the bloodstream and concentrated in the thyroid follicles.
- Oxidation. Iodide is rapidly oxidised to iodine.
- Iodination. Iodination of tyrosine to form mono-iodotyrosine (MIT) and di-iodotyrosine (DIT). The enzyme, thyroid peroxidase, catalyses the oxidation of iodide and iodination of tyrosine. Tyrosine residues are part of the thyroglobulin molecule (glycoprotein) in the colloid. Thyroglobulin is synthesised in the thyroid cells and secreted into the colloid by exocytosis.
- Combination. T3 is formed by combining one MIT and one DIT molecule. T4 is formed by combining two DIT molecules. T4 is stored in the colloid bound to the thyroglobulin molecule. Proteases digest iodinated thyroglobulin, releasing the hormones, T4 and T3, the biologically active agents central to metabolic regulation.

The production of T4 and T3 is regulated by TSH, released by the anterior pituitary, which in turn is controlled by thyrotropin releasing hormone released by the hypothalamus. When the T4 levels are high, TSH production is suppressed forming a negative feedback loop.

In the blood, T3 and T4 are partially bound to thyroxine binding globulin and albumin and only a small fraction of the circulating hormone is free (unbound). The free fraction of the hormone is active. The half-life of T4 is 5-7 days; the half-life of T3 is only 24 hours. T3 is four times more active than the more abundant T4.

What are the drugs used in the management of hyperthyroidism?

The two main group of drugs used in the treatment of hyperthyroidism are antithyroid drugs and beta-blockers.

Antithyroid drugs

◆ Carbimazole. This prevents the synthesis of T3 and T4 by inhibiting oxidation of iodide to iodine, thereby preventing the iodination of tyrosyl residues in thyroglobulin. It can cause bone marrow suppression causing pancytopenia and agranulocytosis. Carbimazole is a prodrug, well absorbed from the gastrointestinal tract and converted to methimazole (active component) in the liver. It usually takes 4-8 weeks for the patient to become euthyroid; the dose is then gradually reduced and continued for 12-18 months. The side effects include rashes, arthralgia and pruritis. Agranulocytosis is a rare side effect.

◆ Propylthiouracil. This inhibits the iodination of tyrosyl residues in thyroglobulin and prevents the peripheral conversion of T4 to T3. It is used if patients are sensitive to carbimazole. It can also cause bone marrow suppression. A euthyroid state is usually achieved after 4-8 weeks of treatment. It has a slightly higher incidence of agranulocytosis compared with carbimazole.

◆ Lugol's iodine. Traditionally this has been used as an adjunct to antithyroid drugs for 10-14 days before a partial thyroidectomy to reduce the vascularity of the gland.

Beta-blockers

These are used to control the symptoms of thyrotoxicosis. Propranolol is most commonly used. It controls the cardiovascular effects and prevents the peripheral conversion of T4 to T3. It is also used in a thyrotoxic crisis to control the sympathetic effects. Propranolol is a non-selective beta-blocker and is relatively contraindicated in patients with cardiac failure and chronic obstructive airway disease.

What are the anaesthetic implications in this patient?

◆ Anaesthetic implications due to the effects of thyrotoxicosis. As she is hyperthyroid at present, she is more prone to cardiovascular complications such as arrhythmias, an exaggerated cardiovascular response to laryngoscopy and surgical stimulation, and peri-operative ischaemic events. There may be precipitation of a thyroid storm in the peri-operative period. This patient most probably has eye signs (she uses methylcellulose drops) and may be more prone to corneal abrasions and pressure injury because of the proptosis.

- Anaesthetic implications due to the effects of goitre. With regard to the airway, a large goitre may cause tracheal deviation or obstruction. It may be worse in the supine position and usually eases in the lateral position. Postoperatively, after the removal of the thyroid gland, tracheomalacia can lead to airway obstruction. There may be involvement of the recurrent laryngeal nerve causing a hoarse voice (unilateral) or stridor (bilateral).
- Anaesthetic implications due to the effect of the sickle cell trait. A sickle crisis may occur in the peri-operative period due to hypoxia, acidosis, and hypothermia.

What investigations would you do to assess her airway?

- Thoracic inlet X-ray with an anteroposterior view to check for tracheal deviation and narrowing. A lateral thoracic inlet view is needed to assess the degree of tracheal compression. The thoracic inlet X-ray may also reveal retrosternal extension of the goitre.
- A CT scan of the neck and thoracic inlet is useful in assessing the site and extent of tracheal obstruction. The diameter of the airway at the narrowest point can be measured which will aid in estimating the size of the ETT.
- An indirect laryngoscopy or fibreoptic nasoendoscopy should be performed to view and document the pre-operative function of the vocal cords.

What could precipitate a sickle cell crisis?

The following factors can precipitate a sickle cell crisis:

- Infection.
- Dehydration.
- Acidosis.
- Hypothermia.

◆ Inadequate analgesia.
◆ Vascular stasis (tourniquets).
◆ Alcohol.
◆ Stress.

What are the types of sickle cell crises you know of?

◆ Vaso-occlusive crisis. This is the most common of all the crises. It is caused by sickling and subsequent obstruction of small vessels. It may present as an acute abdomen, priapism or acute pain in the hands and feet (dactylitis).
◆ Aplastic crisis. This usually follows infection with parvovirus B19, which causes temporary shutdown of the bone marrow.
◆ Sequestration crisis. This occurs mainly in children. There is splenic pooling of red cells causing painful splenomegaly which may lead to hypovolaemia and circulatory collapse.
◆ Haemolytic crisis. This presents as a fall in haemoglobin and a rise in reticulocytes and bilirubin.

What precautions would you take to prevent sickle cell crises in this patient?

The aim is to avoid dehydration, hypoxia, acidosis and hypothermia during the peri-operative period.

An intravenous fluid infusion should be started pre-operatively to avoid dehydration whilst the patient is starved. Administration of oxygen along with sedative premedication avoids hypoxia during the pre-operative period. Pre-oxygenation at induction and meticulous care during positioning to avoid venous stagnation should be taken. The temperature of the patient should be monitored and active warming should be used to prevent hypothermia. During the postoperative period, hydration, adequate analgesia and supplemental oxygen should be continued.

Would you anaesthetise this patient?

This patient should not be anaesthetised for an elective thyroidectomy as she is not in a euthyroid state.

If this patient was clinically euthyroid and had no airway problems anticipated how would you anaesthetise her?

Pre-operatively

Benzodiazepine premedication may be beneficial in reducing anxiety.

Intra-operatively

Monitoring during anaesthesia includes peripheral oxygen saturation using pulse oximetry, continuous ECG and non-invasive blood pressure measurement.

Induction and maintenance of anaesthesia

The cardiovascular response to laryngoscopy can be minimised by using opioids at induction. Local anaesthetic spray to the vocal cords and trachea reduces the pressor response to tracheal manipulation during surgery.

As there are no anticipated airway problems, pre-oxygenation and intravenous induction can be used. Prior to administration of the muscle relaxant the ability to ventilate the lungs should be checked with gentle ventilation through a face mask. An armoured ETT is usually chosen to secure the airway. The eyes should be taped and padded to protect the exophthalmic eye.

If intubation and/or ventilation should prove difficult, manually lifting forward a large goitre may relieve airway obstruction.

The MAC of volatile anaesthetics in patients with thyrotoxicosis may be increased.

The patient should be positioned in the head-up tilt position, with neck extension achieved with a sand bag or a one litre fluid bag placed between the shoulders. Care should be taken to prevent venous obstruction and venous engorgement.

During the intra-operative period factors triggering sickling of red blood cells (RBCs) such as hypothermia, hypovolaemia, hypercarbia and hypoxia should be avoided.

At the end of the procedure the surgeon may request for a Valsalva manoeuvre to be performed to check haemostasis.

Recovery and postoperative period

The trachea should be extubated once the patient is fully awake. While the patient is still 'deep' the ETT can be replaced by an LMA. This enables visualisation of the vocal cord movement via the LMA using a fibreoptic scope, after which the patient is allowed to wake up.

The patient should be monitored in the immediate postoperative period for airway obstruction, thyroid storm, sickle cell crisis and hypocalcaemia. Postoperative analgesia should be provided with regular paracetamol and NSAIDs such as ibuprofen or diclofenac sodium. Opioids such as codeine phosphate and morphine can be administered to manage breakthrough pain when required.

Supplementary oxygen and intravenous fluids should be continued in the postoperative period to prevent dehydration and hypoxia. Sitting the patient up reduces oedema and venous engorgement.

What are the possible postoperative complications that can occur following thyroidectomy?

Postoperative haemorrhage

This may cause swelling of the neck and airway obstruction. If airway obstruction due to a haematoma is suspected, the immediate management involves removal of skin clips or sutures to evacuate the haematoma. Clip removers or stitch cutters should be available at the patient's bed side.

Laryngeal oedema

This may be due to traumatic intubation or extensive neck surgery. Dexamethasone 8mg administered intra-operatively may reduce oedema. It can also be treated with humidified oxygen and nebulised steroids.

Recurrent laryngeal nerve palsy

A bilateral partial injury of the recurrent laryngeal nerves may cause complete airway obstruction. Unilateral injury causes hoarseness of the voice. Intra-operative electrophysiological monitoring of the recurrent laryngeal nerve has been used to reduce injury to the nerve. This technique uses a special ETT with integrated electromyographic (EMG) electrode wires to detect the EMG signs from the laryngeal muscles (vocal cord movement). While placing the ETT in the trachea, care should be taken to ensure that the distal ends of the electrodes are in contact with the vocal cords.

Tracheomalacia

This is a rare but possible complication following thyroidectomy in longstanding or retrosternal goitre. At the end of surgery the surgeon may want to examine the trachea under direct vision for erosion of the tracheal rings. Prior to extubation there should be an air leak around the tracheal tube after deflating the cuff. Airway obstruction due to tracheomalacia may need immediate reintubation and a subsequent tracheostomy.

Hypocalcaemia

Hypocalcaemia may occur due to accidental removal or injury or oedema of the parathyroid glands. This usually occurs 24-36 hours following surgery. The serum calcium should be checked after 24 hours.

Pneumothorax

May occur following surgery for a retrosternal goitre.

Thyroid crisis

A thyroid crisis is rare if hyperthyroidism is controlled pre-operatively.

10 hours postoperatively the patient starts to become agitated and complains of nausea. She is febrile (temperature 39.2°C) and tachycardic. What do you think is the most likely diagnosis and what would you do?

As this patient had a subtotal thyroidectomy 10 hours ago, this is most likely to be a thyroid crisis, also known as thyroid storm. This is a medical emergency and needs urgent treatment as it can be fatal.

Supportive measures

- Ensure and establish an adequate airway, breathing, circulation and administer 100% oxygen.
- Secure venous access and administer cold intravenous fluids (a litre of crystalloid infused rapidly and further IV fluids should be given as required).
- Paracetamol 1g IV or orally should be given 6-hourly to control the temperature.

Specific drug therapy

- Propylthiouracil 600-1200mg given orally or via a nasogastric tube.
- Lugol's iodine (potassium iodide) given orally, or sodium iodide 0.25g IV. It should not be given until an hour after the administration of antithyroid drugs. It acts immediately and prevents the further release of thyroid hormones.
- Esmolol 0.5mg/kg as a bolus dose over one minute, followed by 50-200µg/kg/minute as an infusion, or propranolol 1-5mg IV up to 10mg should be used to control the sympathetic effects.
- Hydrocortisone 100mg IV should be administered every 6-hourly.
- Plasma exchange may be needed.
- Dantrolene has been used with variable success.
- Ionotropes and vasopressors may rarely be required.

A thyrotoxic crisis occurring during the intra-operative period has often been misdiagnosed as malignant hyperthermia and successfully treated with dantrolene.

The clinical features of hyperthyroidism

The classical features of thyrotoxicosis include hyperactivity, weight loss and tremor. The important cardiovascular effects are tachycardia, atrial fibrillation (AF) and congestive cardiac failure.

Table 4.5 Clinical features of hyperthyroidism.	
Symptoms	**Signs**
Weight loss	Goitre
Increased appetite	Tachycardia
Diarrhoea/vomiting	Atrial fibrillation
Palpitation	Exophthalmos
Heat intolerance	Lid lag
Menstrual disturbance	Conjunctivitis
	Pretibial myxoedema

Retrosternal goitre

Retrosternal goitre occurs when the thyroid extends underneath the sternal wall. Retrosternal goitres can cause compression of mediastinal structures leading to dyspnoea and dysphagia. The pressure effect on the superior vena cava impairs the venous drainage from the head and neck region and may cause airway oedema and oedema of the face. The engorgement of the nasal mucosa may result in bleeding during nasal fibreoptic intubation. Small retrosternal goitres may cause more problems than huge visible goitres. The problems associated with very large and retrosternal goitres include difficult intubation, excessive blood loss, prolonged operating time and postoperative tracheomalacia.

Anaesthesia for retrosternal goitre can be challenging, particularly with regard to the airway. The incidence of complications can be greatly reduced by adequate pre-operative assessment and planning. The presence of noisy breathing, dyspnoea and position-related breathing difficulty indicates airway obstruction.

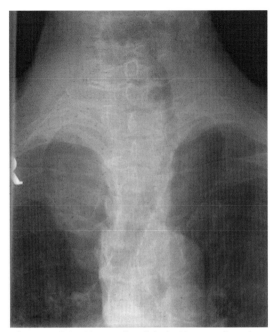

Figure 4.2 Thoracic inlet X-ray showing tracheal deviation.

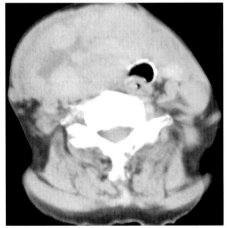

Figure 4.3 CT scan showing tracheal compression and deviation.

The following options for airway management are available when a difficulty is anticipated:

♦ Inhalational induction with sevoflurane. The aim is to maintain spontaneous ventilation until the airway is secured. Premedication with an anti-sialogogue should be considered to dry the secretions in patients with a non-toxic goitre. A nasopharyngeal or oral airway should be immediately available to overcome the airway obstruction at the level of the oropharynx or nasopharynx. In the presence of airway obstruction, inhalation induction may be prolonged. Airway collapse leading to complete airway obstruction may occur as the patient is induced.

♦ Awake fibreoptic intubation. This is the technique of choice when the airway anatomy is distorted. If the patient is in stridor, due to narrowing of the airway, however, passage of the fibreoptic scope may result in complete airway obstruction.

Sickle cell disease

In normal adults the haemoglobin molecule (HbA) consists of four polypeptide chains: two alpha chains and two beta chains. Each alpha chain consists of 141 amino acid residues and each beta chain of 146 amino acid residues. When valine (amino acid) replaces the glutamine (amino acid) at the 6th position of the beta chain of the haemoglobin molecule, abnormal haemoglobin is formed, known as haemoglobin S (HbS).

There are two genes responsible for haemoglobin synthesis. In the heterozygous state (sickle cell trait) there is a mixture of normal gene (HbA) and abnormal gene (HbS). This haemoglobin is known as HbAS. In the homozygous state (sickle cell disease or sickle cell anaemia) both genes are abnormal. This haemoglobin is known as HbSS.

Sickle cell trait

Individuals with a sickle cell trait have no symptoms unless they are exposed to severe hypoxia. Typically they have about 60% HbA and 40% HbS. A sickle cell trait protects against plasmodium falciparum, which causes malaria. The diagnosis of a sickle cell trait is made by a positive sickle cell test and by haemoglobin electrophoresis.

Sickle cell anaemia

Individuals with sickle cell anaemia have 85-95% HbS, the remainder being HbF (foetal haemoglobin). The deoxygenated HbS is 50 times less soluble in blood than deoxygenated HbA. The deoxygenated Hb forms long crystals called tactoids which distort the red blood cell membrane causing the red cell to assume a sickle shape. The sickle cells are susceptible to premature destruction, which causes chronic haemolytic anaemia. Sickled cells result in increased blood viscosity, cause damage to the endothelium and result in vascular injury.

The Sickledex test is a rapid screening tool. It detects the presence of HbS but does not differentiate a sickle cell trait from sickle cell anaemia. Haemoglobin electrophoresis is useful in distinguishing sickle cell anaemia from the trait.

Patients with sickle cell anaemia may require pre-operative blood transfusion prior to major surgery. A conservative transfusion to achieve an Hb around 10g/dL is as effective as aggressive exchange transfusion to reduce HbS below 30%. The optimal transfusion requirement should always be discussed with a haematologist.

Key points

- For elective thyroid surgery the patient should be euthyroid.
- In a large goitre careful airway evaluation should be performed to rule out potential airway obstruction.
- A retrosternal goitre can cause compression of the mediastinal structures.
- In a patient with sickle cell disease, hypoxia, dehydration, hypercarbia and acidosis should be avoided.

Further reading

1. Farling PA. Thyroid disease. *British Journal of Anaesthesia* 2000; 85: 15-28.
2. Vijay V, Cavenagh JD, Yate P. The anaesthetist's role in acute sickle cell crisis. *British Journal of Anaesthesia* 1998; 80: 820-8.
3. Malhotra S, Sodhi V. Anaesthesia for thyroid and parathyroid surgery. *British Journal of Anaesthesia CEACCP* 2007; 7: 55- 8.
4. Howlett TA. Endocrine disease. In: *Clinical medicine*, 6th ed. Kumar P, Clark M, Eds. Philadelphia, USA: Elsevier Saunders, 2005; Chapter 18: 1073-80.

Short case 4.1: Latex allergy

A 25-year-old theatre nurse has presented for elective laparoscopy on a gynaecology list. She is usually fit and well but for the past 6 months has developed an itchy rash on her hands 10-15 minutes after wearing normal theatre gloves.

What do you think is the most likely cause of the rash?

As this patient is a health care professional who gets a rash after wearing gloves, she is most likely to be having a latex allergy.

Who is more prone to develop a latex allergy?

The condition usually occurs in persons who are repeatedly exposed to latex:

- Health care workers; the prevalence may be as high as 17%.
- Rubber industry workers.
- Patients with spina bifida (prevalence may be as high as 60%).
- Patients exposed to repeated bladder catheterisation and multiple operations.
- History of anaphylaxis of uncertain aetiology, especially if associated with previous surgery and hospitalisation.
- Patients who have a fruit allergy to banana, grapes, avocado, tomato, kiwi fruit and chestnuts (they have a cross reactivity with latex).

How does a latex allergy present?

A latex allergy has a wide clinical spectrum ranging from irritant contact dermatitis to life-threatening anaphylaxis.

Irritant contact dermatitis (non-allergic) is due to damage to the skin from an exogenous substance.

Contact dermatitis (Type IV delayed hypersensitivity reaction) is mediated by T-lymphocytes. It is probably a reaction to the anti-oxidants and accelerators used in the manufacturing process of latex rubber.

A Type I hypersensitivity reaction is mediated by IgE and occurs in latex sensitised individuals on re-exposure to latex protein antigens. This may manifest as a full blown anaphylactic reaction.

Type I reactions can be of the following three types:

♦ Contact urticaria.
♦ Asthma and urticaria.
♦ Anaphylaxis.

If it is confirmed that this lady has a latex allergy, what precautions would you take before her operation?

♦ Inform theatre staff.
♦ Ensure that she is first on the operating list.
♦ Ensure latex-free gloves and equipment are used in the anaesthetic room.
♦ Ensure that all latex-containing equipment is removed from the theatre to minimise airborne exposure.
♦ Ensure the availability of resuscitation drugs (epinephrine, atropine, hydrocortisone, intravenous salbutamol) to treat possible anaphylaxis.
♦ Prevent exposure to latex in the recovery area. The patient may be recovered in the theatre and transferred directly to the ward.
♦ The use of premedication with anti-histamines and corticosteroids is controversial.

In the event of anaphylaxis, what would be your management?

The management of anaphylaxis from a latex allergy is similar to the management of anaphylaxis due to any other cause.

Primary therapy

◆ Call for help.
◆ Stop the operation.
◆ Ensure that there is no ongoing exposure to latex particles.
◆ Maintain the airway, give 100% oxygen and lay the patient flat with the legs elevated.
◆ Give epinephrine (adrenaline) 50-100μg intravenously (0.5 to 1ml of 1:10,000) over 1 minute for hypotension with titration of further doses as required. Alternatively, it may be given intramuscularly in a dose of 0.5mg-1mg (0.5 to 1ml of 1:1,000), repeated every 10 minutes according to the arterial pressure and pulse until improvement occurs.
◆ Start rapid intravenous infusion of crystalloids (1L of Hartmann's solution rapidly); 2 to 4L of crystalloids may be required.

Secondary therapy

◆ Give antihistamines (chlorpheniramine 10-20mg by slow intravenous infusion).
◆ Give corticosteroids (100 to 500mg hydrocortisone slow IV).
◆ Bronchodilators may be required for persistent bronchospasm.
◆ Further inotropic or vasopressor support may be needed. An arterial blood gas sample should be obtained and analysed for pH, and acidosis should be corrected. In the postoperative phase, the patient should be monitored in the HDU or ITU for at least 24 hours.

Investigations

Serum tryptase
A blood sample should be collected as soon as possible after the initial management, and about 1 hour and 6 hours after the reaction. Samples should be stored at 4°C if it is possible to analyse them within 48 hours, or at -20°C if there is a delay. The rise in serum tryptase is transient and the concentration usually peaks an hour after the anaphylactic reaction.

Elevated serum tryptase after an anaphylactic reaction indicates mast cell degradation.

Later, all the events should be documented and the patient should be tested for an adverse drug reaction. Once the drug responsible for the event is identified, the patient and the primary care physician should be informed in writing. A medic alert bracelet should be given to the patient. The event should also be reported to the Committee on Safety of Medicines and on the yellow card.

What investigations should be done for a patient with suspected anaphylaxis?

The tests can be classified into two groups: *in vivo* and *in vitro*.

In vivo tests

◆ Intradermal skin tests.
◆ Skin prick tests.

These tests are done with antigen solution and has a risk of provoking local and systemic reactions. The *in vivo* tests should be carried out in a place where resuscitation facilities are available. Intradermal skin tests are done using a more dilute solution compared with that used for a skin prick test. The skin prick test should be done 4-6 weeks after the reaction.

In vitro test

◆ RAST (radio-allergosorbent testing): this is a serological testing of the patient's serum with an antigen polymer complex which carries no risk of provoking local and systemic reactions.

For a limited number of anaesthetic drugs, specific antibodies can be measured (e.g. succinylcholine).

What is the difference between anaphylaxis and an anaphylactoid reaction?

Anaphylaxis is an IgE mediated Type 1 hypersensitivity reaction that results in mast cell activation and release of multiple mediators such as histamine, leukotrienes, tumour necrosis factor (TNF) and various other cytokines.

An anaphylactoid reaction is non-IgE mediated. Certain allergens including drugs can trigger the mast cell cascade directly without involving IgE as the initial mediator. Anaphylactoid reactions therefore do not require prior sensitisation as they are direct mast cell releasers and may produce anaphylaxis-like reactions in a dose-dependent manner.

Clinical features of anaphylaxis

The clinical features of anaphylaxis include tachycardia, hypotension, bronchospasm, cutaneous rashes, urticaria, angioedema, pulmonary oedema, and gastrointestinal symptoms. The severity of reaction may vary from mild urticaria to severe cardiovascular collapse. Cardiovascular manifestation is the most common clinical feature and in about 10% of patients, cardiovascular collapse may be the only feature observed. Factors that lead to reduced endogenous release of catecholamine, such as beta-blockers, spinal and epidural anaesthesia, may increase the severity of the reaction. The clinical diagnosis of anaphylaxis may be difficult due to the wide variation in clinical presentation.

Anaphylaxis referral

Following a suspected anaphylaxis, the patient should be referred to a specialist allergy investigation centre. The relevant referral details should include date and time of the reaction, the presenting clinical features, all the drugs and fluids administered before the event, all the drugs and fluids administered after the event, anaesthetic technique, surgical procedure, response to the treatment and the investigations performed. The contact details of various referral centres are available on www.aagbi.org.

Key points

- ◆ Health care workers are more prone to a latex allergy.
- ◆ There is a wide spectrum of clinical presentation with a latex allergy, the spectrum ranging from irritant contact dermatitis to life-threatening anaphylaxis.
- ◆ Communication with theatre staff to ensure a latex-free environment in the theatre and anaesthetic room is of paramount importance.

Further reading

1. Suspected anaphylactic reactions associated with anaesthesia. The Association of Anaesthetists of Great Britain and Ireland, http://www.aagbi.org/publications/guidelines/docs/anaphylaxis03.pdf.
2. Farley CA, Jones HM. Latex allergy. *British Journal of Anaesthesia CEACCP* 2002; 2: 20-3.
3. Dakin MJ, Yentis SM. Latex allergy: a strategy for management. *Anaesthesia* 1998; 53: 774-81.

Short case 4.2: Wolff-Parkinson-White (WPW) syndrome

A 35-year-old female patient is scheduled on the ENT list for functional endoscopic sinus surgery. During pre-operative assessment she says she has suffered from palpitations for a year.

What is a palpitation?

A palpitation is defined as an increased awareness of one's normal heart beat or the sensation of slow, rapid or irregular heart rhythms.

What are the causes of palpitations?

- Anxiety.
- Exercise.
- Panic attacks.
- Caffeine, alcohol and nicotine.
- Drugs: thyroxine, cocaine, ephedrine, β2 agonists.
- Endocrine disorders: hyperthyroidism, hypoglycaemia, phaeochromocytoma.
- Cardiac causes: can be due to either bradyarrhythmias or tachyarrhythmias.
- The causes of bradyarrhythmias include first, second and third-degree atrioventricular heart block and sick sinus syndrome.

The causes of tachyarrhythmias include atrial, junctional and ventricular tachyarrhythmias.

Table 4.6 The causes of tachyarrhythmias.		
Atrial tachy-arrhythmias	**Junctional tachy-arrhythmias**	**Ventricular tachy-arrhythmias**
Atrial flutter	AV nodal re-entry tachycardia	Ventricular ectopic beats
Atrial fibrillation	Accelerated junctional tachycardia	Ventricular tachycardia
Uni/multifocal atrial tachycardias		

How would you investigate the cause of palpitations?

- History: detailed history including lifestyle and medications.
- Physical examination: heart rate and rhythm, heart sounds and murmur.
- Diagnostic tests:
  - a 12-lead electrocardiogram;
  - ambulatory electrocardiogram monitoring;
  - invasive cardiac electrophysiological study/mapping.

What does the ECG show (Figure 4.4 overleaf)?

It shows sinus rhythm with a heart rate of 75 beats per minute. The P-R interval is short (0.08 seconds). The beginning of the QRS complex is slurred (delta wave) in leads II, III, aVF and V4 to V6. This is most likely to be Wolff-Parkinson-White (WPW) syndrome.

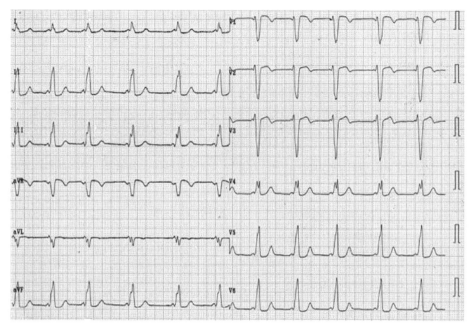

Figure 4.4 ECG.

What is Wolff-Parkinson-White syndrome?

Wolff-Parkinson-White (WPW) syndrome is a condition in which there is an accessory pathway between the atria and ventricles which can electrically bypass the AV node. This causes early depolarisation of the ventricles. This accessory pathway is known as the bundle of Kent. In normal sinus rhythm, conduction takes place through the AV node and partly through the accessory pathway. Because the AV node and the accessory pathways have different conduction speeds, a re-entry circuit can develop, which can cause paroxysmal tachycardia.

What happens when AF develops in a patient with WPW syndrome?

As the accessory pathway lacks the normal rate-limiting properties of the AV node, the onset of AF may produce very rapid ventricular rates via the accessory pathway. This may precipitate ventricular fibrillation. Atrial fibrillation can, therefore, be a potentially dangerous rhythm in WPW syndrome.

Are there any drugs that should be avoided in this syndrome?

Verapamil, digoxin and adenosine may cause preferential block of the AV node which in turn may increase conduction through the accessory pathway.

What are the treatment options in WPW syndrome?

- Drug treatment includes Class Ia anti-arrhythmic drugs (e.g. procainamide), Class Ic anti-arrhythmic drugs (e.g. flecainide), or Class III anti-arrhythmic drugs (e.g. amiodarone).
- Radiofrequency catheter ablation of the accessory pathway.

Pre-excitation syndrome

WPW syndrome is the commonest pre-excitation syndrome. In WPW syndrome the Kent bundle connects the atria and ventricle. There may be more than one accessory pathway bypassing the AV node. In Lown-Ganong-Levine (LGL) syndrome, an accessory pathway connects the atria to the bundle of His. The accessory pathway in LGL syndrome is called James fibres. The classic ECG changes in WPW syndrome include a short PR interval, slurring and slow rise in the initial upstroke of the QRS complex (delta wave), and a widened QRS complex (duration >0.12 seconds). Depending on the location and relative impulse transmission characteristics of the accessory pathway, the ECG morphology may vary from classic changes. In LGL syndrome, the PR interval is shortened but the QRS morphology is normal, as the impulse though the accessory pathway directly activates the His-Purkinje system, without depolarising the ventricle. If the impulse through the accessory pathway and through the AV node arrive simultaneously to the ventricle, the ECG morphology may appear normal.

The treatment of AF associated with WPW syndrome is different from that of standard treatment of AF. The conventional drugs used in the treatment of AF, such as digoxin and beta-blockers, may prolong the impulse transmission through the normal pathway (AV node) and increase the rate of transmission through the accessory pathway with a corresponding increase in ventricular rate. Cardioversion is therefore the treatment of choice for treating AF associated with WPW syndrome.

There is a very small risk of sudden cardiac death (0-4%) in patients with WPW syndrome. The mortality is secondary to associated arrhythmias or mistreatment of the arrhythmias. The patient may present with palpitations or with or without cardiopulmonary compromise. Most often WPW syndrome is diagnosed in children or young adults presenting with arrhythmias. A study published in 2003 suggests that prophylactic radiofrequency ablation of the accessory pathway is beneficial in high-risk asymptomatic patients.

Key points

- In WPW syndrome, an accessory pathway between the atria and ventricle causes early depolarisation of the ventricles.
- AF in WPW syndrome can be potentially dangerous.
- There is a small risk of VF and sudden cardiac death, even in asymptomatic patients with WPW syndrome.
- Verapamil, digoxin and adenosine should be avoided in WPW syndrome.
- Routine electrophysiological testing and radiofrequency ablation should be considered in asymptomatic patients with WPW syndrome.

Further reading

1. Boon NA, Fox KAA, Bloomfield P, Bradbury A. Cardiovascular disease. In: *Davidson's principles and practice of medicine.* London: Churchill Livingstone, 2002; Chapter 12: 407-11.
2. Hemingway JM. Wolf-Parkinson-White syndrome, August 2008; http://www.emedicine.com/emerg/topic644.htm.
3. Pappone C, Santinelli V, Manguso F, *et al.* A randomised study of prophylactic catheter ablation in asymptomatic patients with the Wolff-Parkinson-White syndrome. *New Engl J Med* 2003; 349: 1803-11.

Short case 4.3: Post-tonsillectomy bleeding

You have anaesthetised a 5-year-old child for tonsillectomy on a routine ENT list. After 4 hours, you receive a call from the ward informing you that the child is bleeding from the tonsillar bed. He needs to return to the operating theatre as soon as possible.

What are the main problems presented by this scenario?

- Anxious child and parents.
- Residual effects from previous GA.
- Hypovolaemia.
- Anaemia.
- Full stomach with a risk of aspiration.
- Difficult airway:
  - upper airway oedema from previous surgery and intubation;
  - excessive bleeding obscuring the laryngeal view.

How would you proceed with this case?

Initial assessment and management

Call for help. Assessment should be done on the ward and the patient should be transferred to the operating theatre once stable. The child may be drooling and spitting out blood and is likely to be sitting up. Avoid suctioning except at the front of the oral cavity (suction may cause trauma and exacerbate bleeding). Administer oxygen via a face mask. The parent can hold the mask if it causes distress. Monitor oxygen saturation if possible.

Assess hydration status by measuring the heart rate, respiratory rate, blood pressure, capillary refill, mental status and urine output. A low blood pressure and altered state of consciousness are signs of severe volume depletion. It is easy to underestimate the blood loss because blood may be swallowed or spat out.

Venous access should be obtained with a large-bore cannula, but access may be difficult and intra-osseous infusion of fluids may be necessary.

Initial fluid management

A fluid bolus of 10-20ml/kg should be administered and the response checked. Further fluid management should be guided by the trends in monitoring and an improvement in clinical signs. Colloids or crystalloids can be administered. Blood for a cross-match and FBC should be taken, and the recent anaesthetic chart reviewed.

How would you anaesthetise this child?

Anaesthesia should be induced once haemodynamic stability is achieved, in the presence of senior anaesthetic help and an experienced theatre technician.

Prior to induction, in addition to the standard equipment, a selection of laryngoscope blades, tracheal tubes a half to one size smaller than used previously, and two suction catheters should be available.

Two options are available for induction following pre-oxygenation. They should both achieve rapid control of the airway and prevent pulmonary aspiration:

- Rapid sequence induction in the supine position with the head slightly tilted down. The lateral position should be considered if there is excessive bleeding.
- Gas induction in the supine position with the head down or in the left lateral position. When the level of anaesthesia is deep enough, laryngoscopy is performed. If the cords are visualised, administer succinylcholine and intubate. In a child, tracheal intubation can be performed under deep inhalational induction, but it can worsen hypotension.

In the presence of intravenous access, rapid sequence induction with cricoid pressure is usually preferred. There is a possibility that intubation may be difficult due to the oedema of the upper airway and the presence of blood in the upper airway.

The ENT surgeon should be scrubbed and ready to perform a tracheostomy if necessary.

Fluid resuscitation and the transfusion of blood and blood products should continue intra-operatively and should be guided by the haemoglobin, trends in the monitoring, and clinical signs.

Once haemostasis is achieved, a large-bore nasogastric tube should be passed and the stomach emptied. The remaining blood in the stomach can cause nausea and vomiting and, therefore, a risk of postoperative aspiration.

Dexamethasone 0.1mg/kg IV is useful as an anti-emetic and also reduces airway oedema.

Extubate the child awake and with the neuromuscular block antagonised in the head-down left lateral position.

Postoperatively, the child should be closely monitored for any re-occurrence of bleeding.

How would you calculate the size of the endotracheal tube required for a 4-year-old child?

◆ The size of ETT for a child is calculated using the formula = age/4 + 4.0.
◆ Length of the ETT at lips = age/2+12cm.

How would you calculate fluid requirements for a child?

The volume and rate of intravenous fluid administered depends on the weight of the child and degree of existing fluid deficit.

For children aged 1-8 years, the approximate weight can be calculated based on the formula:

$$weight = (age+4) \times 2,$$
e.g. a 4-year-old child approximately weighs $[(4+4) \times 2] = 16kg$.

(For further details on fluid management refer to SOE1, Short case 1.1.)

Anaesthesia for tonsillectomy

Tonsillectomy is one of the most common surgical procedures among children. These children may have associated obstructive sleep apnoea (OSA). Children with OSA are more likely to develop peri-operative complications such as coughing, desaturation, laryngospasm and airway obstruction. They are more sensitive to the respiratory depressant effects of opioids and benzodiazepines.

Most children do not need pre-operative sedation and it should be avoided in the presence of airway obstruction. Midazolam 0.5mg/kg (maximum 15mg) can be given 30 minutes before induction for those children with significant anxiety. Topical local anesthetic cream such as Ametop or EMLA should be applied to facilitate intravenous induction.

Induction of general anaesthesia can be performed either via the intravenous or inhalational route. With children who have upper airway obstruction it may be difficult to maintain the airway during induction. Either a flexible LMA or a preformed RAE (Ring, Adair and Elwyn) endotracheal tube may be used to secure the airway.

The main benefits of an LMA include protection of the trachea and larynx from blood, smooth emergence and the avoidance of muscle relaxants. The LMA can be left in place during recovery until the patient is awake. It is, however, less secure than a tracheal tube and may impair surgical access.

The tracheal tube provides a more definitive airway and provides good surgical access. Tracheal extubation at a deep plane of anaesthesia leaves the airway unprotected and there is a risk of laryngospasm. Patients should be extubated either deep in the lateral head-down position, or allowed to wake up. The disadvantages of tracheal intubation include the need for muscle relaxation, trauma during laryngoscopy and coughing at extubation.

Intra-operative analgesia can be provided with paracetamol, NSAIDs and opioids such as fentanyl. A combination of regular paracetamol and NSAIDs is commonly used for postoperative analgesia. Further analgesia can be provided with either codeine phosphate or oral morphine. A multimodal approach involving dexamethasone, a 5-HT3 receptor antagonist (ondansetron) and adequate hydration reduces the risk of postoperative nausea and vomiting.

Tonsillectomy can be performed as a day-case procedure with an extended postoperative observation for 4-6 hours. The incidence of post-tonsillectomy bleeding in the first 24 hours is about 0.6% and in the majority this occurs within the first 4-6 hours. The use of diathermy during tonsillectomy is associated with a higher incidence of bleeding as compared with blunt dissection.

Key points

- In a child presenting with a post-tonsillectomy bleed, adequate resuscitation should be established with IV fluids prior to induction of general anaesthesia.
- Bleeding and upper airway oedema may complicate airway management.
- Following tracheal intubation the stomach should be emptied using a wide-bore nasogastric tube.

Further reading

1. Ravi R, Howell T, Anaesthesia for paediatric ear, nose and throat surgery. *British Journal of Anaesthesia CEACCP* 2007; 7: 33-7.

Applied anatomy 4.1: Blood supply to the spinal cord

A 70-year-old male patient has undergone an abdominal aortic aneurysm (AAA) repair. It was a complicated operation and 24 hours afterwards the patient is complaining of weakness in both legs. On examination he has spastic type paraplegia and reduced pain and temperature sensation in both legs.

Clinical Science

What complication of this procedure may result in this clinical picture?

The most likely cause is intra-operative ischaemia of the spinal cord; the neurological examination suggests anterior spinal artery syndrome.

What are the causes of spinal cord ischaemia?

Spinal cord ischaemia can occur in the following conditions and surgical procedures:

◆ Aortic aneurysm repair especially thoraco-abdominal.
◆ Aortic dissection.
◆ Scoliosis surgery.
◆ Laminectomy or spinal decompression procedures.
◆ Profound hypotension secondary to coeliac plexus block.

What is the blood supply to the spinal cord?

There are three main spinal arteries: one anterior and two posterior; all have courses that run parallel to the spinal cord.

Anterior spinal artery

Formed at the foramen magnum by union of the two anterior spinal arteries, it descends in the anterior median sulcus. It is reinforced by a succession of small radicular arteries entering the vertebral canal through the intervertebral foramina from the vertebral, ascending cervical, posterior intercostal and first lumbar arteries. It supplies the anterior two thirds of the cord. The spinal tracts and areas supplied by the anterior spinal artery include the anterior horns, the central grey matter, the lateral horns, lateral spinothalamic tract, anterior spinothalamic tract, spinocerebellar tracts, pyramidal tracts (corticospinal tracts) and extrapyramidal tracts (reticulospinal, olivospinal, vestibulospinal and tectospinal).

Posterior spinal arteries

These arise from the posterior inferior cerebellar arteries at the level of the foramen magnum, one on each side. Each artery is reinforced by small spinal branches from the vertebral, ascending cervical and posterior intercostal arteries. They supply the posterior third of the spinal cord. The dorsal columns (fasciculus gracilis and fasciculus cuneatus) are supplied by the posterior spinal arteries.

Radicular arteries

Most anterior radicular arteries are small; the largest anterior radicular artery is called the artery of Adamkiewicz. It usually arises from the intersegmental branch of the aorta at T9-T11. The site of origin of this artery may vary from T8 to L4. Since it makes a major contribution to the anterior spinal artery, injury to it during aortic and spinal surgery may compromise the blood flow to the lower part of the spinal cord. Posterior radicular arteries are more numerous and are very variable in size.

How would you prevent intra-operative spinal cord ischaemia?

◆ Maintain adequate perfusion of the spinal cord by maintaining mean arterial blood pressure by ensuring adequate intravenous fluids and vasoconstrictors.
◆ Minimise the duration of aortic cross-clamping.

The chance of spinal cord ischaemia is very high in thoraco-abdominal aortic aneurysms (up to 15%) and the following are some of the steps taken to prevent it:

◆ Using partial cardiopulmonary bypass (at 32-34°C) for distal aortic perfusion.
◆ Deep hypothermic circulatory arrest when sequential clamping is impossible.
◆ Monitoring motor evoked potentials and reconstruction of the critical collaterals to spinal arteries.
◆ Pre-operative evaluation using multi-detector row computed tomography or MR angiography to locate the origin of the collateral vessels.
◆ Cerebrospinal fluid drainage reduces the CSF pressure and increases the spinal cord perfusion pressure.

Peri-operative haemodynamic stability is of vital importance for spinal cord protection.

Do you know of any drug undergoing research which may help to achieve neuroprotection?

Erythropoietin has been found to cause brain preconditioning and to induce tolerance to ischaemia in humans. Intravenous administration of erythropoietin has been shown to be safe and beneficial for patients who have suffered an acute stroke.

Anterior spinal artery syndrome

This is caused by ischaemia of the spinal cord as a result of anterior spinal artery insufficiency. It results in a lower motor neurone type of lesion

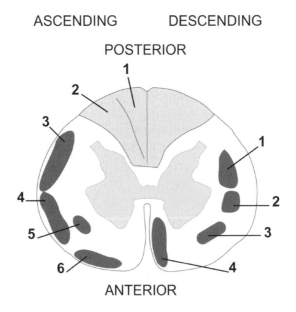

Figure 4.5 Tracts of the spinal cord.

Ascending tracts: 1. Fasciculus gracilis; 2. Fasciculus cuneatus; 3. Posterior spinocerebellar tract; 4. Anterior spinocerebellar tract; 5. Lateral spinothalamic tract; 6. Anterior spinothalamic tract.

Descending tracts: 1. Lateral corticospinal (pyramidal) tract; 2. Tectospinal tract; 3. Vestibulospinal tract; 4. Anterior corticospinal tract.

(spastic paraplegia) with reduced crude touch, pain and temperature sensation below the level of the ischaemia. Joint position sense and vibration are well preserved as they are carried by the posterior columns which are not affected in this syndrome.

Even a short period of spinal cord ischaemia can result in damage to the spinal cord, particularly in the presence of hypotension. The possible mechanisms responsible for anterior spinal cord syndrome during repair of aortic aneurysms include direct occlusion of the anterior radicular artery by the aortic clamp, prolonged hypotension, pre-existing arteriosclerosis of the spinal cord arteries, prolonged aortic cross-clamp, resection of the aorta at the level of the major radicular artery and thrombosis of the major collateral artery.

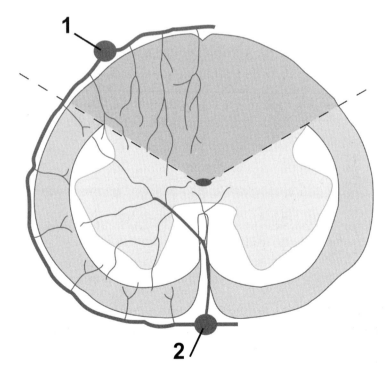

Figure 4.6 Blood supply to the spinal cord.
1. Posterior spinal artery; 2. Anterior spinal artery.

Key points

♦ The artery of Adamkiewicz is the largest radicular artery.
♦ Anterior spinal artery syndrome is a complication which may follow surgical procedures on the thoraco-abdominal aorta. Its occurrence is unpredictable.
♦ Maintenance of adequate perfusion of the spinal cord by maintaining mean arterial blood pressure is of paramount importance.

Further reading

1. Ellis H, Feldman S, Harrop-Griffiths W. *Anatomy for anaesthetists*, 8th ed. Oxford: Blackwell Science Ltd, 2004.
2. Gravereaux EC, Faries PL, Burks JA, Latessa V. Risk of spinal cord ischemia after endograft repair of thoracic aortic aneurysms. *Journal of Vascular Surgery* 2001; 34: 997-1003.
3. Jacobs MJ, Elenbaas TW, Schurink GWH, Mess WH, Mochtar B. Assessment of spinal cord integrity during thoraco-abdominal aortic aneurysm repair. *Annals of Thoracic Surgery* 2002; 74: 1864-6.
4. Jacobs MJ, Mommertz G, Koeppel TA. Surgical repair of thoracoabdominal aortic aneurysms. *Journal of Cardiovascular Surgery* 2007; 48: 49-58.

Applied physiology 4.2: Physiology of pregnancy

A 25-year-old lady is admitted to the labour suite for an elective Caesarean section. All her blood results are normal apart from her haemoglobin which is 9g/dL. She has no history of anaemia and her haemoglobin a year ago was 13g/dL. She is otherwise fit and well and has so far had an uneventful pregnancy.

Can you explain the most likely reason for her low haemoglobin?

One of the most likely causes of her low haemoglobin could be anaemia of pregnancy. In pregnancy there is an increase in RBC volume by about 30% above non-pregnant levels, but at the same time there is a much larger rise of plasma volume, by about 50% above non-pregnant levels. The lesser increase in RBC volume relative to the increase in plasma volume results in physiological anaemia of pregnancy.

What other physiological changes take place during pregnancy?

Most of the physiological changes which take place during pregnancy are due to increased levels of oestrogen, progesterone and hormones derived from the placenta.

Cardiovascular system

- Cardiac output increases (by 40-50% at term) with a large increase in stroke volume (30%), and a small increase in heart rate (25%).
- Blood pressure falls by 5-10mm Hg due to a fall in systemic vascular resistance. There is a greater fall in diastolic blood pressure compared with the systolic blood pressure.
- The baroreceptor reflexes are blunted during pregnancy. Aortocaval compression by the gravid uterus results in reduced venous return and cardiac output.

Haematological system

- Anaemia of pregnancy as described above.
- Progressive rise of white blood cells, which is predominantly polymorphonuclear cells.
- Overall increase in all clotting factors except Factors XI and XIII which decrease.
- Fibrin degradation products are increased.
- Fall in total plasma proteins.
- Fall in plasma cholinesterase by about 20-25%.

Respiratory system

- There is an increase of tidal volume (45%) and a slight increase in rate due to an increase in sensitivity of the respiratory centre to $PaCO_2$ (progesterone effect).

- Minute ventilation increases by 45-50% primarily as a result of an increase in tidal volume.
- Functional residual capacity (FRC) is decreased but there is no change in vital capacity.
- There is an increase in PaO_2 and a decrease in $PaCO_2$ and an increase in pH.

Renal system

- Renal plasma flow and glomerular filtration rate increase.
- More glucose is filtered resulting in glycosuria.
- Water retention in excess of sodium results in a low plasma sodium level.

Metabolic system

- There is resistance to the action of insulin, and this may cause an increase in plasma glucose.
- Plasma albumin level falls, leading to a fall in plasma calcium level, although the ionised calcium concentration remains constant.
- Thyroid gland increases in size but thyroid hormone levels remain at non-pregnant levels.

Gastrointestinal system

- Gastro-oesophageal reflux occurs in the majority of pregnant women, caused by the effects of progesterone on the lower oesophageal sphincter (LOS) pressure, and the enlarging uterus increasing intra-abdominal pressure.
- Gastric volume may be increased and pH may be lower than the non-pregnant state.
- Gastric emptying is normal apart from during labour.

Musculoskeletal system

- Enlarged uterus may cause increased lumbar lordosis. It can stretch the lateral cutaneous nerve and result in meralgia paraesthetica (a sensory loss over the anterolateral aspect of the thigh).

◆ A hormone called relaxin increases the mobility of the sacro-iliac joints, and causes an increase in ligamentous laxity. It may also result in an increased incidence of carpal tunnel syndrome.

What are the anaesthetic implications of these changes?

These physiological changes have implications for both general and central neuraxial anaesthesia.

General anaesthesia

◆ Left lateral tilt by tilting the operation table or by a wedge should be performed to avoid aortocaval compression.
◆ Aspiration prophylaxis should be administered, as there is a high chance of reflux and aspiration. This is achieved by a combination H_2 receptor antagonist (e.g. ranitidine) or a proton pump inhibitor (omeprazole) and 30ml 0.3 molar sodium citrate. These drugs reduce the gastric volume and pH.
◆ Reduced FRC results in hypoxia during induction despite pre-oxygenation.
◆ Increased risk of difficult intubation and the need for a smaller size ETT due to laryngeal oedema and a reduced diameter of the trachea due to mucosal oedema.

Muscle relaxants

Care with the dose of succinylcholine as there is a decrease in the plasma pseudocholinesterase level. There is an increased sensitivity to non-depolarising muscle relaxants.

Central neuraxial blocks

◆ Reduced intervertebral space due to increased lumbar lordosis.
◆ Increased incidence of hypotension.
◆ Reduced dose requirement for subarachnoid block due to reduced CSF volume (as a result of distended vertebral venous plexuses).

What hormones are secreted by the placenta?

◆ Human chorionic gonadotrophin.
◆ Human placental lactogen.

- ◆ Oestrogen.
- ◆ Progesterone.
- ◆ Hypothalamic releasing factors.
- ◆ Hypothalamic inhibitory factors.
- ◆ Thyroid stimulating hormone.
- ◆ Prostaglandins.

Placental transfer of drugs

Drugs administered to the mother may cross the placenta and have effects on the foetus. The ratio of maternal plasma concentration of the drug to the foetal plasma concentration is useful in understanding the effect of a maternally administered drug on the foetus.

The placental transfer of drug depends on the following factors:

- ◆ Molecular weight of the drug.
- ◆ Lipid solubility.
- ◆ Tissue binding.
- ◆ Protein binding.
- ◆ Degree of ionisation (pKa of the drug).
- ◆ pH of the maternal blood.
- ◆ Placental blood flow.
- ◆ Maternal to foetal concentration gradient.

Drugs with molecular weights greater than 500D have incomplete transfer across the human placenta. A high lipid solubility allows the drug to cross the placenta easily. The pKa of a drug determines the fraction of the drug which is non-ionised at physiological pH. Foetal acidaemia will enhance the maternal to foetal transfer of basic drugs such as local anaesthetics and opioids. Most of the intravenous induction agents, volatile anaesthetics and nitrous oxide cross the placenta. Amongst the benzodiazepines, diazepam is highly lipophilic and crosses the placenta easily. Midazolam also readily crosses the placenta reaching a foetal to maternal ratio of 0.76 at 20 minutes. However, the ratio decreases to 0.3 by 200 minutes. All the opioid analgesics cross the placenta readily; a remifentanil infusion results in a foetal to maternal ratio of 0.88 but has no adverse effects on the neonate.

The neuromuscular blocking drugs are quaternary ammonium compounds, are highly ionised and do not readily cross the placenta. A high dose of succinylcholine together with a foetal pseudocholinesterase deficiency may result in neonatal neuromuscular blockade. Anticholinergic drugs, except glycopyrrolate, cross the placenta easily.

Key points

♦ A disproportionate increase in plasma volume compared with the RBC volume accounts for anaemia of pregnancy.
♦ Hormones such as oestrogen and progesterone cause pregnancy-related systemic changes.
♦ A reduced FRC may result in hypoxia during induction despite adequate pre-oxygenation.

Further reading

1. Chang AB. Physiologic changes of pregnancy. In: *Obstetric anaesthesia principles and practice*, 3rd ed. Chestnut DH, Ed. Philadelphia, Pennsylvania, USA: Elsevier Mosby, 2004; Chapter 2: 15-36.

Applied pharmacology 4.3: Non-steroidal anti-inflammatory drugs (NSAIDs)

A 73-year-old lady is admitted for a total knee replacement. She suffers from rheumatoid arthritis and diabetes mellitus. Her current medication includes insulin, GTN and tenoxicam.

What is tenoxicam?

Tenoxicam is a non-steroidal anti-inflammatory drug (NSAID) which is used to treat pain and inflammation in rheumatoid arthritis and other musculoskeletal disorders.

What are NSAIDs?

NSAIDs are a heterogeneous class of drugs grouped together by their common anti-inflammatory, analgesic and anti-pyretic properties. They can be classified based on their chemical structure or by their mechanism of action.

Based on their chemical structure:

- Enolic acids: piroxicam, meloxicam, tenoxicam and phenylbutazone.
- Acetic acid derivatives: diclofenac, ketorolac and indomethacin.
- Salicylic acid derivatives: aspirin.
- Propionic acid derivatives: ibuprofen and ketoprofen.

Based on their mechanism of action:

- Non-specific cyclo-oxygenase enzyme (COX) inhibitors: aspirin, diclofenac, ibuprofen.
- Preferential COX-2 inhibitors: meloxicam.
- Specific COX-2 inhibitors: celecoxib, parecoxib and rofecoxib.

NSAIDs provide analgesia for moderate to severe pain. When used in combination with opioids they have been shown to have an opioid-sparing effect. This results in improved analgesia and a reduction in opioid-related side effects.

What is the mechanism of action of NSAIDs?

Arachidonic acid is a major component of cell membrane phospholipids; the enzyme cyclo-oxygenase converts arachidonic acid to cyclic endoperoxides. The spectrum of prostaglandins formed from cyclic endoperoxide depends on the property of the tissue. In most of the tissues, cyclic endoperoxides are converted to prostaglandins E2, F2 and D2 in response to tissue injury. In platelets the cyclic endoperoxides are converted into thromboxane-A_2 (TXA_2), which causes platelet aggregation, and vasoconstriction. In vascular endothelial cells prostacyclin is produced which inhibits platelet aggregation and causes vasodilatation. NSAIDs act by inhibiting the enzyme, cyclo-oxygenase, thereby preventing the production of thromboxane, prostacyclin and prostaglandins. Aspirin produces irreversible inhibition of the enzyme whereas other NSAIDs produce reversible inhibition.

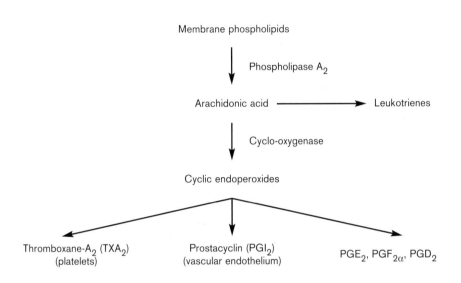

Figure 4.7 Synthesis of prostaglandins.

Describe the different types of COX enzymes

There are two isoforms of the cyclo-oxygenase (COX) enzyme: COX-1 and COX-2. COX-1 (the constitutive form) is responsible for production of TXA_2 in the platelets, PGE_2 in the kidneys and prostacyclin in the endothelial cells and gastric mucosa.

COX-2 (inducible form) forms when tissues are exposed to inflammatory stimuli. It is produced in macrophages, endothelial cells and synovial cells following trauma to the tissues.

Inhibition of COX-1 is responsible for adverse effects produced by NSAIDs and inhibition of COX-2 is responsible for anti-inflammatory and analgesic effects.

What do you understand by the analgesic ladder?

The analgesic ladder is a common framework used to prescribe analgesia in a logical stepwise approach. It was developed by the World Health Organization (WHO) as a three-step pain ladder for relief of cancer pain. It is also widely used in the management of acute postoperative pain. For the treatment of pain there should be prompt oral administration of drugs in the following order: non-opioids (aspirin and paracetamol); then, as necessary, mild opioids (codeine); then strong opioids such as morphine, until the patient is pain free.

What are the adverse effects of NSAIDs?

Most of the adverse effects of NSAIDs are due to the inhibition of COX-1 receptors.

Gastrointestinal system

Prostaglandins play an important role in maintaining gastric mucosal blood flow and in reducing gastric acid secretion. By inhibiting the COX-1 isoenzyme they cause reduction in gastric blood flow and an increase in gastric secretion. This may manifest as dyspepsia, nausea, bleeding from gastric or duodenal vessels and mucosal ulceration. Selective COX-2 inhibitors are associated with a reduced incidence of gastrointestinal complications.

Respiratory system

Some prostaglandins cause bronchodilatation and hence blocking prostaglandin secretion may lead to more arachidonic acid being converted to leukotrienes. This can cause bronchospasm in susceptible individuals. Acute severe asthma may be precipitated in 10-20% of asthmatics when given NSAIDs.

Renal system

NSAIDs impair renal function and can cause acute kidney injury. Renal prostaglandins are important in the maintenance of renal blood flow and glomerular filtration, particularly when the renal blood flow is compromised.

Haematological system

NSAIDs may increase the risk of bleeding by affecting platelet function. NSAIDs can interact with warfarin by displacing it from protein binding sites which may enhance the action of warfarin.

Name some NSAIDs which are selective COX-2 inhibitors

The following drugs are selective COX-2 inhibitors:

◆ Celecoxib (Celebrex).
◆ Parecoxib (Dynastat).
◆ Etoricoxib (Arcoxia).
◆ Valdecoxib (Bexta).
◆ Rofecoxib (Vioxx).

They significantly reduce gastrointestinal complications. They are associated with an increased incidence of thromboembolic events in susceptible patients.

Have you heard about rofecoxib? Why was it withdrawn from the market?

Rofecoxib (Vioxx) is one of the COX-2 inhibitors. It was widely used to treat patients with arthritis and other conditions causing chronic or acute pain. It was withdrawn from the market because of concerns about the increased risk of myocardial infarction and stroke associated with long-term, high-dosage use. The VIGOR (Vioxx GI Outcomes Research) study compared the efficacy and adverse effect profiles of rofecoxib and naproxen, and showed a significant four-fold increased risk of acute myocardial infarction in the rofecoxib group compared with the naproxen group over the 12-month span of the study. This eventually led to the withdrawl of rofecoxib from the market.

COX-2 inhibitors and cardiovascular disease

The selective COX-2 inhibitors were introduced in 1999 as an alternative to conventional NSAIDs in order to minimise the side effects associated with NSAIDs. Numerous initial studies demonstrated the reduced incidence of gastrointestinal side effects. NICE recommended the use of selective COX-2 inhibitors for patients above the age of 65 and for all patients at risk of gastric side effects. Since then there has been clear evidence of increased thromboembolic events associated with the use of selective COX-2 inhibitors.

Selective COX-2 inhibitors adversely affect the prostacyclin: thromboxane A_2 ratio in the vascular wall. Prostacyclin has an anti-thrombotic effect and thromboxane A_2 increases platelet aggregation (thrombotic effect). Selective COX-2 inhibitors inhibit the production of prostacyclin without affecting thromboxane A_2, promoting thombosis and atherosclerosis. Inhibition of prostacyclin in the kidney may lead to sodium and water retention causing hypertension. These biological actions increase the risk of cardiovascular events such as myocardial infarction and stroke in patients with pre-existing cardiovascular disease. Non-selective COX inhibitors may have a cardioprotective effect by inhibiting platelet aggregation.

Key points

◆ NSAIDs primarily exert their effect by inhibiting COX isoenzymes.
◆ Most of the beneficial action of NSAIDs is due to the inhibition of the COX-2 isoenzyme.
◆ Most of the adverse events are due to inhibition of the COX-1 isoenzyme.
◆ There is an increased risk of thromboembolic events with selective COX-2 inhibitors.

Further reading

1. Analgesic drugs. In: *Principles and practice of pharmacology for anaesthetists*, 5th ed. Calvey TN, Williams NE, Eds. Oxford: Blackwell Science Ltd., 2008.

Equipment, clinical measurement and monitoring 4.4: Invasive blood pressure measurement

A 72-year-old patient is to undergo elective AAA repair. He is known to have ischaemic heart disease and hypertension. His regular medications include aspirin, GTN spray, captopril and bendrofluazide.

What intra-operative invasive monitoring will you use?

Intra-arterial blood pressure and central venous pressure monitoring.

What are the components of an invasive arterial blood pressure monitoring system?

The arterial pressure monitoring system includes an arterial cannula, catheter tubing connecting the cannula to the transducer, a transducer, a pressurized flush system, a monitor to display the reading and waveform, and a cable connecting the transducer to the monitor.

How would you choose an arterial cannula, and what are the ideal characteristics?

- Catheter material. Arterial catheters made of Teflon are better as they have a lower risk of thrombosis compared with polyurethane catheters.
- Catheter size. Arterial catheters should be short and wide. A wide cannula has less effect on the natural frequency of the transducer system and less effect on damping.

What is the function of the fluid-filled tubing and what characteristics are preferable?

The purpose of the fluid-filled tubing system is to provide a means of transmitting the pressure generated in the artery to the transducer. Normal saline is used as the flushing fluid. The viscosity of the fluid used influences the natural frequency of the measurement system. Fluids with a viscosity greater than normal saline lead to over-damping. The flushing system is pressurised to 300mmHg and provides a continuous slow flow of heparinised normal saline (3-4ml/hour), to minimise the risk of clot formation in the catheter. The tubing should be non-compliant and should be free from air bubbles. The length should be limited to 122cm and the number of three-way taps should be kept to a minimum. The three-way taps have a narrower lumen than the catheter and can reduce the natural frequency resulting in damping.

What information can you obtain from looking at the arterial trace?

Besides giving beat to beat blood pressure monitoring, the arterial blood pressure trace gives the following additional information:

- Up-slope of the arterial waveform indicates myocardial contractility.
- The position of the dicrotic notch on the down-slope indicates systemic vascular resistance.
- Variation in the arterial pressure waveform during the respiratory cycle during ventilation may indicate hypovolaemia.
- The area under the systolic component of the waveform (from the beginning of upstroke to the dicrotic notch) is an index of stroke volume; the cardiac output can be calculated by multiplying stroke volume by heart rate.

Why should one calibrate the transducer system?

The transducer system needs to be calibrated to obtain an accurate blood pressure reading. Zero calibration eliminates the effect of atmospheric pressure on the measured pressure. For accuracy, the transducer system should be 'zeroed' to a reference point, usually the level of the left ventricle, taken to be the mid-axillary line on the left side.

What is damping?

Damping is the tendency to resist oscillation. It is usually produced by air bubbles, clots, catheter kinking, three-way taps, and narrow, compliant and long tubing.

When the damping coefficient is 1, it is called critical damping. A mass displaced from its equilibrium position will return to the original position without any overshoot.

If the damping coefficient is zero, the system will oscillate indefinitely with undamped natural frequency.

A damping coefficient of 0.67 creates optimal damping. A mass displaced from its equilibrium position will return to its original position quickly, with some overshoot. This is the best compromise that can be obtained between the speed of response and accuracy of the amplitude of the trace (BP reading).

What is the problem with over-damping and under-damping?

An over-damped trace results in under-reading of systolic pressure and over-reading of diastolic pressure.

An under-damped trace results in over-reading of systolic and under-reading of diastolic pressure.

The mean arterial pressure (MAP) remains the same.

How would you test for optimal damping?

Dynamic response of the transducer system can be checked using a fast flush or a 'square wave' test. To perform the square wave test flush the system by applying a pressure of 300mm Hg. This results in a square waveform followed by oscillations.

In an optimally damped system, there will be two or three oscillations before settling to zero.

An over-damped system settles to zero without any oscillations.

An under-damped system oscillates for more than 3-4 cycles before settling to zero.

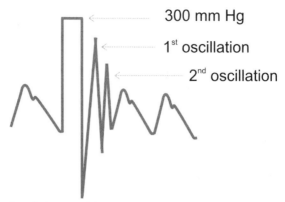

Figure 4.8 Optimal damped trace.

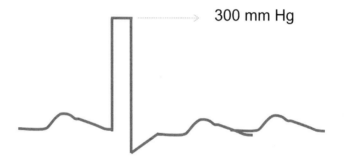

Figure 4.9 Over-damped trace.

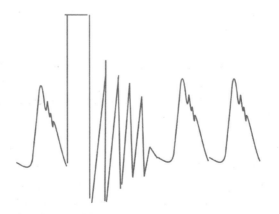

Figure 4.10 Under-damped trace.

What are the complications of invasive blood pressure monitoring?

◆ Haemorrhage and haematoma.
◆ Thrombosis and ischaemia.
◆ Embolism.
◆ Infection.
◆ Aneurysm and AV fistula.
◆ Nerve damage.
◆ Accidental drug administration.

Non-invasive blood pressure measurement

Blood pressure can be measured indirectly using non-invasive methods.

Manual devices

◆ Sphygmomanometer (mercury and aneroid).
◆ Von Recklinghausen oscillotonometer.

Automated devices

◆ Automated oscillometric technique.
◆ Continuous non-invasive blood pressure measurement: Penaz technique (Finapress).

The basic components of a non-invasive device include a cuff with inflatable bladder, a mechanism to inflate and deflate the cuff and a display unit. The Von Recklinghausen oscillotonometer consists of two cuffs, a dial for reading the blood pressure and a control lever. The pulsations in the detecting cuff are amplified and are seen as oscillations on the dial. The needle on the dial will start oscillating when systolic pressure is reached. The maximum oscillation is seen at the mean blood pressure. This does not accurately measure the diastolic pressure.

The DINAMAP (device for indirect non-invasive automated mean arterial pressure measurement) is an automated device; the principle is the same as the Von Recklinghausen oscillotonometer, but it uses a single cuff and instead of bellows, a pressure transducer measures the pressure and oscillations. A microprocessor controls the inflation, deflation, and display of numerical value. A pneumatic pump inflates the arm cuff and a solenoid valve controls the deflation of the cuff.

It is important to select an appropriately sized cuff. The bladder inside the cuff should encircle at least 80% of the arm circumference. The width of the cuff should be 20% more than the diameter of the arm. The cuff should be placed so that the midline of the bladder is over the arterial pulsation. In general a narrow cuff results in over-reading and a large cuff results in under-reading of the actual blood pressure. In obese patients due to the conical shape of the upper arm, cuff placement can be difficult.

Continuous NIBP measurement

The Finapress (FINger Arterial Pressure) device uses a finger cuff and a transducer. The volume of the blood in the finger varies with the cardiac cycle. A small cuff placed around the finger is used to keep the blood volume of the finger constant. An infrared photo-plethysmograph detects changes in the volume of the blood within the finger with each cardiac cycle. A controller system alters the pressure in the cuff accordingly to keep the volume of the finger constant. The applied pressure waveform correlates with the arterial blood volume and, therefore, with the arterial blood pressure. This applied pressure is then displayed continuously, in real time as the arterial blood pressure waveform.

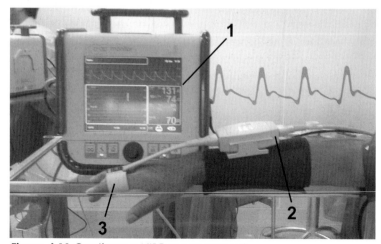

Figure 4.11 Continuous NIBP measurement.
1. Blood pressure reading display; 2. Controller module; 3. Finger cuff.

NIBP is inaccurate at extremes of blood pressure. Non-invasive devices tend to over-read at low blood pressure, and under-read very high blood pressure. As the blood pressure measurement relies on a regular pulse, arrhythmias such as atrial fibrillation can cause inaccurate readings. Movement of the arm, shivering or external pressure, such as someone leaning on the arm, can cause an inaccurate reading. The pressure effects of frequent cuff inflation for a prolonged period can cause nerve damage and petechial haemorrhages.

Key points

♦ Intra-arterial blood pressure monitoring gives beat to beat reading of the blood pressure.
♦ The waveform also gives an indication about other important haemodynamic parameters.
♦ The system should be zeroed at the level of the left ventricle (mid-axillary line) on the left side.
♦ Under or over-damping will give erroneous values, but will not affect the mean arterial pressure.

Further reading

1. Recommendations for standards of monitoring during anaesthesia and recovery. AAGBI guidelines. http://www.aagbi.org/publications/guidelines/docs/standardsofmonitoring07.pdf.
2. Al-Shaikh B, Stacey S. *Essentials of anaesthetic equipment,* 3rd ed. London: Churchill Livingstone, 2007.
3. Davey A, Diba A. *Ward's anaesthetic equipment,* 5th ed. London: Saunders, 2005.

Structured oral examination 5

Long case 5

Information for the candidate

Clinical Anaesthesia

A 56-year-old female patient is scheduled to have an elective craniotomy for clipping of cerebral aneurysms. Six months ago she collapsed at home in the bathroom. She gives a history of headache for the last year. She is a known hypertensive and has smoked 20-30 cigarettes per day for many years. She complains of shortness of breath on climbing one flight of stairs. Cerebral angiography has revealed two aneurysms, one located in the middle cerebral artery measuring 18 x 10 x 10mm and another one in the anterior communicating artery measuring 6 x 5 x 5mm.

History

Her drug history includes amlodipine 10mg o.d., aspirin 75mg o.d., omeprazole 20mg o.d., simvastatin 20mg o.d., a salbutamol inhaler 200µg b.d., and a beclomethasone dipropionate inhaler 200µg b.d.

Clinical examination

She is fully conscious with a GCS of 15.

Table 5.1 Clinical examination.

Weight	105kg
Height	165cm
BMI	38.5
Heart rate	75 bpm
Blood pressure	140/75mmHg
Temperature	37.2°C

Investigations

Table 5.2 Biochemistry.

		Normal values
Sodium	132mmol/L	135-145mmol/L
Potassium	3.8mmol/L	3.5-5.0mmol/L
Urea	4.5mmol/L	2.2-8.3mmol/L
Creatinine	63µmol/L	44-80µmol/L
Blood glucose	5.5mmol/L	3.0-6.0mmol/L

Table 5.3 Haematology.

		Normal values
Hb	18.3g/dL	11-16g/dL
Haematocrit	0.58	0.4-0.5 males, 0.37-0.47 females
RBC	5.9×10^{12}/L	$3.8\text{-}4.8 \times 10^{12}$/L
WBC	7.5×10^9/L	$4\text{-}11 \times 10^9$/L
Platelets	396×10^9/L	$150\text{-}450 \times 10^9$/L
INR	1.0	0.9-1.2
PT	12.0 seconds	11-15 seconds
APTT ratio	1.1	0.8-1.2

Table 5.4 Arterial blood gases whilst breathing room air.

pH	7.34
PCO_2	5.4kPa
PO_2	10.5kPa
SaO_2	95%
BE	1.2mmol/L
HCO_3^-	26mmol/L

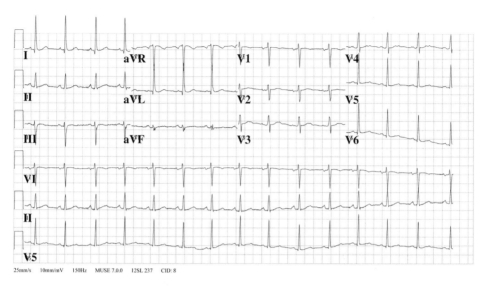

Figure 5.1 ECG.

Examiner's questions

Please summarise the case

This is a 56-year-old, morbidly obese female patient with a history of hypertension, scheduled for craniotomy and clipping of cerebral aneurysms. Her haematology suggests polycythaemia most likely due to smoking and possibly associated obstructive airway disease.

Can you comment on the ECG?

The ECG shows sinus rhythm with a heart rate of 85 per minute. P waves are notched in lead II and are bifid in V1 and V2; the terminal negative component of the P wave is suggestive of left atrial hypertrophy. There are tall R waves in leads I and aVL. The height of the QRS complex in aVL is >11mm suggesting left ventricular hypertrophy (LVH). The other features supporting LVH include tall R waves in lead I and the lateral leads.

Both left ventricular and left atrial hypertrophy can be due to hypertension.

Can you comment on the blood gas result?

The blood gas result indicates a normal pH, a normal $PaCO_2$ value with slightly low PaO_2 and low oxygen saturation which can account for smoking and associated chronic obstructive airway disease.

Why would you say she is morbidly obese? What is the definition of BMI?

Her body mass index (BMI) is 38.5, therefore, she is morbidly obese. BMI is calculated using the formula:

$$BMI = \frac{\text{weight in kg}}{(\text{height in metres})^2}$$

BMI <18.5: underweight.
BMI 18.5-24.9: normal range.
BMI 25.0-29.9: overweight.
BMI 30-34.9: obesity.
BMI 35-54.9: morbid obesity.
BMI >55 super-morbidly obese.

What are the problems associated with obesity?

The problems can be broadly classified into physiological and anatomical.

Respiratory system

Total respiratory compliance is decreased (mainly due to reduced chest wall compliance); it can be as little as 30% of normal. FRC and expiratory reserve volume (ERV) are reduced; FRC decreases steeply with increasing BMI, and can be reduced to such an extent that it can fall within the closing capacity and result in alveolar collapse. As a result there is more rapid desaturation during induction and intubation despite pre-oxygenation. With increasing obesity alveolar ventilation is insufficient to excrete CO_2, and $PaCO_2$ increases (obesity hypoventilation syndrome); these patients often have sleep apnoea. If pulse oximetry saturation is <96% on room air, further investigations including lung function tests and blood gases should be performed. The incidence of obstructive sleep apnoea increases with obesity.

Cardiovascular system

The metabolic demands of increased fatty tissue (increased oxygen consumption and increased carbon dioxide production) result in increased cardiac output and total blood volume. The left ventricular wall thickness increases due to additional cardiac workload. There is increased incidence of ischaemic heart disease, hypertension, cardiomegaly and congestive cardiac failure.

Non-invasive blood pressure (NIBP) monitoring can be inaccurate if the wrong sized cuff is used and placed incorrectly on the arm.

Gastrointestinal system

There may be a greater risk of acid reflux, requiring antacid prophylaxis.

Endocrine and metabolic

Morbidly obese patients have a high incidence of diabetes and hypercholesterolaemia.

Airway

Associated factors such as short neck, limited movement of the atlanto-occipital joint, a large chin, breasts and thoracic fat can lead to a difficult airway both in terms of mask ventilation and endotracheal intubation. Patients with obstructive sleep apnoea, frequently have increased fat tissue in the pharyngeal wall, with a tendency to airway collapse when exposed to negative pressure. Pre-oxygenation should be performed. The traditional intubation position (sniffing the morning air) should be modified to the ramped position with supports under the nape of the neck, and shoulders.

Veins may be hard to find; location of anatomical landmarks for invasive monitoring procedures and regional techniques may also be difficult.

There is an increased risk of deep vein thrombosis (DVT) and pulmonary embolism (PE) in obese patients. Peri-operative DVT prophylaxis using both mechanical and pharmacological methods should be considered in all obese patients.

Positioning

Surgical positioning requires additional manpower and a special operating table may be needed.

Pharmacokinetics

Compared with total body weight there is a smaller proportion of total body water and a greater proportion of body fat. These factors can lead to changes in the proportion of drug distributed to various body compartments, e.g. increased uptake of volatile agents into the fat compartment. Fat-soluble drugs (e.g. benzodiazepines, thiopentone) will have an increased volume of distribution. Drug protein binding is affected by increased levels of lipoproteins. Renal excretion and hepatic excretion of drugs can also be reduced. Relative overdosage can occur when the drug dose is calculated based on the actual weight of the patient.

Postoperative problems include delayed recovery due to the effect of residual anaesthetic agents. Respiratory depression, hypoventilation and desaturation may occur in the recovery room. Late complications such as atelectasis, chest infection, respiratory failure, wound infection and DVT are more common in morbidly obese patients.

What are the causes of polycythaemia?

In this patient, the most likely cause is hypoxia related to heavy smoking and obstructive airway disease.

Other causes include:

- Primary: polycythaemia rubra vera.
- Secondary: high altitude, chronic lung disease, cyanotic congenital heart disease, obstructive sleep apnoea.
- Renal: renal cell carcinoma (hypernephroma).
- Liver: hepatocellular carcinoma, uterine fibroids.

Relative polycythaemia is seen in dehydration and burns.

What are the clinical implications of polycythaemia?

Polycythaemia increases the viscosity of blood such that the patient has an increased risk of DVT and PE. There is an increased risk of cerebrovascular accident (CVA).

What other investigation would you like to see before anaesthetising this patient?

◆ CT of the brain and cerebral angiogram. A CT of the brain will reveal the presence of any intracerebral bleed and a cerebral angiogram is essential to locate the site of the aneurysm.

◆ Lung function tests are useful in assessing the severity of obstructive airway disease as a cause of dyspnoea.

◆ An echocardiogram may be useful in assessing left ventricular function and wall motion abnormalities as a result of myocardial ischaemia.

◆ Carotid Doppler. This patient collapsed 6 months ago; this may be due to a transient ischaemic attack due to carotid insufficiency, resulting in cerebral hypoperfusion.

What are the risk factors associated with subarachnoid haemorrhage (SAH)?

◆ Smoking.
◆ Hypertension.
◆ Alcohol intake and illicit drug abuse.
◆ Pregnancy.
◆ Female.
◆ Age 40-60 years.
◆ Familial conditions, e.g. Marfan's syndrome, Ehlers-Danlos syndrome and polycystic kidney disease.

Which vessels are most commonly involved?

Aneurysms in the anterior cerebral artery (ACA) are most common, followed by the internal carotid artery (ICA) and then the middle cerebral artery (MCA).

What is the pathophysiology of SAH?

Rupture of the aneurysm causes an immediate increase in intracranial pressure (ICP)(Munroe-Kellie doctrine) approaching diastolic pressure in the proximal intracerebral arteries. The increase in ICP causes a decrease in cerebral perfusion pressure (CPP) resulting in reduced cerebral blood flow (CBF). This fall in CBF slows down the bleeding from an SAH, leading to a decrease in ICP, and an improvement in CPP and the neurological condition. The persistent rise in ICP causes vasospasm and thrombi, and may cause hydrocephalus. The CPP can be calculated as follows:

$$CPP = MAP - ICP$$

where CPP = cerebral perfusion pressure, MAP = mean arterial pressure, ICP = intracranial pressure.

How would you anaesthetise this patient? Describe the anaesthetic management of this patient

The main goals include:

- Prevention of aneurysm rupture on induction and intra-operatively.
- Maintenance of adequate CPP and cerebral oxygenation.
- Smooth and rapid emergence from anaesthesia to allow full neurological assessment.
- Use of balanced anaesthesia with muscle relaxation.

Pre-operative assessment

A focused neurological examination should be performed and recorded. Her current drug therapy including amlodipine and bronchodilators should be continued. The blood group and availability of cross-matched blood should be checked. Aspirin should be stopped a week before the surgery to prevent bleeding associated with platelet dysfunction. Aspirin causes irreversible inhibition of platelet cyclo-oxygenase, hence the duration of effect lasts for 7-9 days, the lifetime of platelets.

Sedative drugs and anxiolytics are generally avoided as they may cause respiratory depression and mask the signs of neurological deterioration.

In the anaesthetic room, 1-2mg of midazolam may be given to reduce anxiety.

Monitoring during anaesthesia includes peripheral oxygen saturation using pulse oximetry, continuous ECG, invasive arterial blood pressure, central venous pressure, body temperature (nasopharyngeal), urine output, neuromuscular blockade, blood loss estimation and intermittent blood gases, glucose and haematocrit.

Peripheral venous access should be secured using two large-bore cannulae.

Induction of anaesthesia

Pre-oxygenation followed by smooth induction with limitation of hypertensive response to laryngscopy is essential to avoid rupture of the aneurysms. Intravenous induction can be performed with propofol 1-2mg/kg (ensuring loss of consciousness while maintaining haemodynamic stability) and remifentanil (a bolus of 0.5µg/kg over 1 minute followed by an infusion of 0.25-0.5µg/kg/minute or target controlled infusion [TCI] at 3-8ng/ml), followed by a non-depolarising muscle relaxant (vecuronium 0.1mg/kg or atracurium 0.5mg/kg) to facilitate tracheal intubation.

Maintenance of anaesthesia

Total intravenous anaesthesia with propofol and remifentanil or a volatile agent (desflurane, sevoflurane or isoflurane) and remifentanil is used for maintenance of anaesthesia. Nitrous oxide should be avoided altogether due to the risk of venous air embolism. It increases the ICP without depressing the cerebral metabolism.

Controlled hypotension should be avoided as it decreases regional CBF. In patients with SAH, normal autoregulation is impaired due to cerebral vasospasm.

Mannitol at a dose of 0.5-1g/kg reduces the ICP. The peak effect usually occurs approximately 30-45 minutes after the start of intravenous infusion. Dexamethasone (8-10mg) is administered intravenously to reduce cerebral oedema. A prophylactic anticonvulsant (loading dose phenytoin sodium 15mg/kg) is usually administered during the intra-operative period unless already administered on the ward.

Emergence and recovery

Provided there are no intra-operative complications and the aneurysm is successfully clipped, the patient should be woken up at the end of surgery. This allows neurological assessment and reduces respiratory complications associated with postoperative ventilation. During extubation and recovery, hypertension, coughing, straining and hypercarbia should be avoided. Before discontinuing remifentanil, adequate analgesia is essential, using long-acting opioids (titrated doses of morphine 0.1-0.15mg/kg) and intravenous paracetamol.

Postoperative care

The patient should be monitored in a neurosurgical intensive care unit. Blood pressure should be maintained very close to the normal range (at least within 20% of patient's normal blood pressure). Relative hypervolaemia and relative haemodilution should be maintained in the postoperative period. Neurological observations (level of consciousness, size and reactivity of the pupil, limb movements) along with blood pressure, heart rate, temperature, urine output, sedation score and pain score should be monitored regularly.

Postoperative analgesia includes regular administration of paracetamol 1g (oral or IV) four times a day and codeine phosphate 30-60mg (oral or IM) four times a day. Patient-controlled analgesia (PCA) with morphine or titrated doses of intravenous morphine can also be used whilst monitoring the patient in a neurosurgical ICU or HDU unit.

Management of aneurysmal subarachnoid haemorrhage (SAH)

The neurological injury associated with SAH can vary, and includes unconsciousness, a reduced level of consciousness, focal neurological deficits and isolated cranial nerve palsy.

Investigations

◆ Serum urea and electrolytes. Hyponatraemia is common due to cerebral salt wasting (release of brain natriuretic peptide) or due to the syndrome of inappropriate anti-diuretic hormone (SIADH) resulting from pituitary dysfunction.
◆ A CT scan (non-contrast) may show blood in the ventricles.
◆ Lumbar puncture for analysis of cerebrospinal fluid (CSF) is recommended when SAH is suspected but the CT scan is negative. Blood containing CSF that does not clear during continued flow and presence of xanthochromia is highly suspicious of SAH.
◆ CT angiography or magnetic resonance angiography (MRA), or catheter angiography by direct intracranial catheterisation are useful techniques to delineate the anatomy of intracranial aneurysms.
◆ Transcranial Doppler is recommended for the diagnosis and monitoring of vasospasm.
◆ MRI is relatively insensitive at diagnosing acute SAH.

In a normal scan the third ventricle and the septum between the frontal horns of the lateral ventricle should lie in the midline: the line joining the falx

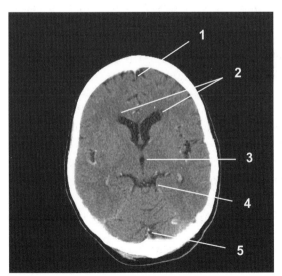

Figure 5.2 Normal CT scan.
1. Midline falx cerebri (anterior); 2. Frontal horns of lateral ventricles; 3. Third ventricle; 4. Basal cistern; 5. Midline falx cerebri (posterior).

cerebri anteriorly and posteriorly. Increased pressure on one side of the cranium can cause midline shift.

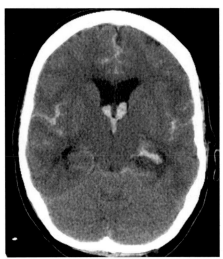

Figure 5.3 CT scan with blood in the subarachnoid space.

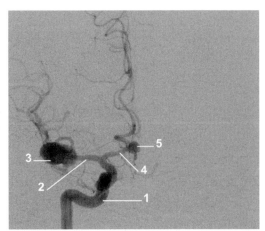

Figure 5.4 Cerebral angiogram delineating the middle cerebral artery and anterior communicating artery aneurysms.

1. Internal carotid artery; 2. Middle cerebral artery; 3. Middle cerebral artery aneurysm; 4. Anterior cerebral artery; 5. Anterior communicating artery aneurysm.

Treatment of SAH

The risk of re-bleeding in untreated ruptured aneurysms is 3%-4% in the first 24 hours, 1%-2% per day in the first month and a long-term risk of 3% per year after three months.

Vasospasm leads to ischaemia and cerebral infarction. This is most common 3-12 days after SAH and occurs in about 25% of patients. Cerebral ischaemia may be worsened by hypovolaemia, reduced MAP, cerebral oedema or hydrocephalus.

Management and prophylaxis of cerebral vasospasm includes administration of nimodipine, mild sedation, positive fluid balance and avoidance of episodes of hypotension.

Nimodipine is a calcium channel blocker, which reduces the incidence of cerebral infarction by one third if given as a prophylactic. The dose is 60mg orally or by nasogastric tube four-hourly. Intravenous infusion of nimodipine is associated with hypotension.

Triple H therapy (hypervolaemia, hypertension and haemodilution) increases cerebral perfusion pressure, reduces viscosity and increases CBF.

ECG abnormalities include T-wave inversion, ST segment depression, a prolonged QT interval and rhythm disturbances. These abnormalities probably result from increased release of catecholamines and increased sympathetic tone associated with injury of the posterior hypothalamus.

Early therapeutic intervention either by clipping or coiling reduces the incidence of cerebral vasospasm and reduces the risk of re-bleeding.

Coiling of the aneurysm has been associated with a slightly lower procedural morbidity and mortality as compared with clipping. In cases of aneurysms with wider necks and large aneurysms, coiling will be less effective compared with clipping.

Grading of cerebral aneurysm

Clinical grading scales are used for standardising the clinical assessment and for estimating the prognosis. The most commonly used scale in the UK is the World Federation of Neurosurgeons (WFNS) Scale.

Table 5.5 WFNS scale.

WFNS Grade	GCS	Motor deficit
I	15	Absent
II	13-14	Absent
III	13-14	Present
IV	7-12	Absent or present
V	3-6	Absent or present

Table 5.6 Hunt and Hess grading scale.

Grade	Clinical features
I	Asymptomatic or minimal headache
II	Moderate to severe headache, no neurological deficit other than cranial nerve palsy
III	Drowsiness, confusion or mild neurological deficit
IV	Stupor, moderate to severe hemiparesis
V	Deep coma and decerebrate rigidity

The higher the clinical grade the more severe will be the pathology with cerebral vasospasm, raised ICP and impaired cerebral autoregulation.

Complications of SAH

The major complications of SAH include re-bleeding, vasospasm and delayed ischaemic deficit, hydrocephalus, seizures, electrolyte imbalance and cardiac dysfunction.

Techniques to attenuate response to laryngoscopy and tracheal intubation

◆ Esmolol: 0.5mg/kg over 30 seconds prior to laryngoscopy.
◆ Alfentanil: 20-30µg/kg one minute prior to laryngoscopy.
◆ Remifentanil: 0.5µg/kg bolus prior to laryngoscopy.
◆ Additional dose of propofol 0.5mg/kg prior to laryngoscopy.
◆ Lidocaine: 1.5mg/kg prior to laryngoscopy.
◆ Ensuring adequate muscle relaxation by monitoring response to neuromuscular stimulation.

Intra-operative fluid therapy

◆ Dextrose-containing solutions should be avoided due to the risk of hyperglycaemia and cerebral oedema.
◆ Normal saline and lactated Ringer's solution can be used. Hyperchloraemic acidosis may develop with an infusion of a large volume of normal saline, and hyponatraemia and brain oedema may develop with a large volume infusion of Hartmann's solution.
◆ Hypertonic saline may have a role, especially in decreasing ICP.

Postoperative analgesia for craniotomy

Pain following craniotomy is a greater problem than previously thought; many patients have moderate to severe pain postoperatively. Codeine phosphate administered intramuscularly has been the main analgesic in managing postoperative pain due to the fear of respiratory depression and the masking of neurological signs with morphine and other opioids. Codeine is less potent than morphine and the clinical effect depends on its demethylation to morphine. Morphine PCA may also provide good analgesia without causing excessive respiratory depression.

Key points

◆ Hypoxia secondary to smoking and obstructive airway disease can result in polycythaemia.
◆ Rupture of a cerebral aneurysm increases intracranial pressure and reduces cerebral perfusion pressure.

◆ Clinical grading of aneurysms is useful in estimating the severity and prognosis.

◆ Triple H therapy increases cerebral perfusion pressure and increases cerebral blood flow.

◆ Many patients experience a moderate degree of pain following craniotomy, and use of opioid analgesics with close monitoring should be considered.

Further reading

1. Dinsmore J. Anaesthesia for elective neurosurgery. *British Journal of Anaesthesia* 2007; 99: 68-74.

2. Priebe H-J. Aneurysmal subarachnoid haemorrhage and the anaesthetist. *British Journal of Anaesthesia* 2007; 99: 102-18.

3. Roberts GC. Post-craniotomy analgesia: current practices in British neurosurgical centres - a survey of post-craniotomy analgesic practices. *European Journal of Anaesthesiology* 2005; 22: 328-32.

4. Stoneham MD, Walters FJ. Post-operative analgesia for craniotomy patients: current attitudes among neuroanaesthetists. *European Journal of Anaesthesiology* 1995; 12: 571-5.

5. Roberts G. A review of the efficacy and safety of opioid analgesics post-craniotomy. *Nurs Crit Care* 2004; 9: 277-83.

6. Peri-operative management of the morbidly obese patient. The Association of Anaesthetists of Great Britain and Ireland, 2007.

7. Lotia S, Bellamy MC. Anaesthesia and morbid obesity. *British Journal of Anaesthesia CEACCP* 2008; 8: 151-6.

Short case 5.1: Malignant hyperthermia

A 9-year-old girl undergoing correction of scoliosis develops tachycardia during the procedure.

What are the causes of tachycardia?

The causes of tachycardia during the intra-operative period can be due to anaesthesia, and patient or surgery-related factors:

- Inadequate analgesia: often associated with hypertension.
- Inadequate depth of anaesthesia: usually associated with hypertension, sweating and lacrimation.
- Muscle relaxation wearing off: there are other signs such as breathing against the ventilator, high airway pressure and inspiratory efforts seen on the capnograph trace.
- Hypovolaemia: this is usually due to blood loss. A rapid assessment of blood loss in the suction and surgical field and the amount of fluid administered will aid in the diagnosis.
- Hypoxia: a systematic approach to checking the inspired oxygen concentration, FGF and patency of airway will aid in the management.
- Hypercarbia: this may be due to hypoventilation or to increased CO_2 production.
- Drugs: accidental or therapeutic administration of anti-cholinergic drugs or catecholamines can cause tachycardia. Anaphylaxis to drugs may manifest as tachycardia.
- Surgical stimulation.
- Malignant hyperthermia (MH): increasing $ETCO_2$ despite adequate ventilation and rapidly depleting carbon dioxide absorber may suggest the diagnosis.

Despite correcting all possible causes, tachycardia persists and the $ETCO_2$ increases. What is the most likely diagnosis?

Malignant hyperthermia is the most likely diagnosis.

How would you manage a malignant hyperthermia crisis?

- Turn off the vaporiser and use high FGF and hyperventilate with 100% oxygen.
- Call for help.
- Stop the surgery if possible.
- Maintain anaesthesia with an intravenous propofol infusion.
- Monitor temperature and start active body cooling measures.
- Administer dantrolene 2-3mg/kg IV initially and then repeat with a dose of 1mg/kg until CO_2 production, tachycardia and temperature are controlled.

- Monitor arterial blood gases, invasive blood pressure, central venous pressure, urine output, haematocrit, platelets, clotting screen and creatine kinase (peaks at 24 hours).
- Acidosis should be treated with sodium bicarbonate and hyperventilation.
- Hyperkalaemia should be treated with sodium bicarbonate, calcium chloride and dextrose insulin infusion.
- Forced alkaline diuresis, aiming for a urine output of >3ml/kg/hour and a urine pH of >7.0 in order to treat myoglobinaemia.
- Disseminated intravascular coagulation (DIC) should be treated with FFP, cryoprecipitate and platelets.
- Cardiac arrhythmias should be treated with magnesium and amiodarone; calcium channel blockers should be avoided.

Once the vital parameters are stable continuation of the surgery may be considered, and postoperatively the patient should be transferred to the ICU.

Late management involves counselling the patient and family regarding the implications of MH and referring the patient to an MH unit for investigation.

How would you confirm the diagnosis of MH?

MH is mainly diagnosed by *in vitro* contracture testing (INVCT). Fresh muscle strips should be taken from the patient's vastus muscle under local anaesthesia. The test involves exposure of muscle strips to halothane and caffeine and measuring the tension generated in the muscle. Muscles from MH-susceptible patients develop higher tension at lower concentrations of halothane and caffeine compared with normal individuals.

DNA testing can be used to complement INVCT. DNA should be screened for mutations in the ryanodine receptor protein (*RYR1*) gene. If the mutation is not present, diagnosis of MH cannot be rejected. Diagnosis should be confirmed by muscle biopsy.

What anaesthetic agents trigger MH?

Triggering agents include all volatile anaesthetics (halothane, enflurane, isoflurane, sevoflurane, desflurane) and the depolarizing muscle relaxant, succinylcholine.

What is the pathogenesis of MH?

Volatile anaesthetics and/or succinylcholine cause a rise in the myoplasmic calcium concentration. The rise in calcium concentration leads to an activation of actin and myosin filaments and explains the rigidity and the masseter spasm, one of the early signs of MH. The raised calcium concentration further leads to stimulation of the energy consuming processes in the skeletal muscle, leading to metabolic acidosis. There is uncontrolled oxidative phosphorylation. The hypermetabolism seen in MH leads to several clinical signs, such as hypertonia, arrhythmia, tachycardia and hyperthermia. Acidosis results from excessive production of CO_2 and lactic acid. Rhabdomyolysis occurs as a result of excessive contractile activity. Laboratory findings include hyperkalaemia, raised creatine kinase and myoglobinuria.

There is a statistically significant association between inheritance of DNA markers for ryanodine receptor protein (RYR1) and MH susceptibility in >60% families. Ryanodine, an alkaloid, binds selectively to the ryanodine receptor, a calcium channel in the sarcoplasmic reticulum. In some families with MH predisposition, no ryanodine receptor defect has been isolated. Because of this heterogenecity it is difficult to diagnose MH based on genetic testing.

What other conditions are associated with MH?

Central core disease and inherited forms of peripheral muscle weakness are associated with MH. Several other neuromuscular diseases and heat stroke may be associated with MH, although true association with these conditions has not been confirmed.

Clinical presentation of malignant hyperthermia

Malignant hyperthermia (MH) is an acute pharmacogenetic disorder, with autosomal-dominant inheritance. Both genetic predisposition and one or more triggering agents are necessary to evoke MH. The prevalence of the genetic MH predisposition is between 1:5,000 to 1:10,000; the incidence of reported MH reactions varies from 1 in 40,000 to 1 in 100,000 anaesthetics.

MH has a wide spectrum of presentation:

♦ Muscle rigidity after succinylcholine. This can be isolated masseter spasm or generalised rigidity. Masseter spasm associated with grossly elevated creatine kinase and myoglobin increases the likelihood of MH.

♦ Classical MH crisis. Apart from masseter spasm, the two most important clinical features are an unexplained increase in $ETCO_2$ and tachycardia due to hypermetabolism. Later, a rise in body temperature can occur which can exceed a rate of more than $1°C$ per ten minutes. Eventually, because of extensive cellular damage, hyperkalaemia, acidosis, increased plasma creatine kinase and myoglobinuria ensues. Arrhythmias and DIC are other features.

♦ Other miscellaneous presentations include postoperative acute renal failure due to myoglobinuria, unexpected cardiac arrest or even death.

The differential diagnosis of MH includes thyroid storm, phaeochromocytoma, infection and sepsis.

In a patient with suspected MH who presents for surgery:

♦ Avoid all triggering agents and use total intravenous anaesthesia.
♦ Consider regional anaesthesia if feasible.
♦ Use a vapour-free anaesthetic machine.

With the above measures prophylactic dantrolene is not necessary. If a vapour-free anaesthetic machine is not readily available, it can be prepared by the removal of vaporisers and flushing through the machine and ventilator with 100% oxygen at maximal flow for about 20-30 minutes.

All intravenous anaesthetics, including ketamine and benzodiazepines, are safe, as are all analgesics and non-depolarising muscle relaxants. Nitrous oxide also has been safely used. Other drugs which can be used include local anaesthetics, neostigmine, atropine and glycopyrrolate.

Key points

◆ Masseter spasm and muscle rigidity following succinylcholine is one of the early signs of malignant hyperthermia.
◆ Malignant hyperthermia should be suspected in the presence of unexplained tachycardia and increasing $ETCO_2$.
◆ The diagnosis of malignant hyperthermia is confirmed by *in vitro* contracture testing.

Further reading

1. Halsall PJ, Hopkins MP. Malignant hyperthermia. *British Journal of Anaesthesia CEACCP* 2003; 3: 5-9.
2. Guideline for management of malignant hyperthermia crisis. http://www.aagbi.org/publications/guidelines/docs/malignanthyp07.pdf.

Short case 5.2: Guillain-Barre syndrome

A 32-year-old male patient is admitted to the ICU with a 2-week history of malaise, fatigue and progressive symmetrical weakness of the lower limbs following a minor upper respiratory tract infection.

What is the most likely diagnosis?

The most likely diagnosis is Guillain-Barre syndrome (GBS), an acute demyelinating polyneuropathy. The differential diagnosis includes polyneuropathy, multiple sclerosis and motor neurone disease.

How would you manage this patient in intensive care?

Immediate assessment of the patient's airway, breathing and circulation should be conducted. A full history and clinical examination should be performed including assessment of neurological status.

What are the treatment options?

The treatment options involve supportive therapy which includes ventilatory support with physiotherapy, and disease modifying treatments which are aimed at reducing inflammation of neural tissues to expedite recovery, such as immunoglobulin administration and plasmapheresis.

Since GBS tends to run as a long and progressive illness with a slow gradual recovery there should be a multidisciplinary team approach involving medical and nursing staff, physiotherapists and occupational therapists.

There is a high incidence of DVT and patients need thromboprophylaxis with low-molecular-weight heparin and gradient compression stockings.

What are the causes of respiratory failure in GBS?

About 25% of patients with GBS require ventilatory support during the course of their illness. The factors contributing to respiratory failure include facial, laryngeal and bulbar weakness, inability to clear secretions due to weakness of the chest muscles and diaphragm, and secondary respiratory infections.

The following are useful in identifying patients with GBS who are at particular risk of respiratory failure:

◆ Vital capacity. Regular monitoring.
◆ Pulse oximetry. Hypoxaemia is a late consequence of neuromuscular respiratory failure.
◆ Clinical clues. Patients who develop bulbar involvement, bilateral facial weakness and rapid disease progression are likely to require intubation and ventilation.

The indications for intubation and ventilation include:

◆ Vital capacity <20ml/kg.
◆ Maximal inspiratory pressure (MIP) <-30cm H_2O.
◆ Maximal expiratory pressure (MEP) <40cm H_2O.
◆ Decrease of >30% of vital capacity.

Non-invasive ventilation is generally not useful in GBS as it does not solve the problem of inability to eliminate secretions due to muscular weakness.

What specific treatment options are available for GBS?

The currently available treatment options for GBS include:

- Intravenous immunoglobulin.
- Plasma exchange.
- Corticosteroids.
- CSF filtration.

Intravenous immunoglobulin and plasma exchange are disease modifying modalities. Immunoglobulin therapy has the advantage of easier administration and fewer side effects, particularly in the elderly, and is generally the initial treatment of choice.

The recommended dose of intravenous immunoglobulin therapy is 0.4mg/kg daily for 5-6 days which should be commenced within 2 weeks of the onset of symptoms.

Plasma exchange has been shown to reduce the duration of ventilator dependence and hospital stay, and leads to earlier mobilisation if commenced within 2 weeks of the onset of illness. It is associated with more significant side effects and contraindications compared with immunoglobulin therapy. Administration is limited to specialist centres. Typically, up to five exchanges are performed substituting 250ml/kg of plasma with 4.5% human albumin solution. Contraindications to plasmapheresis include haemodynamic instability, uncontrolled sepsis and severe haemostatic problems. Side effects include hypotension, hypocalcaemia, coagulation abnormalities and septicaemia.

Although patients with chronic demyelinating neuropathies respond to steroids, most studies fail to show any beneficial effect of using steroids to treat GBS.

What are the side effects of immunoglobulin therapy?

The side effects of immunoglobulin therapy are only seen in a minority of patients and include nausea, fever, headache, a transient rise in liver enzymes, encephalopathy, meningism and malaise. More serious side effects include skin reactions (e.g. erythroderma), hypercoagulability, deterioration in renal function due to renal tubular necrosis, and anaphylaxis.

Contraindications to treatment include IgA deficiency (increased incidence of anaphylaxis) and previous anaphylaxis to immunoglobulin therapy. IgA levels must be checked in all patients prior to administration of immunoglobulin.

Extreme caution must be taken in patients with renal impairment as renal function may deteriorate further with immunoglobulin therapy. Severe congestive cardiac failure is also a relative contraindication.

Clinical features of GBS

Motor dysfunction

Symmetric limb weakness typically begins as proximal lower extremity weakness and ascends to involve the upper extremities, truncal muscles, and head. Respiratory muscle weakness with shortness of breath may be present.

Cranial nerve palsies (III-VII, IX-XII) may be present. Patients may present with facial weakness mimicking Bell's palsy, dysphagia, dysarthria, ophthalmoplegia, and pupillary disturbances. The Miller-Fisher variant is unique in that this subtype begins with cranial nerve deficits.

Lack of deep tendon reflexes is a hallmark sign.

Sensory dysfunction

Paraesthesia usually begins in the toes and fingertips and progresses upward but generally does not extend beyond the wrists or ankles. Pain is most severe in the shoulder girdle, back, buttocks, and thighs, and may occur with even the slightest movements. Loss of vibration, proprioception, touch, and pain distally may be present.

Autonomic dysfunction

Cardiovascular signs may include tachycardia, bradycardia, dysrhythmias, wide fluctuations in blood pressure, and postural hypotension. Urinary retention, paralytic ileus and gastric dysmotility may be present.

Causes of GBS

GBS has been associated with antecedent bacterial and viral infections and vaccinations. Bacterial infections include *Campylobacter jejuni*, *Haemophilus influenzae* and *Mycoplasma pneumoniae*. Viral infections include cytomegalovirus, Ebstein-Barr virus and the human immunodeficiency virus (HIV) during seroconversion.

Anecdotal associations include systemic lupus erythematosus, lymphoma and sarcoidosis.

Investigations

Diagnosis is usually is made on clinical grounds. Investigations are useful to rule out other diagnoses and to assess the functional status and prognosis.

Biochemical screening

- Serum urea and electrolytes. The syndrome of inappropriate anti-diuretic hormone (ADH) (where increased antidiuretic hormone is produced) may occur in association with GBS resulting in hyponatraemia, low plasma osmolality and high urine osmolality.
- Liver function. This is impaired in one third of patients.
- Clotting screen. To rule out abnormal clotting prior to plasmapheresis.
- Antiganglioside antibody. The presence of anti-GM1 antibodies is associated with a poor prognosis.
- Creatinine phosphokinase (CPK) and erythrocyte sedimentation rate (ESR) may be elevated with myopathies or systemic inflammatory conditions.

Lumbar puncture and CSF analysis may show elevated or rising protein levels on serial lumbar punctures. Less than 10 mononuclear cells/mm^3 strongly supports the diagnosis.

Muscle biopsy may help to distinguish GBS from a primary myopathy in unclear cases.

Many different abnormalities may be seen on the ECG, including second-degree and third-degree atrioventricular (AV) block, T-wave abnormalities, ST depression, QRS widening, and a variety of rhythm disturbances.

Most patients (up to 85%) with GBS achieve a full and functional recovery within 6-12 months. Patients may have persistent weakness, areflexia, imbalance, or sensory loss. Some patients may have permanent neurologic sequelae including bilateral foot drop, intrinsic hand muscle wasting, sensory ataxia, and dysaesthesia. The mortality rate is approximately 10%, usually from complications such as cardiac arrest secondary to autonomic dysfunction, sepsis, pulmonary embolism and respiratory infection.

Key points

◆ Guillain-Barre syndrome is characterised by symmetric limb weakness, and begins as proximal muscle weakness of lower limbs.
◆ Improved intensive care management involving a multidisciplinary team approach along with supportive ventilator therapy has reduced the morbidity and mortality associated with Guillain-Barre syndrome.
◆ Intravenous immunoglobulin and plasma exchange are effective in reducing the progression of the disease.
◆ There is insufficient evidence for the benefit of corticosteroids.

Further reading

1. Miller A. Guillain-Barre syndrome. http://www.emedicine.com/ EMERG/topic222.htm.
2. Richards JCK, Cohen AT. Guillain-Barre syndrome. *British Journal of Anaesthesia CEACCP* 2003; 3: 46-9.
3. Winer JB. Treatment of Guillain-Barre syndrome. *Q J Med* 2002: 95: 717-21.

Short case 5.3: Dental anaesthesia

A 6-year-old child presents for extraction of multiple teeth.

How would you anaesthetise this child?

This child needs pre-operative assessment which will include a full history and clinical examination. A detailed history should be elicited from the parents about the child's general health, any previous anaesthetics, current medications/allergies and family history of any anaesthetic problems. The child should be starved, 2 hours for clear liquids and 6 hours for solids and milk. The possible need for any premedication and the anaesthetic induction plan should be established during the pre-operative visit. If the child is unco-operative, oral midazolam 0.5mg/kg about 30 minutes before the induction can be used.

A topical local anaesthetic such as a eutectic mixture of local anaesthetic (EMLA) or Ametop (tetracaine 4% gel) can be used to provide painless intravenous cannulation.

What are the specific problems associated with giving an anaesthetic to this child for dental surgery?

Pre-operative

The child may be emotionally upset because of the hospital environment and may not be co-operative.

Induction

If the child is unco-operative during induction, monitoring and pre-oxygenation may not be possible. Intravenous access can be difficult and inhalational induction may be required. Due to lack of preoxygenation, a reduced FRC and high metabolic rate, the child can rapidly desaturate.

Anaesthetic equipment

Breathing systems and airway devices are different to those used in adults. Drug dosages should be carefully calculated according to body weight.

Intra-operative

With a shared airway during the surgical procedure it is important that an adequate airway is maintained and is protected from blood, secretions and tooth debris. The surgeon should have good access to the mouth. A shared airway requires close co-operation and communication between the surgeon and anaesthetist.

There can be local anaesthetic toxicity due to intravascular injection of local anaesthetic and epinephrine. Lidocaine 2% with epinephrine 1:80,000 concentration is commonly used in dental practice. Each ml of local anaesthetic solution contains 20mg of lidocaine and 12.5µg of epinephrine.

Cardiac arrhythmias

Stimulation of the trigeminal nerve during teeth extraction is an important cause of cardiac arrhythmias, and can be prevented by prior infiltration of local anaesthetic. Anaesthetic factors such as hypoxia, hypercarbia and volatile anaesthetic agents, particularly halothane, can contribute to cardiac arrhythmias.

Recovery and extubation

Again, as with induction, appropriate monitoring and oxygen administration are difficult. Children are more likely to suffer airway complications such as laryngeal oedema and laryngospasm.

How would you induce anaesthesia in this child?

Following pre-operative assessment and checking of all equipment, the choice of induction is either inhalational or intravenous depending on the co-operation of the child. Monitoring includes pulse oximetry, ECG, blood pressure and $ETCO_2$. Sevoflurane, due to its non-irritant property and pleasant smell offers a smooth inhalational induction.

After induction and venous access, the airway is secured using a flexible (armoured) LMA. It is important to discuss the airway management plan with the surgeon.

The advantages of an LMA include ease of placement, avoidance of muscle relaxant and better tolerance in spontaneously breathing patients, leading to a smooth recovery.

The disadvantages include the LMA tube in the oral cavity interfering with surgical access, aspiration of gastric contents and the possibility of dislodgement while inserting and changing the side of the bite block.

The advantages of endotracheal intubation include good airway maintenance, a clear operative field and reduced risk of aspiration.

What are the problems in the immediate postoperative period?

Postoperative problems include pain, postoperative nausea and vomiting, prolonged recovery and laryngospasm. Swallowed blood and nitrous oxide may be contributing factors for postoperative nausea and vomiting.

Are you aware of any recommendations which will help you in planning the anaesthetic management for dental surgery?

The Poswillo report, published in 1990, was compiled by an expert working party on the subject of general anaesthesia, sedation and resuscitation in dentistry. It recommends avoidance of general anaesthesia wherever possible and the use of uniform standards of monitoring and personnel necessary for patient safety. General anaesthesia is safer when administered in hospital rather than the dental surgery.

The General Dental Council in consultation with The Royal College of Anaesthetists published guidance in 1998. Dental surgeons were made professionally responsible for giving a clear explanation of risks involved in general anaesthesia and to suggest alternative methods of pain relief and sedation.

The Royal College of Anaesthetists Standards and Guidelines for General Anaesthesia for Dentistry, published in 1999, defined the situations where general anaesthesia would be indicated.

"Standards for Conscious Sedation in Dentistry: Alternative Techniques", a report from the Standing Committee for Sedation in Dentistry, published in 2007, defines the components of conscious sedation, premises where it can be administered, the team involved in providing the service, patient selection, and qualification and training requirements for the practitioner.

What are the indications for general anaesthesia for dental treatment?

◆ Patients who, because of problems related to age, immaturity or physical/mental disability, are unlikely to allow completion of treatment under local anaesthesia, e.g. children and patients with a learning disability and mental handicap.

◆ A clinical situation where it is not possible to achieve adequate local anaesthesia, e.g. acute infection, allergy to local anaesthesia and failure of local anaesthesia.

◆ Patients in whom a long-term phobia may lead to reactions when awake, e.g. persistent fainting.

What alternative techniques to general anaesthesia are available?

◆ Local anaesthesia.
◆ Local anaesthesia with conscious sedation.
◆ Nitrous oxide and intravenous midazolam.
◆ Oral/transmucosal benzodiazepine.

What is conscious sedation?

It is defined as a technique in which the use of a drug or drugs produces a state of depression of the central nervous system enabling treatment to be carried out, but during which verbal contact with the patient is maintained throughout the duration of sedation.

The standard techniques of providing conscious sedation include:

◆ Inhalational sedation using nitrous oxide.
◆ Intravenous sedation using midazolam alone.
◆ Oral/transmucosal benzodiazepine.

Alternative techniques of conscious sedation include:

◆ Benzodiazepine plus any other intravenous agent with sedative effects (opioid, propofol, ketamine).

- Propofol alone or with any other agent (benzodiazepine, opioid, ketamine).
- Inhalation sedation agents other than nitrous oxide/oxygen alone.
- Combination of routes (intravenous plus inhalational agent).

Chair dental anaesthesia

Chair dental anaesthesia has been practised in general dental practice, community dental clinics, dental hospitals and in hospital outpatient departments, often in locations away from the main theatre complex. It should be limited to patients of ASA categories I and II in a hospital setting. The semi-reclining position referred to as the sitting position is usually used. The main disadvantage of this position is that venous pooling and reduced venous return from lower limbs reduces cardiac output and may cause cerebral hypoperfusion. Debris passing into the oropharynx can cause aspiration and laryngospasm. The benefits include the reduction of passive regurgitation of stomach contents due to the effect of gravity. In a spontaneously breathing patient, respiratory mechanics are better maintained in the sitting position.

Nitrous oxide anaesthesia has been very popular for dental chair anaesthesia. Occupational exposure to nitrous oxide in dental practice can exceed the recommended limits of 100 ppm. Active scavenging and adequate ventilation is essential to minimise the exposure to N_2O. Halothane is associated with a high incidence of ventricular arrhythmias (>30% incidence). Isoflurane is associated with an unexpectedly high incidence of coughing and laryngospasm. Sevoflurane is a suitable alternative to halothane as it has no association with ventricular arrhythmias.

The majority of patients attending for chair dental anaesthesia are children, and anaesthesia is more commonly induced by inhalational route if they are very young. Intravenous induction with propofol is suitable for older children.

During recent years the number of general anaesthetics in dental practices has dramatically decreased and the number of local anaesthetics has increased. More recently, sedation techniques involving sevoflurane and propofol, along with supplementation with fentanyl, have been used.

Key points

♦ The anaesthetic management of a child for teeth extraction involves a detailed pre-operative assessment and preparation.

♦ The shared airway is an important intra-operative consideration with close attention to airway maintenance and airway protection.

♦ The sitting position is a potential cause for morbidity and mortality in chair dental anaesthesia.

♦ The General Dental Council in consultation with The Royal College of Anaesthetists have published guidance for improving safety in dental anaesthesia.

Further reading

1. Standards for conscious sedation in dentistry: alternative techniques. A report from the Standing Committee on Sedation for Dentistry, 2007. http://www.rcseng.ac.uk/fds/docs/SCSDAT%202 007.pdf.

2. Blayney MR, Malins AF. Chair dental anaesthesia. *CPD Anaesthesia* 2001; 3: 91-6.

Applied anatomy 5.1: Phrenic nerve

A 50-year-old male patient and driver of a car is admitted to the emergency department following a road traffic accident. He is conscious but complains of pain over the neck, and shortness of breath. He is maintaining his airway and breathing at a rate of 18 breaths per minute. The following is the chest X-ray taken on admission.

What is the most obvious finding on the chest X-ray overleaf?

The dome of the right diaphragm is elevated; this may be either due to diaphragmatic rupture or right phrenic nerve injury.

How would you confirm this?

♦ Fluoroscopy. Paradoxical upward movement on inspiration suggests diaphragmatic paralysis.

♦ Ultrasound of chest: intact but paralysed diaphragm.

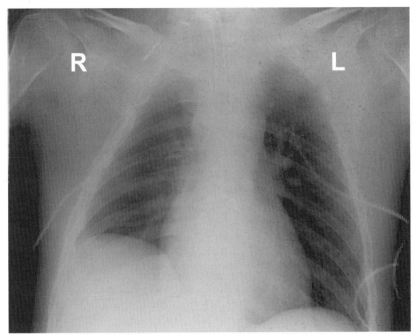

Figure 5.5 Chest X-ray.

♦ CT and MRI scan are useful in distinguishing between diaphragmatic paralysis and diaphragmatic rupture.

Can you list some other causes for paralysis of the diaphragm?

♦ Spinal cord: poliomyelitis, syringomyelia.
♦ Direct injury to phrenic nerve: penetrating injury to neck and thorax, surgery around the neck, thoracic surgery, radiation and tumour.
♦ Iatrogenic: interscalene brachial plexus block, cervical plexus block and internal jugular vein cannulation.
♦ Neurological disorder: multiple sclerosis, Guillain-Barre syndrome, phrenic nerve neuropathy and idiopathic.

Describe the anatomy of the phrenic nerve

The phrenic nerve is the motor nerve of the diaphragm, derived mainly from the anterior ramus of C4 with contributions from C3 and C5. It contains motor and sensory fibres, and carries proprioception from the central diaphragm, pleura and pericardium.

In the neck

It descends to the root of the neck, running obliquely across the front of the scalenus anterior, and beneath the sternocleidomastoid and the inferior belly of the omohyoid muscles.

At thoracic inlet

It passes in front of the first part of the subclavian artery, then between it and the subclavian vein, and as it enters the thorax it crosses the internal mammary artery near its origin.

Within the thorax

It descends nearly vertically in front of the root of the lung, and then between the pericardium and the mediastinal pleura, to the diaphragm. It then divides into branches which pierce the muscle, and are distributed to its under surface. The relations of the phrenic nerve differ on each side.

On the right the phrenic nerve has a short and more vertical course, descending on the lateral side of the right brachiocephalic vein, superior vena cava and right atrium. It pierces the central tendon of the diaphragm, just lateral to the inferior vena-caval opening.

On the left it has a longer course, passing down between the left subclavian artery and left common carotid artery, crossing the aortic arch (anterior to vagus nerve), descending anterior to the lung root, and then along the left ventricle. It pierces the dome of the diaphragm about 1cm lateral to the attachment of the fibrous pericardium.

Describe the anatomy of the diaphragm

The diaphragm is the musculotendinous partition separating the thorax from the abdomen and is a principal muscle of respiration.

It has a central tendinous part and a peripheral muscular component. The peripheral component can be divided into three parts:

- The vertebral part arises from the upper lumbar vertebrae from two crura and from the lateral and medial arcuate ligaments. The right crus arises from the bodies of the upper three lumbar vertebrae (L1-L3) and the left crus from the first two lumbar vertebrae (L1-L2). The median ligament links the right and left crurae. The medial arcuate ligament is the thickened upper edge of the psoas fascia. The lateral arcuate ligament is the thickening of quadratus lumborum fascia.
- The costal part arises from the inner surface of the six lowest ribs and their costal cartilages.
- The sternal part arises from the back of the xiphisternum.

The central tendinous part is the tough aponeurosis near the centre of the dome, merging with the connective tissue of the pericardium.

What are the various openings in the diaphragm?

There are three openings:

- The caval opening at the level of the 8th thoracic vertebra; this transmits the inferior vena cava and the right phrenic nerve.
- The oesophageal opening at the level of the 10th thoracic vertebra; this transmits the oesophagus, the gastric branches of the vagus nerves and gastric vessels.
- The aortic opening at the level of the 12th thoracic vertebra; this transmits the aorta, the thoracic duct and the azygos vein.

What is the nerve supply of the diaphragm?

The motor supply arises from the phrenic nerve. The sensory supply for the central part comes from the phrenic nerve (sub-diaphragmatic pain is referred to the shoulder tip which shares sensory innervations of C5). The peripheral area receives sensory innervation from the lower intercostal nerves.

The diaphragm

The diaphragm is the principal muscle of respiration. Superiorly, the base of the lung within the pleural sac and heart within the pericardial sac lie on the upper surface of the diaphragm. Inferiorly, on the right side lie the liver, the right kidney and the suprarenal gland; on the left side lie the left lobe of the liver, gastric fundus, spleen, left kidney and suprarenal gland.

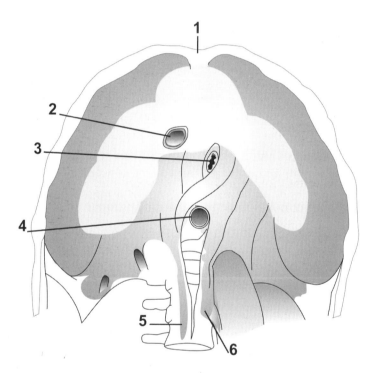

Figure 5.6 Inferior surface of the diaphragm.
1. Xiphoid process; 2. Inferior vena cava; 3. Oesophagus; 4. Aorta; 5. Right crus of diaphragm; 6. Left crus of diaphragm.

During quiet respiration the diaphragm is mainly involved, and inspiration is assisted by the weight of the liver attached to the under surface of the diaphragm.

During inspiration the diaphragm contracts, descends downwards and increases the vertical diameter of the thoracic cavity. The elevation of the 3rd, 4th, 5th and 6th ribs leads to an increase in the anteroposterior and transverse diameters of the thorax. The elevation of the 8th, 9th, and 10th ribs is accompanied by a lateral and backward movement, leading to an increase in the transverse diameter of the upper part of the abdomen. Deep inspiration is assisted by the scalene muscles, sternocleidomastoid, trapezius, serratus anterior, pectoralis, and latissimus dorsi, producing a greater increase in the anteroposterior and vertical diameter of the thorax.

Expiration is produced by the relaxation of the diaphragm and elastic recoil of the lungs. During forced expiration the abdominal muscles contract and force the diaphragm upwards.

Spinal cord injury at the level of C2 and C3 causes respiratory tetraplegia. If the injury is at C4 and below, some phrenic nerve function is preserved. If it is below the level of C6, the diaphragmatic function is fully preserved. The diaphragm contributes to 75% of respiratory function during quiet breathing.

The position of the diaphragm in the thorax depends upon three main factors:

- The elastic retraction of the lung tissue, tending to pull it upward.
- The pressure exerted on its under surface by the viscera, which depends on the position of the patient; in the erect posture it is displaced downwards, and displaced upwards while lying down.
- The intra-abdominal tension due to the abdominal muscles.

Normally the right dome of the diaphragm is higher than the left due to the pressure exerted by the liver. During quiet respiration the diaphragm moves only about 1.5cm but during deep inspiration this can be increased to nearly 10cm. During deep inspiration, in a chest X ray, the diaphragm lies at the level of the 6th rib anteriorly and at the level of the 10th rib posteriorly.

With a hiatus hernia, the weakness of the oesophageal hiatus may allow upward sliding of the lower oesophagus and stomach into the chest interfering with the normal anti-reflux mechanism. The diagnosis can be confirmed by endoscopy and barium meal.

Key points

- The phrenic nerve is derived mainly from the anterior ramus of C4 with contribution from C3 and C5.
- The diaphragm is the principal muscle of respiration; it has a central tendinous part and a peripheral muscular part.
- The diaphragm has three openings at the level of the 8th, 10th and 12th vertebrae transmitting the inferior vena cava, oesophagus and aorta, respectively.

Further reading

1. Diaphragm and phrenic nerve. In: *Gray's anatomy,* 39th ed. Standring S, Ed. London: Elsevier Churchill Livingstone, 2005; Chapter 64: 1081-6.
2. Ellis H, Feldman S, Harrop-Griffiths W. *Anatomy for anaesthetists,* 8th ed. Oxford: Blackwell Science Ltd, 2004.

Applied physiology 5.2: Pre-eclampsia

A 32-year-old, previously well primigravida presents to the antenatal clinic at 26 weeks of gestation with lethargy and upper abdominal discomfort. On clinical examination she weighs 78kg and her height is 164cm. Her blood pressure is 155/95mm Hg, and she has bilateral oedema of the ankles. Urine dipstick shows protein of 2+.

What is the most likely diagnosis?

Pre-eclampsia is the most likely diagnosis, although this should be confirmed by further blood pressure measurement and by measuring the 24-hour protein excretion in the urine.

What is pre-eclampsia?

It is a multi-organ disease developing after the 20th week of gestation. The main features are hypertension and proteinuria. Hypertension is defined as a sustained systolic blood pressure ≥140mm Hg or a diastolic blood pressure ≥90 mm Hg. Proteinuria is defined as ≥300mg of protein in a 24-hour urine sample or two specimens of urine collected ≥4 hours apart with ≥2+ on the protein reagent strip.

The plasma uric acid is elevated in women with pre-eclampsia. A concentration of more than 360μmol/L is associated with pre-eclampsia.

Oedema is not essential for the diagnosis.

What is the cause of pre-eclampsia?

The precise cause is unknown. A genetic predisposition is likely and an autoimmune reaction against the placenta may be involved. It occurs in 2-3% of all pregnancies, with most cases occurring in the first pregnancy.

The other risk factors include:

◆ History of pre-eclampsia. A personal or family history of pre-eclampsia increases the risk of it developing.
◆ Age. The risk of pre-eclampsia is higher in pregnant women who are older than 35.
◆ Obesity. The risk of pre-eclampsia is greater.
◆ Multiple pregnancies. Pre-eclampsia is more common in women who are pregnant with twins, triplets or other multiples.
◆ Gestational diabetes. Women who develop gestational diabetes have a higher risk of developing pre-eclampsia as the pregnancy progresses.
◆ Pre-existing hypertension. Pre-existing high blood pressure, diabetes, kidney disease or lupus increases the risk.

Can you explain the pathophysiology of pre-eclampsia?

It is a disease caused by the feto-placental unit, affecting virtually all maternal organ systems. The common pathological features include endothelial damage and dysfunction of the vascular system in the placenta, kidneys and brain.

In normal pregnancy, the endothelium, the internal elastic lamina and the muscular layer of the spiral arteries are invaded by trophoblasts. This transforms the high resistance arterial system into a low resistance high volume system which meets the needs of the foetus and placenta. Endogenous vasodilators such as prostaglandin I_2 (PGI_2) and nitric oxide predominate.

In pre-eclampsia there is failure or incomplete trophoblastic invasion of spiral arteries resulting in narrowing of the arteries and a high resistance vascular bed. This leads to placental ischaemia. Due to the abnormal endothelium, there is increased permeability. Endogenous vasoconstrictors (thromboxane A_2) predominate, resulting in platelet aggregation, activation of the coagulation cascade and fibrin deposition in the blood vessels. The normal function of the endothelium, including its role in the maintenance of the fluid compartment, prevention of intravascular coagulation, vasodilator response and maintenance of inflammatory response, is altered.

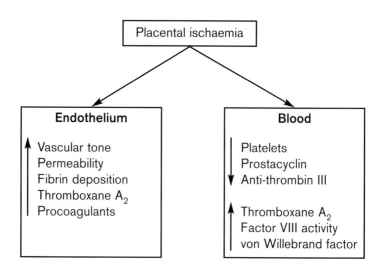

Figure 5.7 Major initiating changes in the placenta and vascular bed.

Multi-system changes

Pathophysiological changes involve most of the body's systems, resulting in multi-organ dysfunction.

Respiratory system

◆ Pulmonary oedema occurs in about 3% of patients with pre-eclampsia and eclampsia due to reduced colloid oncotic pressure and increased capillary permeability.
◆ Oedema may also affect the pharynx and larynx.

Cardiovascular system

◆ Systemic vascular resistance (SVR) is increased.
◆ Sympathetic activity is increased.
◆ Increased response to circulating catecholamines and angiotensin II.
◆ Blood pressure is increased.
◆ Blood volume/plasma volume is reduced resulting in haemoconcentration.
◆ Cardiac output is decreased.
◆ Poor correlation between CVP and PCWP.
◆ Decreased colloid oncotic pressure and leaky vasculature resulting in pulmonary oedema.

Haematological system

◆ Platelet activation, increased platelet consumption and low grade DIC.
◆ Thrombocytopenia occurs in 15-30%.
◆ Reduced platelet function.
◆ Reduced anti-thrombin III.

Renal system

◆ Glomerular filtration rate (GFR) is reduced due to renal ischaemia.
◆ Proteinuria due to increased permeability.
◆ Urate clearance is reduced causing an increase in serum uric acid levels.
◆ Renal clearance is reduced.

Hepatic system

♦ Fibrin deposition in hepatic sinusoids.
♦ Subcapsular haemorrhage.
♦ Periportal necrosis.
♦ Reduced drug metabolism.
♦ Spontaneous liver rupture (rare but fatal).

Nervous system

♦ Vasospasm, cerebral ischaemia and cerebral oedema.
♦ Hypertensive encephalopathy with an increased risk of intracranial haemorrhage.
♦ Visual disturbances in the form of photophobia, diplopia and blurred vision mostly due to ischaemia of the posterior cerebral arteries or oedema of the occipital cortex.

Foetus

♦ Reduced uteroplacental perfusion leads to a high incidence of intra-uterine growth retardation, small for date infants and perinatal mortality. Placental abruption is more common in mothers with pre-eclampsia.

What is severe pre-eclampsia?

Severe pre-eclampsia is defined as one of the following occurring after the 20th week of gestation:

♦ Severe hypertension with systolic blood pressure >160mmHg or diastolic blood pressure >110mm Hg.
♦ Proteinuria >5g per 24 hours.
♦ Oliguria <400ml per 24 hours.
♦ Cerebral irritability with headache, visual disturbance.
♦ Epigastric or right upper quadrant pain.
♦ Pulmonary oedema.

In this section of applied physiology, the pathophysiology of pre-eclampsia is discussed. This topic can, however, be discussed as a short case and also in an applied pharmacology section with relevance to drug therapy in pre-eclampsia and eclampsia.

HELLP syndrome

This is an acronym for Haemolysis, Elevated Liver enzymes and Low Platelets. It is associated with DIC and placental abruption and may progress to multi-organ failure. It involves a combination of hepatic ischaemia with peri-portal haemorrhage and necrosis, haemolytic anaemia and thrombocytopaenia. It occurs in severe pre-eclampsia and may occasionally present in the absence of hypertension and proteinuria. The main clinical features include abdominal pain with nausea and vomiting. As well as DIC the complications of HELLP syndrome include renal failure, pulmonary oedema, pleural effusion and respiratory distress.

Management of pre-eclampsia

The management plan of pre-eclampsia includes early diagnosis, control of blood pressure, timely delivery of the foetus and prevention of eclampsia and other complications. Fluid management should be guided by urine output and central venous pressure. Patients with pre-eclampsia are usually volume depleted but they also have a tendency to develop pulmonary oedema. The aim of fluid therapy is to maintain urine output >0.5ml/kg/hour.

Epidural analgesia is the preferred choice for labour as it offers beneficial effects in controlling blood pressure and improving placental perfusion. Regional anaesthesia is contraindicated if the platelet count is less than 50 x 10^{12}/L. It is safe to perform regional anaesthesia if the platelet count is greater than 100 x10^{12}/L, but if the platelet count is between 50 x 10^{12}/L and 100 x10^{12}/L, regional anaesthesia can be considered if the remaining coagulation parameters are normal.

Problems relating to general anaesthesia include an increased risk of difficult intubation, and cardiovascular instability associated with intravenous induction agents, laryngoscopy and tracheal intubation. Facial oedema, tongue oedema and voice changes are warning signs of airway oedema. Pre-operatively, the upper airway can be assessed using fibreoptic nasendoscopy.

During the postpartum period pre-eclampsia may worsen. In some cases it is only diagnosed after delivery. The management of pre-eclampsia should therefore be continued after delivery.

Drugs used in the management of pre-eclampsia include labetolol, methyldopa, nifedipine, hydralazine and magnesium sulphate.

Magnesium sulphate is effective in reducing the progression of pre-eclampsia to eclampsia. The main mechanism by which magnesium works is by antagonism of calcium. Magnesium reduces calcium transport into the cell by inhibiting calcium transport via the voltage-gated N-methyl-D-aspartate (NMDA) channel. It is a direct vasodilator and decreases the catecholamine release from the adrenal medulla and adrenergic neurones. It also acts as an anti-arrhythmic by reducing SA and AV nodal conduction. At the neuromuscular junction it reduces the membrane excitability by reducing pre-synaptic acetylcholine release and also by decreasing the sensitivity of the postsynaptic membrane. It depresses the central nervous system and acts as an anticonvulsant.

It is administered as a loading dose of 4g over 10-15 minutes followed by an infusion of 1-2g/hour.

(Refer to SOE1: Long case 1 for the side effects of magnesium therapy.)

Key points

- Pre-eclampsia is a multi-organ disease characterised by hypertension and proteinuria.
- The important pathological feature is failure of the trophoblastic invasion of spiral arteries.
- Magnesium sulphate is effective in preventing the progression of pre-eclampsia to eclampsia.

Further reading

1. Mushambi MC, Halligan AW, Wiiliamson K. Recent developments in the pathophysiology and management of pre-eclampsia. *British Journal of Anaesthesia* 1996; 76: 133-48.
2. Hart E, Coley S. The diagnosis and management of pre-eclampsia. *British Journal of Anaesthesia CEACCP* 2003; 3: 38-42.
3. The Magpie trial collaboration group. Do women with pre-eclampsia, and their babies, benefit from magnesium sulphate? The Magpie trial: a randomised placebo-controlled trial. *Lancet* 2002; 359: 1877-90

Applied pharmacology 5.3: Remifentanil

Can you name some drugs in addition to IV induction agents and muscle relaxants that are used to obtund the cardiovascular response to laryngoscopy?

The drugs that can be used for reducing cardiovascular response to laryngoscopy include:

- Opioids with a short duration of action: alfentanil 30µg/kg, fentanyl 3µg/kg and remifentanil in a bolus dose of 0.5µg/kg over 60 seconds.
- Local anaesthetics: lidocaine 1.5mg/kg.
- Beta-blockers: esmolol at a dose of 0.5mg/kg.

Describe the pharmacology of remifentanil

Remifentanil is a potent ultra-short-acting opioid. It is a mu-opioid agonist and a piperidine ester that is susceptible to rapid hydrolysis by red cell and tissue esterases. The metabolism of remifentanil is not affected by plasma cholinesterase or concomitant administration of anticholinesterase drugs. It is available as 1mg, 2mg and 5mg lyophilized powder in 3, 5 and 10ml vials, respectively, to be diluted prior to use to a concentration of 20-250µg/ml.

During general anaesthesia it is used as an infusion at a dose of 0.02-2.0µg/kg/minute following a loading dose of 0.5-1µg/kg administered over 60-90 seconds. Recently, a target controlled infusion programme has been introduced, and adequate analgesia for surgery has generally been achieved with target blood remifentanil concentrations in the range of 3-8ng/ml. A target concentration of up to 15ng/ml has been used for more stimulating surgery.

Pharmacokinetics

Remifentanil is extremely fat-soluble with a steady state volume of distribution of 30 litres. Its terminal half-life is less than 10 minutes. However, the context sensitive half-life is 3-5 minutes, irrespective of the duration of infusion. Since its action is terminated by rapid metabolism rather than redistribution, it has an extremely rapid clearance of around 3L/minute.

It is metabolised by non-specific esterases to an acid metabolite (carboxylic acid) and by N-dealkylation to a second metabolite. Carboxylic acid is the main metabolite; it is also a mu opioid agonist but has only 0.02% activity of the parent compound. The PKa of remifentanil is 7.1; it is 80% ionised compared with fentanyl which is only 9% ionised.

Pharmacodynamics

It produces analgesia, due to its action on mu-receptors.

Respiratory system

It produces chest wall rigidity and dose-dependent respiratory depression. It depresses the hypoxic drive as well as ventilator response to carbon dioxide.

Cardiovascular system

It produces a dose-dependent decrease in heart rate, blood pressure and cardiac output. It decreases blood pressure by about 30% when combined with a propofol infusion. As with fentanyl, it exerts central vagotonic action. These effects may be marked in patients on beta-blockers.

Central nervous system

It reduces global CBF and ICP but preserves cerebral auto regulation.

What are the pharmacokinetic implications in elderly patients?

They have a reduced volume of distribution, resulting in a higher initial concentration. They have increased sensitivity and reduced clearance. Therefore, both the bolus dose and rate of infusion should be reduced by approximately 50%.

What is context sensitive half time?

It is the time taken for the effect site concentration to decrease by 50% after the end of an infusion of varying duration. The 'context' refers to the duration of the infusion. After prolonged infusion remifentanil does not accumulate.

What are the advantages of remifentanil in clinical practice?

♦ Rapid titration for various levels of surgical stimulation to provide analgesia.
♦ It can be used to induce controlled hypotension when indicated, to produce a relatively bloodless operating field for microscopic surgery, e.g. middle ear surgery and neurosurgical procedures.
♦ Does not require dose reduction in renal/hepatic disease.
♦ Predictable recovery on cessation of infusion due to rapid metabolism.
♦ Reduces MAC of volatile agents.

What are the disadvantages of remifentanil in clinical practice?

♦ Does not provide any postoperative analgesia. Postoperative analgesia should be provided either in the form of long-acting opioids or appropriate regional analgesia.
♦ Cannot be used as a sole agent for anaesthesia.
♦ Dedicated intravenous access is necessary, and the intravenous line should be flushed after stopping the infusion to prevent a bolus effect.

What are the side effects of remifentanil?

- Dose-dependent bradycardia.
- Skeletal muscle rigidity.
- Respiratory depression.
- Pruritus.
- Dizziness.
- Nausea.

Clinical uses of remifentanil

Remifentanil has been used in neurosurgery, and head and neck surgery, as sedation during local anaesthesia and as a sedative and analgesic agent in intensive care.

Induction and airway control

Remifentanil reduces the haemodynamic response to tracheal intubation when used alongside neuromuscular blocking agents. Tracheal intubation can be performed without using a neuromuscular blocking agent when remifentanil is used alongside propofol. A target concentration 8-10ng/mL is recommended to produce satisfactory intubation.

Head and neck surgery

In middle ear surgery remifentanil has been used to induce modest hypotension to facilitate microscopic surgery. It also facilitates the use of positive pressure ventilation without further doses of muscle relaxants, which enables the surgeon to use a nerve stimulator to identify the facial nerve. In microlaryngeal surgery it suppresses the cardiovascular response to laryngeal surgery and enables the early return of airway reflexes with a predictable recovery.

Neurosurgery

In neurosurgery the use of remifentanil facilitates rapid recovery and neurological assessment in the early postoperative period. During the intra-operative period, the dose can be titrated to the variable intensity of painful stimuli.

Cardiac surgery

Remifentanil suppresses the intra-operative stress response and enables a rapid recovery, provided appropriate methods of pain relief are used for postoperative analgesia. During hypothermic cardiopulmonary bypass, the volume of distribution increases, but the rate of elimination decreases due to hypothermia.

Intensive care

In neurosurgical intensive care, rapid and predictable awakening after discontinuing an infusion allows neurosurgical assessment, thus allowing a clear differentiation between brain dysfunction and over-sedation.

Since remifentanil is metabolised organ-independently by non-specific esterases, it can be used as a sedative in intensive care patients with organ dysfunction especially in the presence of renal and hepatic impairment.

Bariatric surgery

Remifentanil has a small volume of distribution which does not increase much in obese patients. Rapid recovery is essential for obese patients, particularly in patients with obstructive sleep apnoea.

Other uses

Remifentanil is used for sedation during awake fibreoptic intubation. It has also been used as PCA for labour analgesia.

Key points

- Remifentanil is a potent ultra-short-acting opioid.
- Remifentanil has a constant context sensitive half-life of 3-5 minutes, irrespective of the duration of infusion.
- Remifentanil has a predictable onset and offset of effect due to its unique pharmacokinetics.

Further reading

1. Wilhelm W, Kreuer S. The place of short-acting opioids: special emphasis on remifentanil. *Crit Care* 2008; 12 (suppl 3): S5.
2. Kindler CH, Schumacher PG, Schneider MC, Urwyler A. Effects of intravenous lidocaine and/or esmolol on hemodynamic responses to laryngoscopy and intubation: a double-blind, controlled clinical trial. *J Clinical Anaesth* 1996; 8: 491-6.
3. Servin FS, Billard V. Remifentanil and other opioids. *Handbook of experimental pharmacology* 2008; 283-11.

Equipment, clinical measurement and monitoring 5.4: Monitoring the depth of anaesthesia

A 50-year-old female patient presents for a laparoscopic cholecystectomy. During the pre-operative visit you discover that she is very worried because she experienced awareness during a Caesarean section about 30 years ago.

What measures would you take to prevent awareness?

Maintaining adequate depth of anaesthesia throughout the surgical procedure and monitoring depth of anaesthesia can reduce the risk of awareness.

How would you monitor depth of anaesthesia?

Depth of anaesthesia can be monitored by:

- Clinical signs.
- Clinical experience.
- Lower oesophageal contractility.
- Isolated forearm technique.
- Frontalis electromyogram.
- Monitoring electroencephalogram (EEG) with various techniques such as evoked potentials, compressed spectral array and bispectral analysis.

Clinical signs such as blood pressure, heart rate, sweating and tears (PRST) do not correlate accurately with the depth of anaesthesia. The signs of sympathetic stimulation can be altered by other drugs including remifentanil and beta-blockers administered during the peri-operative period.

Clinical experience is very important, but MAC values for volatile agents do not relate accurately with the depth of anaesthesia. There is also individual variation in the dose of anaesthetic required. The effect produced by an intravenous drug depends on the concentration delivered to the central nervous system rather than the dose administered.

Lower oesophageal contractility is controlled by the autonomic nervous system. With increasing depth the frequency and amplitude of the lower oesophageal contractions decrease but there is a wide variability between patients.

The frontalis muscle is innervated by visceral efferent fibres of the facial nerve. The electromyogram shows decreasing activity with increasing depth of anaesthesia. There is variation between patients, and the technique cannot be used in paralysed patients.

The isolated forearm allows the patient to move the arm on command but it is limited by the duration of time an arterial tourniquet is applied.

What is the role of EEG as a monitor of the depth of anaesthesia?

The four commonly recognised bands in EEG include α (8-13Hz), β (>13Hz), δ (<4Hz) and θ (4-7Hz). With increasing depth of anaesthesia there is a decrease in the fast activity and progressive increase in amplitude of the EEG signal with some intravenous agents causing burst suppression. Burst suppression is characterised by alternate periods of normal to high amplitude activity changing to low amplitude or even isoelectricity, rendering the EEG inactive in appearance. The burst suppression ratio represents the proportion of isoelectric EEG signal in an epoch. The EEG waveform can be analysed either using the time domain method where voltage changes over time are examined or the frequency domain method where frequency changes over time are examined.

There are several practical problems using an unprocessed EEG in clinical practice. A large quantity of data obtained from EEG is too complex to interpret. The precise pattern of the EEG varies with the anaesthetic agent. The EEG is affected by various pathophysiological events such as hypoxia, hypotension and hypercarbia. The electrical equipment used in the operating theatre also interferes with EEG recording.

What are the various modifications to the EEG that have been used to monitor depth of anaesthesia?

The information contained in the EEG can be condensed and simplified using fast Fourier transformation in its component sine waves. The processed EEG can be further analysed with respect to three features:

◆ Frequency distribution.
◆ Power contained in different frequencies.
◆ Phase relationship between waves of different frequencies.

Compressed spectral array is a three-dimensional picture with amplitude on the y-axis, frequency on the x-axis and time on the z-axis. To do this several segments of EEG activity are recorded and the 'power' contained within different frequencies (α, β, δ and θ) is calculated.

As the depth of anaesthesia increases, the 'power' shifts to the lower frequencies and, hence, becomes a guide to assessment of the degree of cerebral suppression. From the power spectrum the median and 95th percentile (spectral edge) frequencies can be derived. However, some studies do not find any correlation between spectral edge frequency and depth of anaesthesia.

The median frequency claims to be a more reliable indicator of depth of anaesthesia, and has been used to provide a closed loop feedback control during total intravenous anaesthesia.

The disadvantage of power spectral analysis is that it ignores the phase information contained in the EEG.

What are evoked potentials?

Evoked potentials are the responses to auditory, somatosensory and visual stimuli. The auditory evoked potential (AEP) is the EEG response to a sound stimulus. The waveform consists of a series of positive and negative waves, representing the passage of electrical activity from the cochlea to the brain stem, the primary auditory cortex and the frontal cortex.

The waveform of the AEP can be divided into three parts depending on the latency of response in relation to the timing of the stimulus. The waves originating from the brain stem appear at 1-10ms, early cortical or mid-latency waves (10-100ms) and late cortical waves (>100ms).

The changes in the mid-latency auditory evoked potentials (Pa and Nb waves) reflect the hypnotic component of anaesthesia. With increasing depth of anaesthesia there is a progressive increase in the latency, and a reduction in the amplitude of the mid-latency auditory evoked potentials.

The somatosensory evoked potentials can be recorded by stimulating any peripheral nerve. The median and ulnar nerves have been frequently studied. A constant current stimulation is applied to the median nerves through a pair of electrodes to produce fine touch stimulation. The recording electrodes can be placed above the seventh cervical vertebra to record responses from the dorsal column, nucleus cuneatus and medial lemniscus. The electrodes placed above the somatosensory cortex on the scalp will record the responses from the thalamus and primary sensory cortex.

The visual evoked potential is defined as the response to visual stimuli using short flashes of light of approximately 12µs. The recording electrodes are placed over the occiput. They are less reliable than the AEP, but have been used to monitor function during surgery for lesions involving the pituitary gland, optic nerve and chiasma.

Bispectral index

The bispectral index monitor displays a real time EEG acquired from the frontotemporal montage and generates a single value (Bispectral Index Score) which measures the depth of anaesthesia. The value displayed is a complex parameter, composed of a combination of time domain, frequency domain and high order subparameters. The Bispectral Index Score (BIS) represents an integrated measure of cerebral activity.

In recent years, a great effort has been made to provide a simplified interpretation of the EEG in order to provide a reliable indictor of depth of anaesthesia. The processed EEG variables have their own limitations, and are not simple enough to be used in routine clinical practice. They do not quantify all the information available in the EEG. Even compressed spectral array ignores the phase information. The bispectral index is a method of signal processing that quantifies the degree of phase coupling between the components of EEG signal.

An algorithm was developed by studying various components of EEG in thousands of patients undergoing anaesthesia with many different anaesthetic techniques and correlating the EEG pattern with clinical measures of anaesthetic depth. The monitor generates a BIS value on a continuous scale of 0 to 100, using a higher order statistical analysis (the bispectrum) of the EEG. The BIS value decreases with decreasing level of consciousness: 100 represents normal cortical activity and 0 represents no cortical activity. BIS values of 40-60 imply an adequate depth of anaesthesia. As the BIS value decreases below 70, the probability of explicit recall decreases dramatically. At a value below 60, a patient has an extremely low probability of consciousness.

In clinical practice, maintenance of anaesthesia in the majority of patients is provided by volatile anaesthetic agents. The potency of volatile agents is compared using MAC equivalents. Maintaining end-tidal anaesthetic concentration at 0.7 MAC is likely to prevent the incidence of awareness. Some early trials have revealed that titrating the end-tidal concentration of volatile agent to maintain the BIS value between 40-60 reduces the amount of volatile agent used.

The B-aware trial showed the reduced risk of awareness among high-risk surgical patients. The B-unaware trial published in 2008, was unable to demonstrate the benefit of BIS-guided protocol.

Key points

- The clinical signs do not correlate accurately with the depth of anaesthesia.
- The EEG is too complex to interpret and is not suitable as a monitor of depth of anaesthesia in routine clinical practice.

- The BIS monitor displays a single value as depth of anaesthesia. It measures the hypnotic effects of volatile and intravenous anaesthetic agents.
- The role of the BIS monitor in reducing the risk of awareness is not well established.

Further reading

1. Rampil IJ. A primer of EEG signals processing in anaesthesia. *Anesthesiology* 1998; 89: 980-1002.
2. Thronton C, Sharpe RM. Evoked responses in anaesthesia, review article. *British Journal of Anaesthesia* 1998; 81: 771-81.
3. Bailey AR, Jones JG. Patients' memories of events during general anaesthesia. Review article. *Anaesthesia* 1997; 52: 460-76.
4. Miller A, Sleigh JW. Barnard J, *et al.* Does bispectral analysis of the electroencephalogram add anything but complexity? *British Journal of Anaesthesia* 2004; 92: 8-13.
5. Myles PS, Leslie K, McNeil J, *et al.* Bispectral index monitoring to prevent awareness during anaesthesia: the B-Aware randomised controlled trial. *Lancet* 2004; 363: 1757-63.
6. Avidan MS, Zhang L, Burnside BA, *et al.* Anesthesia, awareness and the bispectral index. *The New England Journal of Medicine* 2008; 358: 1097-108.

Structured oral examination 6

Long case 6

Information for the candidate

History

A 68-year-old male is scheduled for an inguinal hernia repair. His past medical history includes chronic obstructive airway disease and a cerebrovascular accident occurring 6 years ago from which he has fully recovered. He is an alcoholic, drinking 2-3 pints of strong cider every day. He has smoked 20 cigarettes a day for the last 40 years. Current medication includes a salbutamol inhaler 200µg b.d. and a beclomethasone dipropionate inhaler 200µg b.d.

Clinical examination

Table 6.1 Clinical examination.

Weight	64kg
Height	171cm
Heart rate	76 bpm
Respiratory rate	16/min
Blood pressure	160/85mmHg
Temperature	37.1°C

Cardiovascular system
First and second heart sounds are normal, with no audible murmur.

Respiratory system
On auscultation scattered wheeze and basal crackles are heard.

Investigations

Table 6.2 Biochemistry.

		Normal values
Sodium	130mmol/L	135-145mmol/L
Potassium	4.9mmol/L	3.5-5.0mmol/L
Urea	9.7mmol/L	2.2-8.3mmol/L
Creatinine	118μmol/L	44-80μmol/L

Table 6.3 Haematology.

		Normal values
Hb	10.7g/dL	11-16 g/dL
Haematocrit	0.43	0.4-0.5 males, 0.37-0.47 females
RBC	4.75 x 10^{12}/L	3.8-4.8 x 10^{12}/L
WBC	5.5 x 10^9/L	4-11 x 10^9/L
Platelets	234 x 10^9/L	150-450 x 10^9/L
MCV	106.4fL	80-100fL
MCHC	33.2g/dL	31.5-34.5g/dL
INR	1.1	0.9-1.2
PT	10.4 seconds	11-15 seconds
APTT ratio	1.1	0.8-1.2

Table 6.4 Liver function tests.

		Normal values
Total protein	60g/L	64-79g/L
Albumin	32g/L	34-48g/L
Bilirubin	24μmol/L	4-25μmol/L
Alanine transaminase (ALT)	95 IU/L	10-50 IU/L
Alkaline phosphatase	248 IU/L	30-120 IU/L
Gamma-GT	210 IU/L	10-50 IU/L

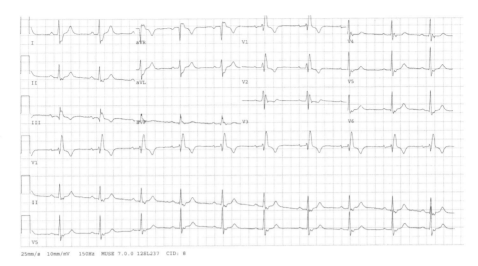

25mm/s 10mm/mV 150Hz MUSE 7.0.0 12SL237 CID: 8

Figure 6.1 ECG.

Examiner's questions

Please summarise the case

This is a 68-year-old male patient scheduled for a hernia repair with significant comorbidities. The main problems include:

- Chronic alcoholism with impaired liver function.
- Heavy smoking with COAD.
- Anaemia.
- Cerebrovascular disease with previous CVA.

What are the abnormal findings in the haematology results?

It shows a low haemoglobin with increased MCV and normal MCHC, suggesting macrocytic normochromic anaemia.

What are the causes of macrocytic anaemia?

- Vitamin B12 and folate deficiency.
- Liver dysfunction.

- ◆ Hypothyroidism.
- ◆ Drugs, e.g. methotrexate and zidovudine.
- ◆ Alcohol excess.
- ◆ Pregnancy.
- ◆ Bone marrow infiltration.

What are the causes of vitamin B12 deficiency?

- ◆ Pernicious anaemia.
- ◆ Post-gastrectomy.
- ◆ Dietary deficiency.
- ◆ Disease of the terminal ileum, e.g. Crohn's disease.

Vitamin B12 binds to intrinsic factor in the stomach, and is carried to the specific receptors on the surface of the mucosa of the ileum where it is absorbed. Intrinsic factor is essential for the absorption of vitamin B12; it is secreted by gastric parietal cells. Following gastrectomy and in pernicious anaemia, absence of intrinsic factor results in Vitamin B12 deficiency.

What are the causes of a microcytic anaemia in an alcoholic patient?

- ◆ Upper GI bleed due to oesophageal varices and gastritis.
- ◆ Poor diet.

What are the abnormal findings in the ECG?

The heart rate is 60 per minute; sinus rhythm. There is right bundle branch block, inverted T waves in leads V1 and V2, and ST depression in leads I and aVL.

Comment on the biochemistry results

The renal function tests show marginally elevated urea and creatinine. Liver function tests reveal an elevated gamma-GT. This and the increased MCV could be due to excessive alcohol intake.

What are the systemic effects of alcohol abuse?

Gastrointestinal system

Excessive alcohol intake can lead to pancreatitis, gastritis, fatty deposition in the liver, alcoholic hepatitis and hepatic cirrhosis. Advanced hepatic cirrhosis leads to portal hypertension, oesophageal varices and haemorrhoids.

Cirrhosis is irreversible liver damage. There is a loss of normal hepatic architecture with fibrosis and nodular regeneration. In severe liver impairment, plasma cholinesterase activity may be reduced. Chronic alcoholism induces microsomal oxidising enzymes, which may affect the metabolism of drugs.

Metabolic system

Acute alcohol intake delays gastric emptying, and leads to impaired glucose tolerance and hypoglycaemia. Electrolyte abnormalities (hypokalaemia and hypomagnesaemia) and hypoalbuminaemia are associated with chronic alcoholism.

Cardiovascular system

Arrhythmias, conduction defects and dilated cardiomyopathy may occur in chronic alcoholics.

Central nervous system

Effects include depression, antisocial behaviour, Wernicke's encephalopathy, Korsakoff's psychosis and acute withdrawal syndrome. The clinical features of Wernicke's encephalopathy include confusion, ataxia and ophthalmoplegia. Korsakoff's psychosis is characterised by amnesia and confabulation (production of false memories).

An acute withdrawal syndrome can occur in chronic alcoholics when alcohol is withdrawn suddenly. Clinical manifestation include generalised tremors, nightmares, hallucinations, tachycardia, arrhythmias and agitation. A small percentage of patients with alcohol withdrawal may present with delirium tremens, a life-threatening emergency characterised by hyperthermia, tachycardia, hypertension and grand mal seizures.

Haematological system

Thrombocytopaenia, leukopenia, anaemia and reduced synthesis of clotting factors (II, V, VII, IX and XIII) can lead to deranged coagulation.

Endocrine system

Decreased adrenocortical response to stress and decreased serum levels of testosterone.

Immune system

Alcohol affects the immune system and leucocyte function. There is an increased postoperative complication rate in heavy drinkers, often due to wound infection, urinary tract infection and pneumonia.

How might a patient with alcoholic hepatitis present?

The patient may present with hyperthermia, tachycardia, tachypnoea, anorexia, diarrhoea and vomiting. Clinical examination may reveal jaundice, tender hepatomegaly and ascites.

How would you identify a patient suffering with chronic alcoholism?

Screening tests

Increased MCV and increased levels of gamma-glutamyl transpeptidase.

Questionnaire

Two yes responses to the following questionnaire indicate that the respondent should be investigated further:

♦ Have you ever felt you needed to cut down on your drinking?
♦ Have people annoyed you by criticizing your drinking?
♦ Have you ever felt guilty about drinking?
♦ Have you ever felt you needed a drink first thing in the morning to steady your nerves or to get rid of a hangover?

How would you optimise this patient prior to his hernia repair?

Following a detailed history and clinical examination every attempt should be made to correct all metabolic derangements prior to surgery.

The patient should be encouraged to reduce the amount of alcohol intake or, if possible, to have a period of alcohol abstinence. This reduces postoperative morbidity and improves cardiovascular and immune function.

The benefits of cessation of smoking should be discussed. Cessation for even 12-24 hours prior to surgery improves the oxygen-carrying capacity of haemoglobin.

Anaemia should be corrected with nutritional supplements of vitamin B12 and folate. Serum magnesium levels should be checked and corrected.

Bronchodilator therapy should be continued and should be administered in nebulised form (salbutamol 5mg q.d.s.) for 24-48 hours prior to the surgery.

This patient is now in the best possible medical condition for surgery. The surgical decision is in favour of an open mesh repair. What are the anaesthetic options?

The options are:

♦ Local anaesthesia - field block.
♦ Regional anaesthesia (spinal or epidural) anaesthesia.
♦ General anaesthesia.

What are the benefits of regional anaesthesia?

♦ The systemic effects of general anaesthetics are avoided.
♦ It causes minimal physiological disturbance.
♦ The use of local anaesthesia is associated with early recovery and absence of drowsiness and sedation.
♦ It provides postoperative analgesia.
♦ It facilitates early discharge and a reduced duration of postoperative stay.

What are the disadvantages?

♦ Lack of patient co-operation.
♦ The patient may experience some sensation and discomfort, particularly during traction of the peritoneum.
♦ The technique is not suitable for large hernias and those with an incarcerated bowel.

Explain how you would perform a local anaesthesic block for an inguinal hernia repair

The local anaesthetic technique should provide anaesthesia to the skin over the incision site, the hernial sac and the deeper tissues. This is achieved by blocking the following three nerves:

♦ Iliohypogastric nerve (L1).
♦ Ilioinguinal nerve (L1).
♦ Genitofemoral nerve (L1 and L2).

Monitoring

Peripheral oxygen saturation using pulse oximetry, continuous monitoring of ECG and non-invasive blood pressure monitoring should be established.

Position

The patient should lie supine.

Asepsis

The inguinal region and scrotal area should be cleaned with antiseptic solution and covered with sterile drapes.

Landmarks

Anterior superior iliac spine and pubic tubercle.

Technique

A skin weal is raised 2cm medial to the anterior superior iliac spine. A regional block needle (short bevelled) is inserted perpendicular to the skin; a click is felt as it pierces the external oblique aponeurosis. 10ml of local anaesthetic is injected under the aponeurosis in a fanwise fashion, following negative aspiration.

Another skin weal is raised lateral to the pubic tubercle; 5ml of local anaesthetic is injected laterally and another 5ml is injected towards the umbilicus.

A subcutaneous infiltration is performed at the incision site with 10ml of local anaesthetic solution (0.25% levobupivacaine or 1% lidocaine with 1:200,000 epinephrine).

What are the complications of this block?

- Intravascular injection leading to local anaesthetic toxicity.
- Intraperitoneal injection.
- Femoral nerve block.

Postoperatively the patient develops hallucinations. What is the likely diagnosis?

As this patient is a heavy alcoholic, this can be due to delirium tremens.

What other signs might you expect with delirium tremens?

Tachycardia, hypotension, tremors, hallucination and convulsions.

How would you treat delirium tremens?

- Assess and manage the airway, breathing and circulation. Administer 100% oxygen.
- Check pulse, blood pressure, saturation and monitor ECG.
- Diazepam 2.5mg IV.
- The specific treatment is chlordiazepoxide 250mg, orally 6-hourly.
- Tachycardia can be treated with beta-blockers.
- Blood glucose should be checked and hypoglycaemia treated with 50% dextrose.
- Haloperidol 10-20mg IV can be given for hallucinations.
- Chlormethiazole (Heminevrin) 0.8% can be given as an IV infusion in the intensive care unit. It should be administered at a rate of 40-80mg (5-10ml) per minute for the initial 5-10 minutes and then gradually reduced to 4-8mg (0.5-1ml) per minute. It may cause respiratory depression and possibly addiction.
- Intravenous vitamin B and C (Pabrinex), administered 8-hourly.
- Thiamine 100mg as an IV infusion.
- Blood glucose should be monitored regularly and hypoglycaemia should be treated.
- In some resistant patients it may be necessary to give an intravenous infusion of ethanol 5% or an alcoholic drink.
- The patient may need to be monitored in a critical care environment due to haemodynamic instability.

Nerve supply to the inguinal region

The sensory supply to the inguinal area is derived from the lumbar plexus via the following three nerves:

- Iliohypogastric nerve (L1).
- Ilioinguinal nerve (L1).
- Genitofemoral nerve (L1 and L2).

The iliohypogastric and ilioinguinal nerves arise from the lumbar plexus within the psoas muscle, then pierce the transverse abdominis muscle to lie between the transverse abdominis and internal oblique near the iliac crest. The iliohypogastric nerve divides into lateral and anterior cutaneous branches. The anterior branch supplies the skin over the hypogastric region. The ilioinguinal nerve enters the inguinal canal to accompany the spermatic cord in males and the round ligament in females.

The genitofemoral nerve descends obliquely over the psoas muscle, dividing into genital and femoral branches. The genital branch follows the spermatic cord through the inguinal canal and supplies the cremaster muscle and skin over the scrotum or labia majora. The femoral branch supplies the skin over the femoral triangle.

The skin and muscles over the lower part of the abdomen are supplied by the last thoracic (subcostal) nerve.

Smoking and anaesthesia

Smoking is an important risk factor for ischaemic heart disease, cerebrovascular disease, peripheral vascular disease and lung cancer. It is also linked to oral, bladder and stomach cancer. Cigarette smoke contains potent carcinogens such as polycyclic aromatic hydrocarbons and nitrosamines. Smoking also increases the risk of postoperative surgical problems, such as anastomotic leak, wound infection and flap necrosis. The following are the major adverse effects of smoking.

Respiratory system

There is an increase in carbon monoxide (CO) levels in smokers, which has a two-fold effect. It reduces the amount of haemoglobin available for oxygen carriage and because CO shifts the oxyhaemoglobin disassociation curve to the left it reduces the ability of haemoglobin to release oxygen to the tissues. CO also inhibits cytochrome oxidase, which is needed for the final oxygen-dependent synthesis of ATP in the mitochondria.

Smoking increases the irritability of the upper airways leading to an increased risk of coughing, breath holding and laryngospasm during induction and recovery of anaesthesia. The impaired mucociliary clearance increases the risk of peri-operative respiratory infection.

Smoking causes chronic bronchitis and obstructive airway disease with a resultant decrease in FEV1 by approximately 60ml per year. There is also an increase in the closing volume and the degree of shunt under anaesthesia.

Cardiovascular system

There is an increased incidence of hypertension, ischaemic heart disease and cerebrovascular disease in smokers. Smokers have a higher resting plasma catecholamine level which makes them prone to an exaggerated sympathetic response to desflurane anaesthesia. ECGs in smokers are more likely to show ST segment depression under general anaesthesia, indicating impaired coronary perfusion. This coupled with the hypoxaemic effects of CO leads to a reduction in myocardial oxygen supply during the peri-operative period.

Haematological system

Smokers may have a degree of polycythaemia due to chronic hypoxaemia, which leads to hypercoagulability. In addition, there is an enhancement of platelet function and increase in fibrinogen levels. These contribute to an increased risk of central and peripheral arterial thromboses.

Gastrointestinal system

There is an increased risk of peptic ulcer disease, gastro-oesophageal reflux and Crohn's disease.

Table 6.5 Benefits of cessation of smoking.

Time of cessation	Effects
More than a year	Reduction in lung cancer, COAD, ischaemic heart disease, cerebrovascular disease
5-6 months	Reduction of postoperative complications
1 month	Possible decrease in postoperative respiratory complications
2-10 days	Improvement in upper airway reactivity
12-24 hour	Clearance of carbon monoxide

Key points

- Chronic alcohol abuse can affect several systems and significantly increase peri-operative morbidity.
- Delirium tremens can be a life-threatening emergency.
- Smoking is an important risk factor for ischaemic heart disease, cerberovascular disease, peripheral vascular disease and lung cancer.
- Cessation of smoking for 5-6 months prior to surgery reduces postoperative respiratory complications.

Further reading

1. Moppett I, Curran J. Smoking and surgical patient. *British Journal of Anaesthesia CEPD reviews* 2001; 4: 122-4.
2. Dunn J, Day CJE. Local anesthesia for inguinal and femoral hernia repair. http://www.nda.ox.ac.uk/wfsa/html/u04/u04_012.htm.

Short case 6.1: Septic shock

Define sepsis

Sepsis is defined as infection together with the systemic manifestation of infection. A suspected or documented infection in the presence of some of the following is defined as sepsis:

- Temperature >38.3°C or <36°C.
- Heart rate >90 bpm.
- Tachypnoea: respiratory rate >20 or $PaCO_2$ <4.4kPa.
- WBC count >12 x 10^9/L or <4 x 10^9/L.
- Altered mental status.
- Hyperglycaemia (plasma glucose 140mg/dL or 7.7mmol/L) in the absence of diabetes.

What is severe sepsis?

Severe sepsis is defined as sepsis plus sepsis-induced organ dysfunction or tissue hypoperfusion.

Sepsis-induced hypotension is defined as a systolic blood pressure (SBP) <90 mm Hg or mean arterial pressure <70 mm Hg or a decrease in SBP >40 mm Hg below the normal for age in the absence of other causes of hypotension.

What is septic shock?

Septic shock is defined as sepsis-induced hypotension persisting despite adequate fluid resuscitation.

What are the typical thresholds for identification of organ dysfunction in severe sepsis?

The following parameters indicate presence of organ dysfunction in severe sepsis:

- Sepsis-induced hypotension.
- Lactate greater than 2mmol/L.
- Urine output <0.5mL/kg/hr for more than 2 hours despite adequate fluid resuscitation.
- Acute lung injury (ALI) with PaO_2/FIO_2 <250 in the absence of pneumonia as the infection source.
- ALI with PaO_2/FIO_2 <200 in the presence of pneumonia as the infection source.
- Creatinine >2.0mg/dL (176.8µmol/L).
- Bilirubin >2mg/dL (34.2µmol/L).
- Platelet count <100 x 10^9/L.
- Coagulopathy (INR >1.5).

What are the principles of management of severe sepsis?

Principles include:

◆ Early goal-directed resuscitation.
◆ Investigations to identify the source of sepsis.
◆ Treatment of infection.
◆ Organ support.

Severe sepsis management bundles are a distillation of the concepts and recommendations found in the practice guidelines published by the Surviving Sepsis Campaign in 2004. They are designed to allow teams to follow the timing, sequence, and goals of the individual elements of care, in order to achieve the goal of a 25% reduction in mortality from severe sepsis. There are two bundles or packages of care for managing patients with severe sepsis: the sepsis resuscitation bundle and the sepsis management bundle. Each bundle has four to eight elements of care.

What are the elements of the sepsis resuscitation bundle?

The goal is to perform all indicated tasks within the first 6 hours following the onset of severe sepsis:

◆ Measure serum lactate.
◆ Obtain blood cultures prior to antibiotic administration.
◆ Administer a broad-spectrum antibiotic, within 3 hours for admissions arriving through the emergency department and within 1 hour of non-emergency department admissions.
◆ In the event of hypotension and/or a serum lactate >4mmol/L:
  - administer an initial bolus of 20ml/kg of crystalloid or an equivalent colloid;
  - administer vasopressors for hypotension not responding to initial fluid resuscitation, to maintain mean arterial pressure (MAP) >65 mm Hg and urine output ≥0.5mL/kg/hour.

♦ In the event of persistent hypotension despite fluid resuscitation (septic shock) and/or lactate >4mmol/L:
  - achieve a central venous pressure (CVP) of 8-12 mm Hg;
  - achieve central venous oxygen saturation (ScvO$_2$) of >70% or mixed venous oxygen saturation (SvO$_2$) of >65%. To achieve this, a further fluid challenge, transfusion of red blood cells (to maintain a haematocrit ≥30%) and/or IV infusion of dobutamine may be required.

What are the elements of the sepsis management bundle?

This consists of four tasks to be completed within 24 hours of presentation for patients with severe sepsis or septic shock:

♦ Administer low-dose steroids for septic shock in accordance with a standardised intensive care unit policy.
♦ Administer drotrecogin alpha (a recombinant human activated protein-C) in accordance with a standardised intensive care unit policy.
♦ Maintain glucose control >70mg/dL (4.3mmol/L), but <150mg/dL (8.3mmol/L).
♦ Maintain a median inspiratory plateau pressure (IPP) <30cm H$_2$O in mechanically ventilated patients.

What is the role of recombinant human activated protein-C (rhAPC) in sepsis?

According to the Surviving Sepsis Campaign, adult patients with sepsis-induced organ dysfunction associated with a clinical assessment of high risk of death, with an acute physiology and chronic health evaluation (APACHE) II >25 or multiple organ failure, should receive rhAPC if there are no contraindications.

What are the contraindications for rhAPC?

The following are contraindications for patients receiving rhAPC:

♦ Active internal bleeding.

- Recent (within 3 months) haemorrhagic stroke.
- Recent (within 2 months) intracranial/intraspinal surgery/severe head trauma.
- Trauma patients with an increased risk of life-threatening bleeding.
- Presence of an epidural catheter.
- Known or suspected intracranial neoplasm or mass lesion.
- Known hypersensitivity to rhAPC (drotrecogin alpha).
- Acute pancreatitis without a proven source of infection.
- Pregnancy.
- Advance directive or patient, family, or physician favour to withhold aggressive treatment.
- Patient is not expected to survive >28 days because of an uncontrollable medical condition.
- Patient is moribund with perceived imminent death within 24 hours.

Key points

- Early management of severe sepsis is based on the guidelines produced by the Surviving Sepsis Campaign.
- The Surviving Sepsis Campaign resuscitation bundle should be completed within the first 6 hours.
- The Surviving Sepsis Campaign management bundle should be completed within the first 24 hours.

Further reading

1. Dellinger RP, Levy MM, Carlet JM, *et al.* Special article - Surviving Sepsis Campaign: International guidelines for management of severe sepsis and septic shock. *Critical Care Medicine* 2008; 36: 296-327.

Short case 6.2: Myasthenia gravis

A 25-year-old female patient presents for thymectomy. She was diagnosed with myasthenia gravis 6 months ago.

What is myasthenia gravis?

Myasthenia gravis is a rare autoimmune disorder causing weakness of skeletal muscles. It predominantly affects young females. 15% of patients have a thymoma.

What is the pathophysiology?

The proposed mechanism for muscle weakness involves polyclonal IgG antibodies directed against the post-synaptic acetylcholine receptors (AChR) at the neuromuscular junction (NMJ). These AChR antibodies reduce the number of functional receptors by blocking the attachment of acetylcholine molecules, increasing the number of degradation receptors and by complement-induced damage to the NMJ.

What is the clinical presentation of myasthenia gravis?

Due to the reduced AChR density there is a decrease in the amplitude of action potentials in the post-synaptic region resulting in failure of initiation of muscle contraction.

The patient may present with the following clinical features:

- The muscle weakness is accentuated by exercise and relieved with rest.
- Diplopia and ptosis may occur due to involvement of eye muscles.
- Generalised weakness of facial and limb muscles.
- Bulbar weakness may be present.
- Patients may present with a myasthenic crisis (respiratory muscle weakness leading to respiratory failure) associated with trauma and infection.

Table 6.6 Classification of myasthenia gravis.	
Type I	Ocular signs and symptoms only
Type IIA	Generalised mild muscle weakness responding well to therapy
Type IIB	Generalised moderate muscle weakness responding less well to therapy
Type III	Acute fulminating presentation or respiratory dysfunction
Type IV	Myasthenic crisis requiring artificial ventilation

What conditions are associated with myasthenia gravis?

In addition to thymoma, it is associated with the following conditions:

+ Endocrine: hyper/hypothyroidism.
+ Musculoskeletal: rheumatoid arthritis, polymyositis.
+ Haematology: pernicious anaemia.
+ Dermatology: psoriasis, vitiligo.

How would you confirm the diagnosis of myasthenia gravis?

+ History and clinical examination.
+ Serology: anti-AChR antibody is found in up to 80% of patients. Anti-striated muscle antibodies are found in 50% of patients who are anti-AChR antibody negative.
+ Electromyography: repetitive nerve stimulation at 3Hz results in a progressive decrease in the amplitude of the compound muscle action potential. A single fibre electromyogram of affected muscle (obtained at muscle biopsy) is a more sensitive test.
+ Pharmacological testing: Tensilon test.
+ Imaging: chest X-ray and CT scan to rule out thymoma.
+ Thyroid function tests: to differentiate from thyrotoxiosis as a cause of muscle weakness.

What is the Tensilon test?

This is used as a primary diagnostic test and also to differentiate a myasthenic crisis from a cholinergic crisis in patients being treated with anti-cholinesterases. It involves intravenous administration of edrophonium, an ultra-short-acting anti-cholinesterase. In a myasthenic crisis, an improvement is seen following edrophonium administration, whereas it worsens in a cholinergic crisis.

Edrophonium binds reversibly to the ionic site of the cholinesterase with no interaction with the esteratic site. Initially, 2mg of edrophonium is injected slowly, intravenously. If no adverse effects are seen (bradycardia or AV block), a further dose of 8mg of edrophonium is administered and a blinded observer tests the strength of the involved muscle group before and after edrophonium. Patients with myasthenia gravis show a marked improvement in muscle power after 30 seconds which is sustained for approximately 5 minutes.

What are the treatment modalities for myasthenia gravis?

♦ Anticholinesterase therapy. Anticholinesterase delays the degradation of acetylcholine and improves the neuromuscular transmission. Pyridostigmine is the commonly used drug. Onset of action is within 30 minutes with a peak effect seen in 2 hours.
♦ Immunosuppressant therapy. Prednisolone is started at a dose of 20mg/day and gradually increased to 60mg/day. Other immunosuppressants include azathioprine (1-2mg/kg/day) and cyclosporine (5mg/kg/day).
♦ Thymectomy is indicated in those patients with thymoma and may be beneficial for most patients with myasthenia gravis.
♦ Plasma exchange reduces the level of anti-AChR antibodies and produces a short-term remission.
♦ Intravenous immunoglobulin also produces short-term improvement.

How would you anaesthetise this patient for thymectomy?

Pre-operative management

Airway examination is important as a large thymoma may cause compression of the trachea. A CT scan of the chest is useful in assessing the degree and site of tracheal compression or deviation. Spirometry (FVC and FEV1) and blood gas analysis would be useful in assessing the respiratory function. The patient may also have other associated diseases such as thyrotoxicosis and rheumatoid arthritis. Blood should be cross-matched.

The patient should be admitted at least 48 hours prior to surgery and should receive chest physiotherapy. Sedative pre-medication should be avoided. Anticholinesterase therapy should be stopped on the morning of the surgery but steroids should be continued.

Indications for postoperative ventilation include:

- FVC <2.9L.
- Grade III or IV myasthenia gravis.
- Duration of myasthenia gravis >6 years.

Intra-operative management

Monitoring
An arterial line is useful for monitoring blood pressure and blood gases. Neuromuscular monitoring is essential as patients with myasthenia gravis are sensitive to non-depolarising neuromuscular blockers.

Airway management
Based on the pre-operative airway assessment, an appropriate airway management plan should be formulated. A range of airway equipment including a rigid bronchoscope and smaller size endotracheal tubes should be available. An awake, fibreoptic-guided intubation under local anaesthesia may be preferred in the presence of airway obstruction. The endotracheal tube should be placed distal to the obstruction.

Neuromuscular blockade
If succinylcholine is used, patients may show initial resistance requiring further doses which is then followed by phase II blockade. Tracheal intubation can be performed under deep inhalational anaesthesia or by using a combination of propofol and remifentanil IV infusion. The dose of non-depolarising neuromuscular blocker should be reduced. About 1/10th of the normal dose (2.5-5mg of atracurium) should provide adequate muscle relaxation for tracheal intubation.

The surgery is usually performed via a median sternotomy. Reversal of neuromuscular blockade with anticholinesterases may increase the risk of a cholinergic crisis.

Postoperative management

The patient should be managed in an intensive care or high dependency unit. Postoperative ventilation is unnecessary in the majority of patients. A nasogastric tube is useful for early administration of anticholinesterases. The postoperative analgesic regimen should include a multimodal approach involving infiltration of local anaesthetic, regular paracetamol, NSAIDs and parenteral opioid in the form of PCA morphine.

Myasthenic syndrome

Myasthenic syndrome (Eaton-Lambert syndrome) is characterised by proximal myopathy. It can be associated with small cell carcinoma of the bronchus. Muscle weakness is due to a reduced release of acetylcholine from presynaptic nerve terminals. Anticholinesterase drugs are not effective in myasthenic syndrome. Patients are sensitive to the effects of both succinylcholine and non-depolarising muscle relaxants.

Key points

◆ Myasthenia gravis is a rare autoimmune disorder causing weakness of skeletal muscles.
◆ Anti-AChR antibodies are found in up to 80% of patients.
◆ Patients with myasthenia gravis are extremely sensitive to non-depolarising neuromuscular blocking drugs and resistant to succinylcholine.

Further reading

1. Thavasothy M, Hirsch N. Myasthenia gravis. *British Journal of Anaesthesia CEPD review* 2002; 2: 88-90.
2. Myasthenia gravis. In: *Anesthesia and co-existing disease*, 4th ed. Stoelting RK, Dierdorf SF. Philadelphia: Churchill Livingstone, 2002; Chapter 26: 522-8.

Short case 6.3: Epidural abscess

You are planning to provide epidural analgesia for postoperative pain relief in a patient undergoing hemicolectomy.

Name the complications of epidural anaesthesia

They can be classified as immediate and delayed complications.

Immediate

◆ Hypotension.
◆ Local anaesthetic toxicity.
◆ Total spinal anaesthetic block.
◆ Accidental dural puncture.
◆ Failure of block.

Delayed

◆ Epidural haematoma.
◆ Infection: meningitis, epidural abscess.
◆ Neurological damage.

What precautions would you take to prevent infection whilst performing an epidural block?

The following precautions should be taken:

◆ Maximal sterile precautions (mask, cap, sterile gloves, gown and large sterile drape).
◆ The skin should be disinfected with chlorhexidine (0.5%) in ethanol (80%).
◆ Insert the needle and catheter gently to minimise the risk of haematoma.
◆ Use a sterile transparent dressing over the site of epidural insertion.
◆ Use a pre-prepared infusion bag of local anaesthetic solution for epidural infusion.
◆ Ensure that a bacterial filter is used.

What are the risk factors for the development of an epidural abscess?

Diabetes mellitus and intravenous drug abuse are two common risk factors. Compromised immunity, procedures around the epidural space and the presence of systemic infection can also contribute.

Compromised immunity

Diabetes mellitus, steroid or other immunosuppressive therapy, malignancy, pregnancy, IV drug abuse, HIV and alcoholism may cause reduced immunity.

Technical procedures

Epidural abscess may develop secondary to a surgical procedure involving instrumentation on the spine. Factors such as difficulty in locating the epidural or subarachnoid space, multiple needle passes, poor aseptic technique, prolonged epidural catheterisation and coagulation disorders leading to haematoma formation may increase the risk of local infection.

Presence of systemic infection

This can occur as a result of haematogenous spread from respiratory, urinary and soft tissue infections. Intravenous drug abusers and patients with indwelling vascular catheters have an increased risk of systemic infection. An epidural abscess may result from contiguous spread from psoas, paraspinal or retropharyngeal abscesses.

What are the clinical features?

The clinical features of an epidural abscess are due to the effect of an enlarging mass and surrounding inflammation, leading to compression of nerve roots and spinal cord. The classic triad of back pain, fever and neurological deficit occurs in <20% of patients at the time of diagnosis. Back pain is the most common symptom in patients with an abscess at the lumbar or thoracic region. An abscess at the cervical region may present with neck stiffness. When untreated the progression of clinical features include nerve root irritation, motor weakness, sphincter incontinence, sensory changes and paralysis.

Clinical examination may reveal the following clinical signs:

◆ Increased body temperature.
◆ Tenderness over the spine.
◆ Meningism.
◆ Motor weakness.
◆ Diminished or absent sensation.
◆ Diminished or absent reflexes.

What investigations would you perform to confirm the diagnosis?

◆ Haematology. A full blood count may show leucocytosis, thrombocytopenia and an increased ESR. Blood cultures may grow the infecting organism.
◆ Radiology. An MRI scan is recommended urgently as the most accurate diagnostic screening tool. A CT scan with IV contrast may demonstrate the abscess.
◆ An X-ray of the spine may demonstrate bony pathology such as osteomyelitis.
◆ Blood culture to identify the causative organisms
◆ Culture and Gram staining of abscess fluid.

What measures would you take to help identify early diagnosis of an epidural abscess?

◆ Regular inspection of the epidural site.
◆ Regular assessment of lower limb motor power.
◆ Use of a low concentration of local anaesthetic (0.1-0.125% bupivacaine, levobupivacaine or ropivacaine) to avoid complete motor block.

Management of epidural abscess

The incidence of epidural abscess after central neuraxial block according to the literature varies from 1:1000 to 1:100,000. The overall mortality following epidural abscess varies between 10-16%. Thoracic lesions tend to produce more severe long-term neurological disability than lumbar lesions. Early diagnosis is important in order to reduce the neurological disability.

A patient may present with signs and symptoms suggestive of an epidural abscess a few days following epidural or spinal anaesthesia.

Treatment includes:

◆ Early surgical decompression; the commonest procedure is a posterior laminectomy.
◆ Antibiotics. Prolonged antibiotic therapy for 6-12 weeks is indicated, and should be guided by culture and sensitivity. An empirical antibiotic therapy (while waiting for the culture results) should cover most commonly implicated organisms such as *Staphylococcus aureus* and Gram-negative bacilli. Mycobacteria (tuberculosis) are common among immunocompromised patients. Third generation cephalosporins (ceftriaxone and ceftazidine) offer Gram-positive and Gram-negative coverage and CNS penetration. A tuberculous abscess may respond well to non-surgical treatment with anti-tuberculosis drugs.

Key points

◆ The classic triad of epidural abscess is back pain, fever and neurological deficit.
◆ Diabetes mellitus and intravenous drug abuse are the two common risk factors for epidural abscess.
◆ Early diagnosis and surgical decompression is essential in order to reduce the neurological disability.

Further reading

1. Grewal S, Hocking G, Wildsmith JAW. Epidural abscess, review article. *British Journal of Anaesthesia* 2006; 96: 292-302.

Applied anatomy 6.1: Coeliac plexus block

A 65-year-old male patient presents with severe upper abdominal pain. He has been diagnosed with carcinoma of the pancreas with bony metastases about 2 months ago. His current analgesics include paracetamol 1g t.d.s., codeine phosphate 60mg q.d.s. and morphine sulphate 100mg per day.

What other options are available for managing pain in this patient?

◆ Medical management: increasing the dose of morphine, switching the opioid to others such as oxycodone, considering the use of transdermal fentanyl or buprenorphine patches.
◆ Interventional management: splanchnic nerve block and coeliac plexus block.

What are the indications for a coeliac plexus block?

It is indicated for the relief of chronic pain originating from non-pelvic intra-abdominal organs, due to malignant or inflammatory pathology. It is most commonly used to treat chronic abdominal pain associated with carcinoma of the pancreas. It provides good pain relief in about 80% of patients. It can be performed during surgery to provide postoperative pain relief.

Are there any contraindications to perform a coeliac plexus block?

Apart from patient refusal, generic contraindications include clotting abnormality and local/systemic infection. It is unsafe to perform the block in the presence of a large aortic aneurysm.

Describe the anatomy of the coeliac plexus

The coeliac plexus is the largest major autonomic plexus supplying the upper abdominal organs. It is situated at the level of the first lumbar vertebra. It lies posterior to the stomach and pancreas, and anterior to the crura of the diaphragm and abdominal aorta (**P**osterior to **P**ancreas and **A**nterior to **A**orta). The inferior vena cava lies lateral to the plexus on the right side.

The sympathetic supply to the upper abdominal organs originates from the following nerves: the greater splanchnic nerve, the lesser splanchnic nerve and branches of the vagus nerve.

The greater splanchnic nerve formed by branches from the fifth to ninth or tenth thoracic ganglia descends obliquely on the vertebral bodies, pierces the ipsilateral crus of the diaphragm and ends mainly in the coeliac ganglion.

The lesser splanchnic nerve is formed by the rami of the ninth and tenth (sometimes tenth and eleventh) thoracic ganglia, pierces the crus of the diaphragm along with the greater splanchnic nerve and ends in the aortic-renal plexus.

Branches of the vagus nerve (parasympathetic) also contribute to the coeliac plexus.

How would you perform a coeliac plexus block?

The block is performed using radiological guidance (X-ray screening or CT scan) in an area with resuscitation facilities.

Intravenous access and basic monitoring are essential. The procedure is performed with the patient in the prone position. Sedation may be considered. Intravenous fluids are required to reduce the risk of hypotension following the procedure.

The technique normally involves two needle insertions, one on each side at the L1 level. The needle entry point is just below the tip of the 12th rib (about 7.5cm from the midline). Using radiological guidance in two planes, the needle is advanced until it hits the side of the L1 vertebral body. The needle is withdrawn and redirected forwards until it is placed in the anterolateral aspect of the body of the L1 vertebra. Radio-opaque contrast is injected to confirm the correct placement of the needle and to rule out epidural spread/intravascular placement. After careful negative aspiration the medication is injected.

More recently, the anterior approach under CT or ultrasound guidance has been described.

What are the neurolytic chemicals in current clinical use for coeliac plexus block?

◆ For non-malignant pain: approximately 15ml 0.5% or 15-20ml 0.25% bupivacaine on each side.

◆ For malignant pain: 20ml 4-6% aqueous phenol or 50% alcohol on each side.

What are the complications of coeliac plexus block?

◆ Due to loss of sympathetic tone, a coeliac plexus block causes dilatation of the upper abdominal vessels and venous pooling which leads to hypotension. This can be exacerbated by pre-existing dehydration.

◆ Diarrhoea may be seen due to unopposed parasympathetic influence following sympathetic block.

◆ Injury to the aorta or inferior vena cava by the needle may result in bleeding and a retroperitoneal haematoma.

◆ Intravascular injection can be prevented by checking the needle position with radio-opaque dye.

◆ Trauma to the pancreas, liver, stomach and bowel.

◆ Paraplegia can result either due to direct injury to the spinal cord or due to injection of phenol into the anterior spinal artery.

Key points

◆ Coeliac plexus block is used in chronic pain management to treat pain from non-pelvic abdominal viscera, most commonly for pain originating from carcinoma of the pancreas.

◆ The coeliac plexus is situated at the level of the first lumbar vertebra - posterior to the pancreas and anterior to the aorta.

◆ Minor complications include hypotension and diarrhoea; major complications include paralysis and autonomic dysfunction.

Further reading

1. Waldman SD. Celiac plexus block. In: *Innovations in pain management.* Weiner RS, Ed. Orlando, FL: PMD Press, 1990: 10-5.
2. Davies DD. Incidence of major complications of neurolytic coeliac plexus block. *J R Soc Med* 1993; 86: 264-6.

Applied physiology 6.2: Cerebral circulation

What is normal cerebral blood flow?

The average cerebral blood flow is about 50ml/100g/minute of brain tissue (~15% of cardiac output). Grey matter receives more blood flow than white matter (grey matter: 80ml/100g/minute, white matter: 20ml/100g/minute). The adult human brain weighs approximately 1.3kg and receives 12-15% of cardiac output. The total intracranial blood volume is about 150ml.

What is the arterial blood supply to the brain?

The arterial supply of the brain is derived from the internal carotid and vertebral arteries. The internal carotid artery terminates by dividing into the anterior and middle cerebral arteries. Two vertebral arteries join to form the basilar artery which divides into the two posterior cerebral arteries.

The circle of Willis is the interconnection between the internal carotid arteries and the basilar artery, and provides collateral blood supply if one of the vessels is occluded. Anteriorly, the two anterior cerebral arteries are joined by the anterior communicating artery. Posteriorly, the two posterior cerebral arteries are joined to the ipsilateral internal carotid artery by the posterior communicating artery.

What is the venous drainage of the brain?

Venous sinuses lie between the two layers of the dura mater. The superior sagittal sinus (found along the attached edge of the falx cerebri which divides the hemispheres) drains into the right transverse sinus. The inferior sagittal sinus (found along the free edge of the falx cerebri) drains into the straight sinus (found in the tentorium cerebelli) and then into the left transverse sinus. The transverse sinuses merge into the sigmoid sinuses before forming internal jugular veins.

Deeper structures drain via the two internal cerebral veins which join the great cerebral vein (of Galen), which drains into the inferior sagittal sinus. The cavernous sinuses (on either side of the pituitary fossa) drain into the transverse sinuses.

How is cerebral blood flow (CBF) regulated?

Flow is determined by the following equation:

$$Q = P/R$$

where Q = flow, P = pressure, R = resistance.

CBF is therefore proportional to the cerebral perfusion pressure (CPP) and inversely proportional to resistance in the cerebral vasculature.

Cerebral perfusion pressure is the difference between the mean arterial pressure (MAP) and central venous pressure (CVP). If the intracranial pressure (ICP) is greater than CVP then CPP = MAP - ICP.

The resistance in the cerebral vasculature is influenced by:

* Autoregulation.
* PaO_2 and $PaCO_2$.
* Neural control.

Autoregulation is the process by which cerebral blood flow is maintained at a relatively constant level despite variation in the perfusion pressure. Cerebral blood flow changes proportionately with cerebral metabolic rate. Local products of metabolism such as K^+, H^+, lactate and adenosine may have an effect on the cerebral vasculature. Cerebral functional state (sleep, awake state, epilepsy), anaesthetics and temperature can regulate cerebral blood flow.

$PaCO_2$ and PaO_2 can alter CBF. A PaO_2 less than 6.7kPa increases CBF. A $PaCO_2$ in the range of 4 to 11kPa increases CBF; the relationship between CBF and $PaCO_2$ is linear.

Both sympathetic and parasympathetic innervations of cerebral blood vessels may have some role in maintaining autoregulation.

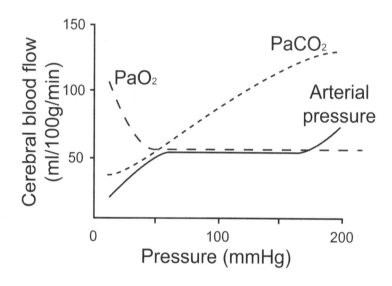

Figure 6.2 The effect of PaO_2 and $PaCO_2$ on CBF.

Cerebral blood flow is constant over a wide range of mean arterial pressures (60 to 140 mmHg). This curve shifts to the right in hypertensive patients.

How would you measure cerebral blood flow?

Cerebral blood flow can be measured using the following techniques:

♦ Kety-Schmidt technique.
♦ Transcranial Doppler ultrasonography.

- ◆ Positron emission tomography (PET).
- ◆ Scintillography and single photon emission computed tomography (SPECT) scanning.

The Kety-Schmidt method is an application of the Fick principle using inhaled nitrous oxide. The Fick principle states that the amount of substance taken up by an organ in unit time is equal to the product of blood flow through the organ and the concentration difference of the substance across the organ.

$$\text{Blood flow to any organ} = Qx / [Ax\text{-}Vx]$$

where Qx = amount of substance taken up by the organ, Ax = arterial concentration, Vx = venous concentration in the jugular venous bulb.

Hence, CBF is equal to the quantity of substance taken up by the brain/ arteriovenous concentration difference.

Nitrous oxide is used as the diffusible tracer. The subject breathes 10% N_2O for 10 minutes, during which time paired peripheral arterial and jugular venous bulb samples are taken. The speed at which the arterial and venous curves equilibrate is a measure of nitrous oxide delivery to the brain.

Transcranial Doppler ultrasonography gives a measure of the velocity of red cells flowing through large cerebral arteries, most commonly the middle cerebral artery. The velocity can give an index of flow provided that the diameter of the artery remains constant.

PET monitors the uptake of 2-deoxyglucose, which is labelled with a positron emitter.

Scintillography and SPECT scanning use radioactive xenon to trace regional blood flow, with or without enhancement by CT or MRI.

What are the effects of anaesthetic drugs on CBF?

◆ All intravenous induction agents reduce cerebral metabolic rate ($CMRO_2$) and as a result CBF falls. The exception is ketamine, which increases MAP and leads to a rise in blood flow.
◆ Volatile anaesthetics cause cerebral vasodilatation and have a dose-dependent effect on cerebral autoregulation. Other than sevoflurane all other volatile agents above 1.5 minimum alveolar concentration (MAC) abolish autoregulation (autoregulation is preserved up to 2 MAC with sevoflurane). Nitrous oxide increases CBF and $CMRO_2$.
◆ Opiates can indirectly affect CBF because of their effect on $PaCO_2$.
◆ Cerebral steal. Cerebral vasodilatation diverts the blood away from focal areas of damaged brain in which autoregulation is lost; this is produced when volatile anaesthetics, sodium nitroprusside and glyceryl trinitrate, are used.
◆ Inverse steal. Vasoconstriction associated with hyperventilation may divert blood from normal to damaged brain, where vasoconstrictor responses have been lost. This may be seen with hypocapnia and thiopentone.

What is the Monro-Kelly doctrine?

The skull is a rigid box with a fixed volume. Intracranial pressure is a function of blood flow, the amount of brain tissue (and oedema), and cerebrospinal fluid. An increase in total volume due to any of the physiological components or a space-occupying lesion results in an increase in intracranial pressure.

Arterial supply to the brain and spinal cord

The arterial supply of the brain is derived from the internal carotid and vertebral arteries. The internal carotid artery (ICA) arises from the bifurcation of the common carotid artery, ascends in the neck and enters the carotid canal of the temporal bone. The subsequent course of the internal carotid artery is described in three parts: the petrous part ascends the carotid canal and enters the cranial cavity via the foramen lacerum; the cavernous part ascends to the posterior clenoid process and then turns anteriorly to the side of the sphenoid within the cavernous sinus; and the cerebral part leaves the cavernous sinus, pierces the dura mater and terminates by dividing into the anterior and middle cerebral arteries. The ophthalmic artery arises from the internal carotid as it leaves the cavernous sinus. The posterior communicating artery runs backwards from the ICA and anastomoses with the posterior cerebral artery (terminal branch of the basilar artery).

The anterior cerebral artery (ACA) is the smaller of the two terminal branches. The anterior communicating artery (branch of the ACA) joins the two anterior cerebral arteries. The two ACAs travel together in the great longitudinal fissure, along the upper border of the corpus callosum to anastomose with the posterior cerebral artery. The ACA gives rise to cortical and central branches. The cortical branches (orbital, frontal and parietal) supply the motor and somatosensory cortices representing the lower limb.

The middle cerebral artery (MCA) is the larger terminal branch of the internal carotid artery. It runs in the lateral cerebral fissure, then postero-superiorly on the insula, dividing into cortical and central branches. The cortical branches of the MCA supply the motor and somatosensory cortices representing the whole of the body except the lower limb, auditory area and the insula.

The vertebral artery arises from the subclavian artery; it ascends upwards through the transverse foramen of the cervical vertebra and enters the cranial cavity through the foramina magnum. It then runs upwards and medially along the anterolateral aspect of the medulla. At the junction of the medulla and pons two vertebral arteries unite to form the basilar artery. The basilar artery terminates by dividing into two posterior cerebral arteries. The vertebral artery and its major branches (vertebrobasilar system) provide blood supply to the upper part of the spinal cord, the brain stem, cerebellum and occipital lobe.

The anterior spinal artery arises from the distal part, near the end of the vertebral artery. It descends anterior to the medulla oblongata and unites with the anterior spinal artery from the other side to form a single anterior spinal artery.

The posterior inferior cerebellar artery is the largest branch of the vertebral artery. It travels downwards into the cerebellar vallecula and divides into medial and lateral branches.

The posterior spinal artery arises from the posterior inferior cerebellar artery; occasionally it may directly arise from the vertebral artery.

The anterior inferior cerebellar artery arises from the lower part of the basilar artery and runs posterolaterally. The superior cerebellar artery arises from the distal part of the basilar artery.

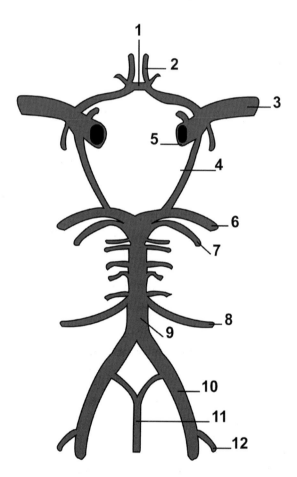

Figure 6.3 Arterial supply to the brain and spinal cord.
1. Anterior communicating artery; 2. Anterior cerebral artery; 3. Middle cerebral artery; 4. Posterior communicating artery; 5. Internal carotid artery; 6. Posterior cerebral artery; 7. Superior cerebellar artery; 8. Anterior inferior cerebellar artery; 9. Basilar artery; 10. Vertebral artery; 11. Anterior spinal artery; 12. Posterior inferior cerebellar artery.

Key points

♦ The circle of Willis is an interconnection between internal carotid arteries and basilar artery, providing collateral circulation.

♦ Cerebral blood flow is autoregulated, remaining constant within a range of MAP (80-140 mm Hg) and changes in proportion to the cerebral metabolic rate.

Further reading

1. Vascular supply and drainage of the brain, In: *Gray's anatomy*, 40th ed. Standring S, Ed. London: Churchill Livingstone, 2008: 247-56.

Applied pharmacology 6.3: Respiratory pharmacology

A 32-year-old, obese female patient who is a known asthmatic, is scheduled for dental extraction. Following pre-oxygenation, general anaesthesia is induced with propofol, fentanyl and rocuronium. Soon after induction she develops severe bronchospasm.

How would you manage intra-operative bronchospasm?

♦ Administer 100% oxygen and confirm the correct placement of the tracheal tube.

♦ Stop administration of agents which irritate the respiratory tract (e.g. isoflurane, desflurane) and increase the depth of anaesthesia using sevoflurane or intravenous propofol.

♦ Exclude the breathing system or airway obstruction.

♦ Exclude pneumothorax.

♦ Administer bronchodilators; a salbutamol inhaler, if immediately available, can be used in one of the following ways:

- disconnect the breathing system at the endotracheal end and discharge 2-4 puffs of salbutamol directly into the tube, reconnect the system and ventilate. Most of the drug is likely to be deposited in the tracheal tube so this method is inefficient;

- place the inhaler canister into the barrel of a 50ml Leur lock syringe and replace the plunger. Attach the syringe to manometer tubing (infusion tubing) placed down the endotracheal tube and discharge 2-4 puffs by pressing the syringe plunger;
- using an appropriate T-piece adapter and external source of oxygen, 5mg of salbutamol can be given by a nebuliser into the breathing system between the breathing filter and endotracheal tube.
- ◆ Intravenous salbutamol 250μg by slow bolus followed by a 5-10μg /minute infusion.
- ◆ Intravenous hydrocortisone 100mg.
- ◆ In extreme cases where there is no response to all the above measures, intravenous epinephrine may be used.

What is salbutamol?

It is a ß2-agonist used to treat both acute and chronic bronchial asthma.

Describe the mechanism of action of ß2-agonists

The ß2-receptor is a trans-membrane receptor linked to the adenyl cyclase enzyme via a trans-membrane G-protein. When these receptors are stimulated the adenyl cyclase enzyme is activated, catalysing the conversion of ATP to cAMP. cAMP activates protein kinase A, which catalyses the phosphorylation of intracellular proteins involved in controlling smooth muscle tone. It also increases intracellular calcium by inhibiting release of intracellular calcium stores.

What are the side effects of selective ß2-agonists?

At low doses ß2 effects predominate, but at higher doses ß1 effects occur causing cardiovascular effects such as tachycardia, positive inotropy, hypertension and arrhythmias. Other side effects include tremors, agitation and hypokalaemia.

What are the various routes in which salbutamol can be administered?

It can be administered orally, intravenously, by inhalation or by nebulisation.

What are the factors that determine the clinical effect when administered by inhalation?

The main benefit of administering the drug by inhalation is the reduced systemic absorption and side effects.

The amount of drug reaching the target site depends on the:

◆ Particle size of the aerosol.
◆ Velocity at which it is released from the device.
◆ Inhalational technique of the patient.
◆ Size of the airway.

What is theophylline?

It is a methylxanthine derivative, a less potent bronchodilator than the β2-agonists and has a greater potential for cardiovascular side effects. The mechanism of action includes:

◆ Phosphodiesterase enzyme inhibition.
◆ Antagonism of adenosine receptors.
◆ Reduction of calcium influx into smooth muscle cells.

The phosphodiesterase enzyme is responsible for degradation of cAMP. By inhibiting the phosphodiesterase enzyme, theophylline increases cAMP. It is available as an oral tablet and administered at a dose 200-600mg t.d.s.

Aminophylline is converted to theophylline. It is administered as a loading dose of 5-7mg/kg over 30 minutes followed by an infusion at a rate of 0.5mg/kg/hr. It has a very narrow therapeutic range of 10-20mg/L. The beneficial effects can be seen at levels lower than 10, but toxic effects can also be seen at levels lower than 20. These include tachycardia, agitation, convulsion, altered gut motility and hypokalaemia.

Theophyllines are metabolised by the liver; changes in hepatic metabolism due to disease and age, or induction of the cytochrome P-450 system can alter clearance and plasma levels.

What is the rationale for using corticosteroids in asthma?

Corticosteroids do not have any direct effect on smooth muscle relaxation. Due to their profound anti-inflammatory effect, they reduce mucosal swelling. The anti-inflammatory effects of glucocorticoids include modulation of cytokine production and marked reduction in the accumulation of basophils, eosinophils and other leukocytes. Inhaled corticosteroids result in better symptom control, less use of supplemental drugs such as β2-agonists, improved lung function and decreased bronchial hyperactivity.

What limits the use of corticosteroids in asthma?

Use is restricted by the side effects. These include protein catabolism, thinning and bruising of the skin, myopathy, and the typical Cushingoid appearance. Metabolic side effects include glucose intolerance, fluid retention, adrenal suppression and osteoporosis. Other side effects include cataracts, gastric bleeding, an increased risk of infection and psychosis.

Inhaled steroids (beclomethasone, budesonide and fluticasone) are commonly used to treat asthma, as they reduce the systemic side effects.

During an acute episode of asthma, oral prednisolone (40-60mg per day) can be used for a short period of 5 days. Chronic use of systemic steroids is reserved for patients who do not respond to combined therapy of inhaled steroids, β2-agonists, inhaled anti-cholinergics and oral leukotriene antagonists.

Anti-inflammatory drugs

Cromolyn sodium and nedocromil sodium inhibit release of histamine from broncho-alveolar mast cells and mediator release from airway epithelial cells. They are mainly used in the prophylaxis of asthma.

Leukotriene antagonists and lipo-oxygenase inhibitors

Leukotrienes are synthesised from arachidonic acid, which is released from membrane phospholipids by phopholipase A2. Zileuton is a lipo-oxygenase inhibitor which inhibits the conversion of arachidonic acid to leukotriene A4. Montelukast and zafirlukast are cysteinyl-leukotriene receptor antagonists which prevent the binding of leukotriene D4 to the cysteinyl-leukotriene receptor.

Montelukast is rapidly absorbed following oral administration and is mainly metabolised in the liver. It reduces inflammation and associated bronchospasm. Montelukast is mainly used in the maintenance therapy of asthma. The dose in adults is 10mg per day. There are very few adverse effects associated with inhibition of leukotriene synthesis. Montelukast and zafirlukast may rarely produce eosinophilia and vasculitis.

Doxapram

Doxapram is a non-specific respiratory stimulant; it acts on the peripheral chemoreceptors and the respiratory centre to increase the tidal volume and respiratory rate.

In anaesthesia it is used for reversing postoperative respiratory depression without antagonising opioid analgesia. In critical care it has been used for treating Type 2 respiratory failure. A meta-analysis has shown that the use of doxapram is only marginally superior to placebo in preventing blood gas deterioration in COAD and has been superseded by non-invasive ventilation.

The dosage is an IV bolus of 0.5-1mg/kg which is effective for 5-12 minutes. It can be used as an infusion at a rate of 1.5-4mg/minute.

Side effects are due to an increase in catecholamine release, which may cause tachycardia, hypertension and arrhythmias. Other side effects include agitation, hallucinations and convulsions.

It is contraindicated in patients with acute asthma and upper airway obstruction. It should be used with great caution in patients with ischaemic heart disease, hypertension and thyrotoxicosis.

Key points

♦ β2-agonists are used in bronchial asthma for acute exacerbation as well as maintenance therapy.

♦ At low doses, β2 agonists have a bronchodilator effect but at higher doses the β1 action can result in cardiovascular side effects.

♦ Doxapram is a non-specific respiratory stimulant with a short duration of action.

Further reading

1. Emla C. Bronchodilators, corticosteroids and anti-inflammatory agents. In: *Anaesthetic pharmacology - physiologic principles and clinical practice.* Evers AS, Maze M, Eds. Philadelphia: Churchill Livingstone, 2004: 703-16.
2. British guidelines on the management of asthma. http://www.sign.ac.uk/pdf/qrg101.pdf.

Equipment, clinical measurement and monitoring 6.4: Magnetic resonance imaging

A 30-year-old female patient has had a diagnostic laparoscopy. During the immediate postoperative period she developed grand mal seizures. Her past history include intermittent headaches for the past 6 months.

What are the likely causes for seizures in this patient?

♦ Neurological system: cerebrovascular accident, intracranial space occupying lesion, epilepsy.

♦ Respiratory system: hypoxia, hypercapnia.

♦ Metabolic system: electrolyte disturbances (hyponatraemia), hypoglycaemia, uraemia, liver failure.

♦ Infective causes: meningitis, respiratory infection, urinary tract infection, sepsis.

♦ Drugs: local anaesthetic toxicity, withdrawal effects from alcohol abuse.

What radiological investigation would you like to do?

A CT scan of the brain or MRI scan of the brain.

What are the problems with monitoring in an MRI scanner?

Electrocardiogram (ECG)

ECG artifacts can occur in the MRI scanner. Maximum voltage charges are induced in any column of conducting fluid (blood within the aorta) when the fluid flow is 90° to the field (supine patient in MR scanner). The superimposed potentials are greatest in ST segments and T waves of leads I, II, V1 and V2, and increase with field strength. Also, spike artifacts that mimic R waves are often produced due to the changing magnetic fields of the imaging gradients. Because of these changes it is difficult to monitor ischaemic changes. ECG changes mimicking hyperkalaemia may be induced. In patients highly susceptible to ischaemia, a 12-lead ECG pre- and post-MRI is recommended. The voltage induced in ECG wires is a potential for electric shock and burns.

Blood pressure monitoring

The monitor can be placed away from the magnetic field with the help of extended tubing. MR-approved monitoring systems based on an automated oscillometric method are less affected by electromagnetic interference. The monitor must be outside the 50 Gauss line.

If invasive blood pressure monitoring is used, conventional disposable transducers may function adequately outside the 50 Gauss line. Increasing the length of the tubing between the arterial cannula and transducer may reduce the natural frequency of the system and cause a damping effect on the arterial blood pressure trace.

Ideally the length of the tubing should be limited to 120cm; increasing the length reduces the natural frequency of the system and causes damping.

Capnography

The monitor can be placed outside the magnetic field by increasing the length of the sampling line, though this will increase the transit time, resulting in a delay of up to 20 seconds in obtaining the capnograph signal.

Pulse oximeter

Severe burns to extremities have been caused by induction of current within a loop of cable. This may be avoided by placing the probe on the extremity distal to the magnet, keeping its cable free of coils, and protecting the digits with clear plastic wrap.

MRI-compatible pulse oximeters use heavy fibreoptic cables, which do not overheat and cannot be looped.

CVP lines

PA catheters with conductive wiring can cause micro-shock. Melting of a thermistor in the PA catheter has been reported. Padding should be placed between cables and the patient's skin, and any loops in the cable should be avoided.

What precautions would you take to minimise ECG artifacts?

Several MRI-compatible ECG systems are currently available, utilising ECG electrodes made of carbon graphite, which have lower resistance, eliminate ferromagnetism and minimise the radiofrequency interference. These systems use co-axialised cables to avoid any coils.

What are the problems related to the use of anaesthetic equipment?

Most scanners use 0.5-1.5 Tesla magnets (about 10,000 times the earth's magnetic field). Near the scanner, the magnetic field exerts a powerful attraction on ferromagnetic materials which can become projectiles.

MRI-compatible anaesthetic machines are available, made largely of stainless steel, brass, aluminium and plastic. MRI-compatible equipment functions normally in the MRI environment. The pilot balloon of the tracheal tube should be firmly secured as it contains a metal spring.

Plastic battery-operated laryngoscopes may be used for tracheal intubation. The airway can be secured using a conventional laryngoscope before the patient is moved into the scanner. Medical gas cylinders constructed from aluminum should be used in the MRI suite. Vaporizers, however, are affected little by the magnetic field and function accurately.

What are the problems related to infusion pumps?

Intravenous infusion pumps should be placed outside the 100 Gauss line. Most of them contain ferromagnetic circuitry, which can malfunction in the presence of a high magnetic field. Long extension tubing may be needed.

Are there any special precautions you need to take with patients?

Patients with cardiac pacemakers require special consideration as they will malfunction in fields over 5 Gauss. Most implants (metal prosthesis, etc.) are non-ferrous, although some surgical clips (e.g. on an intracranial aneurysm) and wires may be magnetic. Metal foreign bodies are likely to be ferrous.

Effect of MRI on staff

A screening questionnaire should be used for all staff to avoid staff carrying any ferromagnetic objects and jewellery to the MRI room and also to identify staff who have pacemakers or metal implants. Pregnant staff should not work in the MRI scanner during the first trimester. If the magnet is shut down in an emergency, release of helium gas can lead to a potentially hypoxic environment.

Noise levels of 85 dB, equivalent to light road work, can be generated by the scanner. Ear plugs are recommended for staff working in the MRI room.

A remote monitoring facility will allow the anaesthetic team to remain outside the scanning room once the patient's condition is stable.

A Gauss is a unit of magnetic field strength. The SI unit of magnetic field strength is the Tesla (1 Tesla = 10,000 Gauss).

Key points

◆ Because of ECG artifacts occurring during MRI, monitoring ischaemic changes is difficult.
◆ MRI-compatible equipment should be used during the procedure.
◆ Ferromagnetic materials are attracted by the strong magnetic field.

Further reading

1. Provision of anaesthetic services in magnetic resonance units. http://www.aagbi.org/publications/guidelines/docs/mri02.pdf.
2. Peden JC, Twigg SJ. Anaesthesia for magnetic resonance imaging. *British Journal of Anaesthesia CEPD review* 2003; 4: 97-101.

Structured oral examination 7

Long case 7

Information for the candidate

History

A 42-year-old male with a history of manic depression is scheduled for full dental clearance. In the past he has been treated with electroconvulsive therapy (ECT). His current medication includes imipramine 50mg o.d., venlafaxine 75mg o.d. and lithium carbonate 300mg o.d. He also gives a history of polyuria. He has seen a nephrologist and is on treatment for hypertension. He smokes 15-20 cigarettes per day and lives alone.

Clinical examination

On examination, he is unkempt, has ankle oedema and an expiratory wheeze with crackles at the left base. His HR is 90 bpm and BP is 170/110mmHg.

Investigations

Table 7.1 Biochemistry.		
		Normal values
Sodium	131mmol/L	135-145mmol/L
Potassium	4.2mmol/L	3.5-5.0mmol/L
Urea	19.8mmol/L	2.2-8.3mmol/L
Creatinine	200μmol/L	44-80μmol/L
Lithium level	0.7mmol/L	0.5-1.0mmol/L

Table 7.2 Haematology.

		Normal values
Hb	13.2g/dL	11-16g/dL
Haematocrit	0.46	0.4-0.5 males, 0.37-0.47 females
RBC	4.1×10^{12}/L	$3.8\text{-}4.8 \times 10^{12}$/L
WBC	13.2×10^{9}/L	$4\text{-}11 \times 10^{9}$/L
Platelets	245×10^{9}/L	$150\text{-}450 \times 10^{9}$/L
INR	1.0	0.9-1.2
PT	12.5 seconds	11-15 seconds
APTT ratio	1	0.8-1.2

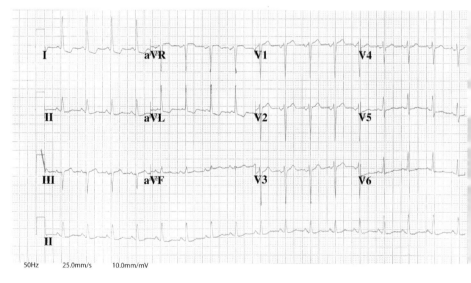

50Hz   25.0mm/s   10.0mm/mV

Figure 7.1 ECG.

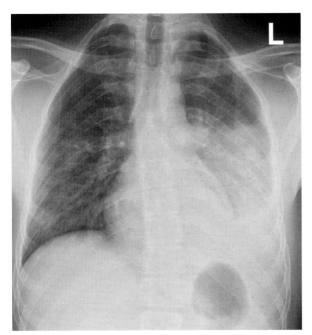

Figure 7.2 Chest X-ray.

Examiner's questions

Describe the main issues which might make anaesthesia problematic

These are:

- Uncontrolled hypertension.
- Chest X-ray suggestive of left lower lobe consolidation.
- Renal impairment.
- Narrow therapeutic/toxic ratio for lithium and its drug interactions.
- Difficulty with communication and obtaining consent.
- Postoperative nursing and analgesia.

Can you tell me about this patient's current medication?

His current medication includes:

◆ Lithium carbonate.
◆ Imipramine, a tricyclic antidepressant (TCA).
◆ Venlafaxine, a selective serotonin reuptake inhibitor (SSRI).

How does lithium act?

Lithium (carbonate or citrate) is a mood-stabilising drug and is mainly used for prophylaxis in patients with repeated episodes of mania and depression. It is also the drug of choice for acute mania in the absence of severe hyperactivity.

In excitable cells, lithium mimics sodium and enters cells via fast voltage gated channels. Unlike sodium it cannot be pumped out by Na^+/K^+ ATPase leading to intracellular accumulation. It decreases the release of neurotransmitters both centrally and peripherally.

What problems can lithium pose to the anaesthetist?

Lithium can pose problems for the anaesthetist in two different ways:

◆ Problems due to toxic effects:
  - it has a narrow therapeutic/toxic ratio. The normal therapeutic range for lithium is 0.5-1.0mmol/L. Toxicity occurs when the serum lithium concentration exceeds 1.5mmol/L. The signs of toxicity include tremor, ataxia, dysarthria, gastrointestinal disturbance, confusion and convulsions. It should therefore be stopped 24-72 hours before major surgery and the lithium level measured in the pre-operative period. As >95% of lithium is excreted by the kidney, urea and electrolyte levels should be monitored. This man has some renal impairment so is more susceptible to lithium toxicity;
  - lithium interacts with thyroid function and can produce hypothyroidism;

- long-term use of lithium can cause nephrogenic diabetes inspidus and reduced creatinine clearance. Nephrogenic diabetes insipidus produces symptoms such as polyuria and polydypsia.
- Problems due to drug interactions:
  - lithium enhances the effects of muscle relaxants;
  - it antagonises the effects of neostigmine;
  - an increased risk of toxicity when given with metronidazole;
  - an increased risk of toxicity when given with ibuprofen and diclofenac;
  - an increased risk of ventricular arrhythmias when administered with amiodarone;
  - the excretion of lithium is reduced by loop and thiazide diuretics leading to an increased risk of toxicity.

Serum lithium levels, urea, creatinine, TSH and thyroxine levels should be checked regularly.

What happens if lithium is stopped abruptly?

In a patient with a bipolar disorder, abrupt discontinuation of lithium increases the risk of relapse of mania. Lithium treatment should be gradually discontinued over at least 4 weeks to reduce this risk and preferably over a period of up to 3 months, particularly if the patient has a history of manic relapse (even if they have been commenced on another drug to treat mania).

How would you stop lithium in a patient having a major elective operation?

It is wise to stop lithium treatment for 24 hours pre-operatively, provided serum electrolytes are normal. Treatment should usually be resumed soon after the operation.

What are the possible causes of this man's renal dysfunction?

There could be two possible reasons:

- Uncontrolled hypertension.
- Long-term lithium use.

What are the major groups of antidepressants that you know of and how do they act?

The following are the major types of antidepressant drugs:

- Tricyclic antidepressants (TCAs).
- Monoamine oxidase inhibitors (MAOIs).
- Selective serotonin reuptake inhibitors (SSRIs).
- Serotonin and norepinephrine reuptake inhibitors (SNRI).
- Atypical agents such as lithium.

TCAs

Tricyclic antidepressants are tertiary amines (e.g. amitritptyline, imipramine and dothiepin) and are chemically related to phenothiazines. They block the neuronal uptake of norepinephrine and serotonin thereby increasing the concentration of these neurotransmitters in the synapse. They have minimal influence on dopaminergic synapses, and do not affect muscarinic acetyl choline and histamine receptors.

The side effects include sedation and anticholinergic effects (tachycardia, blurred vision, dry mouth, delayed gastric emptying and urinary retention). They also cause orthostatic hypotension and cardiac arrhythmias, and increase the duration of atrial and ventricular depolarisation. This is manifested by an increased PR and QT interval and wide QRS complexes on the ECG.

Tricyclic antidepressants may exaggerate the effect of sympathomimetic drugs, increasing the risk of arrhythmias and a possible hypertensive crisis. They also increase both the respiratory depressant effect of narcotics and the central effects of anticholinergic drugs, which may lead to 'central anticholinergic syndrome'.

MAOIs

Monoamine oxidase (MAO) causes de-amination of neurotransmitters. MAOIs inhibit MAO and increase the level of amine neurotransmitters.

There are two types:

◆ Irreversible MAOIs: phenelzine and tranylcypromine.
◆ Reversible MAOIs: moclobemide, which causes less potentiation of amines.

SSRIs

These cause selective inhibition of neuronal uptake of serotonin. (fluoxetine, citalopram, paroxetine). They do not have anticholinergic effects and have little effect on norepinephrine uptake. Fluoxetine is a potent inhibitor of hepatic cytochrome P_{450} enzymes. It potentiates the effect of other drugs which are metabolised by hepatic cytochrome P_{450}enzymes (e.g. tricyclic antidepressants).

Would you discontinue the use of TCAs or MAOIs pre-operatively?

MAOIs are usually discontinued 2 weeks before surgery and substituted with a TCA, but one should balance the risk of suicide in patients with severe depressive illness with the potential benefits of stopping the drug. Advice should be sought from a psychiatrist regarding modification of treatment during the peri-operative period. Current review of literature reveals that adverse drug interactions only occur in a minority of patients and that anaesthesia can be safely administered in these patients.

What is a 'cheese reaction'?

Gastrointestinal MAO usually inhibits dietary amines from entering the tissues, but when patients are on MAOIs it can cause a reaction with food rich in tyramine (cheese, certain red wines, pickled herring) or rich in dopamine, such as broad beans. This can occur for as long as 2 weeks after the last dose of MAOI. The most serious effects of this interaction are convulsions and hyperpyrexic coma (particularly after narcotics). This is called a 'cheese reaction'.

How would you manage intra-operative haemodynamic instability due to MAOIs?

Indirectly acting sympathomimetic agents depend on MAO for their metabolism, so if given with MAOIs can produce severe hypertension.

Those patients presenting for surgery and on MAOIs should not be given pethidine or any indirect adrenergic agonist such as ephedrine. Direct adrenergic agonists can be used as they depend on catechol O-methyl transferase (COMT) as well as MAO for their metabolism. They do not produce such an exaggerated hypertensive response as indirect agents. TCAs can be safely continued up to the day of surgery.

What is serotonin syndrome?

It is a potentially life-threatening adverse drug reaction that can occur following therapeutic drug use, inadvertent interactions between drugs, or the recreational use of certain drugs. It is a result of excess serotonergic activity produced at serotonin receptors, either peripherally or centrally. It is characterised by restlessness, sweating, tremor, shivering, muscle spasms, hyperthermia, confusion, convulsions and, ultimately, death.

It occurs classically with the combination of MAOIs and SSRIs. In its milder form it is treated by discontinuation of the drugs; in its more severe form it constitutes a medical emergency and requires symptomatic treatment, often in an intensive care unit.

What is neuroleptic malignant syndrome and how does it differ from serotonin syndrome?

Neuroleptic malignant syndrome (NMS) is a life-threatening, neurological disorder most often caused by an adverse reaction to neuroleptic or antipsychotic drugs. The clinical features of NMS and serotonergic syndrome are very similar. This can make the differentiation very difficult. The classical features of NMS are hyperthermia and muscle rigidity.

Why does he have polyuria?

The most likely cause for polyuria in this patient is lithium-induced diabetes insipidus (DI). It is characterised by excretion of large amounts of diluted urine.

In general, DI is caused either by a deficiency of ADH (cranial), or by an insensitivity of the kidneys to that hormone (nephrogenic). Lithium reduces the sensitivity of renal tubules to ADH. Patients with DI will have a raised plasma osmolality and a large volume of dilute urine.

To distinguish between the two forms of DI, the desmopressin stimulation test can be used. Desmopressin is administerd as an injection or a nasal spray. If the test results in a reduction of urine output and increases osmolarity, the pituitary production of ADH is deficient, and the kidneys respond normally. If the DI is due to renal pathology, the test does not change either urine output or osmolarity.

Can you read the chest X-ray in a systematic way?

This is a postero-anterior view of a chest X-ray in a male patient. It is an erect, centralised film with adequate exposure of lung fields, but the film is over penetrated as the intervertebral disc spaces are visible through the cardiac shadow. The chest X-ray can be interpreted in the following systematic way:

- A = airway: trachea in midline.
- B = bones: no obvious bony defects seen.
- C = cardiac silhouette: shape of heart and cardiothoracic ratio is within normal limit.
- D = diaphragm: left diaphragm is not clearly seen.
- E = effusion/empty space: no pneumothorax.
- F = fields (lungs): there is a homogeneous shadow in the left lower and mid zone of the lung field.
- G = gastric air bubble: this is present indicating that the X-ray is taken in an erect posture.
- H = hilar region: there is bilateral peri-hilar congestion.

The most probable diagnosis is pneumonia with consolidation of the left lower lobe and cardiac failure.

Can you comment on the ECG?

The ECG shows sinus rhythm with a heart rate of 100 bpm, the axis is normal and there is left ventricular hypertrophy (height of QRS in aVL is 14mm). It also shows ST depression in leads I, aVL and V6.

Would you anaesthetise this patient?

No, he has poorly controlled hypertension, renal dysfunction and lithium-induced diabetes insipidus. He also has a chest infection which needs to be treated prior to surgery. Further investigations and treatment will be guided by a detailed history and clinical examination. His further management requires a multidisciplinary team approach involving a consultant anaesthetist, psychiatrist and renal physician.

Once he has been optimised how would you anaesthetise him?

Pre-operatively

Tricyclic antidepressants and antihypertensive medications should be continued on the day of surgery. This patient may also require anxiolytics, such as temazepam, on the day of the surgery, as premedication.

Intra-operatively

Monitoring during anaesthesia includes peripheral oxygen saturation using pulse oximetry, continuous ECG and non-invasive blood pressure measurement.

Induction of anaesthesia

Following pre-oxygenation anaesthesia can be induced using an intravenous induction agent. As this patient needs full dental clearance, a nasal intubation may be required. It is important to discuss the airway management plan with the surgeon. A throat pack should be inserted to prevent soiling of the airway from blood and debris. The temperature should be monitored during the peri-operative period. Anaesthesia should be maintained with oxygen and a volatile agent (isoflurane, desflurane or sevoflurane) with or without nitrous oxide. Maintenance fluids should be supplemented intravenously during the intra-operative period to maintain adequate hydration. Due to impaired renal function excessive use of intravenous fluids should be avoided. Infiltration of local anaesthetic provides postoperative analgesia.

Lidocaine 2% with epinephrine 1:80,000 is usually given by the surgeon. In this patient, epinephrine should be best avoided as it may result in cardiac arrhythmias due to the presence of tricyclic antidepressants.

Recovery and extubation

After completing the procedure the pharynx should be suctioned and the throat pack removed. After reversing the neuromuscular blockade the trachea should be extubated when the patient is awake.

Postoperative analgesia can be provided with regular paracetamol and weak opioids such as codeine phosphate. In view of the impaired renal function, NSAIDs should be avoided.

Tricyclic (TCA) overdose

The toxic effects of TCAs are due to the anticholinergic effects, inhibition of norepinephrine and serotonin reuptake, and blockade of fast sodium channels in myocardial cells, resulting in membrane-stabilising effects. The major effects are due to cardiovascular instability and CNS toxicity.

Clinical features of TCA overdose

Cardiovascular system
Hypotension, tachycardia, bradycardia and asystole may develop. Prolongation of the QT interval can lead to ventricular dysrhythmias (ventricular tachycardia and ventricular fibrillation, and impaired conduction resulting in heart blocks).

Central nervous system
Agitation, excitability, muscle rigidity, delirium, seizures and coma. Anticholinergic effects include a dry mouth, flushing, mydriasis, blurred vision and urinary retention. Other effects include respiratory and/or metabolic acidosis.

Management of TCA overdose

The management of tricyclic overdose is mainly supportive. Initial measures include supporting the airway, administration of 100% oxygen and supporting the circulation. Tracheal intubation and ventilatory support may be required in the presence of CNS depression, impending respiratory failure and uncontrolled seizures.

Continuous ECG and SpO_2 monitoring along with non-invasive or invasive blood pressure monitoring should be established.

Activated charcoal should be administered as soon as possible. If the patient presents within an hour of taking drugs, gastric lavage may be useful.

Seizures should be treated with benzodiazepines.

As tricyclics have a large volume of distribution and a high level of protein binding, haemodialysis is not effective.

Treatment of cardiac arrhythmias includes supportive measures to correct acidosis, and intravenous fluids to correct hypovolaemia. Class IA, class IC, class II, and class III anti-arrhythmic drugs should be avoided. Class IA and IC drugs block sodium channels and prolong depolarisation. Class II drugs (beta-blockers) depress myocardial contractility and worsen the hypotension. Class III drugs (amiodarone, sotalol) prolong the repolarisation (QT interval). Class IB drugs (phenytoin and lidocaine) and magnesium are useful in treating arrhythmias.

Sodium bicarbonate therapy may be used to correct the acidosis. Tricyclic-specific fragment binding antigens (FABs) have been shown to reverse the cardiotoxicity in animal studies.

Key points

◆ Lithium has a very narrow therapeutic/toxic ratio.
◆ The serum lithium, urea, creatinine, TSH and thyroxine levels should be checked regularly.
◆ Dental procedures involve a shared airway. It is important to safeguard the airway to protect it from blood, secretions and tooth debris.

Further reading

1. NICE guidelines for management of hypertension. http://www.nice.org.uk/nicemedia/pdf/CG034NICEguideline.pdf.
2. Standards and guidelines for general anaesthesia for dentistry, February 1999. Royal College of Anaesthetists http://www.rcoa.ac.uk/docs/dental.pdf.
3. Psychiatric disease and substance abuse. In: *Anesthesia and co-existing disease*, 4th ed. Stoelting RK, Dierdorf SF, Eds. Philadelphia: Churchill Livingstone, 2002; Chapter 29: 629-54.
4. Central nervous system. In: *Pharmacology for anaesthesia and intensive care*, 2nd ed. Peck TE, Williams M, Hill SA. Cambridge: Cambridge University Press, 2003; Chapter 18: 271-83.

Short case 7.1: Carotid endarterectomy

A 68-year-old male patient is scheduled for coronary artery bypass grafting (CABG). During the pre-operative assessment he is found to have a 90% stenosis of his right carotid artery and is now scheduled for carotid endarterectomy under local anaesthetic.

What comorbidities would you expect in a patient presenting for carotid endarterectomy?

These patients are often elderly with significant cardiovascular comorbidities and peripheral vascular disease:

◆ Central nervous system: cerebrovascular disease with transient ischaemic attacks and stroke.
◆ Cardiovascular: ischaemic heart disease and hypertension.
◆ Respiratory: COAD and chest infection.
◆ Endocrine: diabetes and hypothyroidism.
◆ Renal system: impaired renal function.
◆ Pharmacology: they are likely to be on medications such as aspirin and other antiplatelet drugs (dipyridamole, clopidogrel).

The risk factors for ischaemic stroke include systemic hypertension, smoking, hyperlipidaemia, diabetes mellitus and excessive alcohol consumption.

What is the incidence and what are the risks of carotid artery disease?

Significant carotid artery disease increases the risk of ischaemic stroke. Approximately 1% of the British population over the age of 75 years will die as a result of carotid artery disease each year. The rate of peri-operative stroke has been reported as 7%. Peri-operative mortality from myocardial infarction as well as stroke is 5% for symptomatic and 3% for asymptomatic carotid stenosis.

What are the indications for carotid endarterectomy?

- Symptomatic patients with greater than 70% stenosis: clear benefit was found in the North American Symptomatic Carotid Endarterectomy Trial (NASCET).
- Syptomatic patients with 50-69% stenosis: benefit is marginal and appears to be greater for male patients.

What are the anaesthetic options for carotid endarterectomy?

The options are:

- Local infiltration.
- Cervical epidural: not widely used in the UK.
- Deep cervical plexus block.
- Deep cervical and superficial cervical plexus block.
- Superficial cervical plexus block with local infiltration.
- General anaesthesia.

The GALA trial is an ongoing multicentre randomised trial assessing the relative risks of stroke, cardiac events and death following carotid endarterectomy under general or local anaesthesia. It was also designed to assess whether the type of anaesthesia influences peri-operative morbidity and mortality. Some of the non-randomised studies have suggested the potential benefit of regional anaesthesia in reducing the risk of peri-operative stroke.

What nerves do you need to block for the surgery?

The main nerves that need to be blocked for this operation are C2, C3, C4, branches of the trigeminal nerve, supplying the submandibular region, and carotid sheath infiltration.

How would you perform a deep cervical plexus block?

The deep cervical plexus can be blocked with a single level (Winnie) or injection of local anaesthetic at three levels (Moore).

Monitoring

Peripheral oxygen saturation using pulse oximetry, continuous ECG monitoring and invasive blood pressure monitoring should be established.

Position

The patient lies supine, with their head resting on a pillow and turned opposite to the side of surgery.

Asepsis

The area around the neck should be cleaned with antiseptic solution and draped with sterile drapes.

Landmarks

The mastoid process (corresponds to the level of C1) and transverse process of C6 (Chassaignac tubercle) at the level of the cricoid cartilage should be marked. A line is drawn between the two points (mastoid process and Chassaignac tubercle). A second line is drawn, 1cm posterior and parallel to the first line. The C2 transverse process lies 1-2cm caudal to the mastoid process on the second line; the C3 transverse process lies 1-2cm below the C2 transverse process; the C4 transverse process lies 1-2cm below the C3 transverse process.

Technique

Lidocaine 1% is infiltrated into the skin at the levels of the C2, C3 and C4 transverse processes (0.25ml at each space). A short bevelled 22G needle is then inserted at each level, aiming slightly posteriorly and caudad, to reduce the risk of intrathecal or intra-arterial injection. The needle is advanced until either the transverse process is encountered, or paraesthesia is elicited. After careful aspiration, 3ml of plain bupivacaine 0.5% is injected at each site. Eliciting paraesthesia may increase efficacy of the block but may also increase the risk of undesirable consequences, including postoperative dysaesthesia and intrathecal or intra-arterial injection, as a consequence of further needle manipulation.

What are the complications of a deep cervical plexus block?

- Subarachnoid injection.
- Epidural injection.
- Intravascular injection.
- Local haematoma.
- Phrenic nerve palsy.
- Transient recurrent laryngeal nerve palsy.
- Horner's syndrome (ptosis, miosis, anhydrosis, enophthalmos).
- Stellate ganglion block.

How would you perform superficial cervical plexus block?

This may be performed in conjunction with a deep cervical plexus block.

Position

The patient lies supine, with their head resting on a pillow and turned opposite to the side of surgery.

Landmarks

The posterior border of the sternocleidomastoid muscle is identified by asking the patient to raise his/her head and the midpoint is marked. The external jugular vein usually crosses the muscle 1-2cm below this point.

Technique

Using a 22G needle, 20ml of local anaesthetic (LA) solution is injected between the skin and muscle in an upward and downward direction at the above point. The LA should ideally spread along the posterior border of the muscle.

Complications (rare)

◆ Damage to the superficial nerves.
◆ Local haematoma.
◆ Intravenous injection of local anaesthetic.

A systematic review in the *British Journal of Anaesthesia* (2007) of complications of superficial and deep cervical plexus block for carotid endarterectomy concluded that superficial cervical plexus block is safer than deep cervical plexus block. There was a higher rate of conversion to general anaesthesia with the deep and combined block and it may have been influenced by the higher incidence of direct complications due to these blocks, but may also suggest that the superficial/combined block provides better analgesia during surgery.

The surgeon has opened the artery and the patient becomes confused and develops a reduced level of consciousness; what would you do?

A patient who was previously fully conscious who suddenly becomes confused and has a reduced level of consciousness may be suffering from reduced blood flow to the same side cerebral hemisphere. The main aim should be to improve blood flow as soon as possible.

The possible options are:

◆ Use a shunt to divert blood flow above the level of the clamp (performed by the vascular surgeon).
◆ Increase blood pressure and rely on collateral circulation.
◆ Convert to general anaesthesia.

How would you monitor cerebral functions?

Cerebral function monitoring enables early detection of inadequate cerebral perfusion during cross-clamp. There are many ways of monitoring cerebral function:

◆ Awake patient. An awake patient is able to communicate with symptoms of inadequate cerebral perfusion.
◆ Carotid artery stump pressure. A needle or cannula is inserted into the common carotid artery and connected to a transducer to measure the mean pressure before cross-clamping. A mean pressure less than 50mmHg has been reported to be a reliable predictor of ischaemia.
◆ Transcranial Doppler monitoring. This assesses blood flow velocity and emboli in the middle cerebral artery and also helps to asses shunt function.
◆ Near infrared spectroscopy measures oxygenation in the cerebral hemisphere. It is based on the principle that light near the infrared region is transmitted through biological tissues.
◆ EEG monitoring has proved to be a sensitive indicator of cerebral ischaemia, but specificity is limited due to similar changes associated with hypothermia, hypotension and general anaesthesia. EEG monitoring equipment is expensive, cumbersome and is difficult to interpret.
◆ Cerebral function monitoring. This is a form of processed EEG. It filters the EEG input from a single channel and displays the average voltage.
◆ Somatosensory-evoked potentials. This is electrical activity recorded from the CNS following repeated peripheral stimulation. This is not commonly used.

What are the postoperative complications which may be seen following carotid endarterectomy?

◆ Hypertension. This can cause a neurologic deficit by causing hyperperfusion syndrome and possibly leading to an intracerebral bleed.
◆ Hypotension.
◆ Myocardial infarction.
◆ Stroke (usually embolic).
◆ Bleeding - possibly causing airway obstruction.

◆ Cranial nerve injury.
◆ Damage to the carotid body.

General anaesthesia versus regional anaesthesia for carotid surgery

The proposed benefits of regional anaesthesia include the ability to monitor neurological function, reduced shunt usage and reduced postoperative hospital stay. The GALA trial, a large multicentre trial, compared general anaesthesia (GA) versus local anaesthesia (LA) for carotid surgery. The main findings of this trial were:

◆ GA was associated with a slightly higher risk of peri-operative stroke, myocardial infarction, and death, as compared with LA but this was not statistically significant.
◆ LA is associated with a reduced rate of shunt insertion.
◆ Deep cervical plexus block was associated with an increased occurrence of complications in comparison with superficial cervical plexus block.
◆ Blood concentrations of norepinephrine and systolic blood pressure were higher in patients operated under LA possibly indicating high anxiety or insufficient block.
◆ No difference in the duration of surgery, time spent in critical care units, or the overall length of stay in hospital.
◆ No difference in quality of life at about 1 month after surgery.

Key points

◆ Regional anaesthesia with awake patients may be one of the best ways of monitoring cerebral function during carotid endarterectomy.
◆ A recent systematic review of complications of superficial and deep cervical plexus block suggests that superficial cervical plexus block is safer than deep cervical plexus block.

Further reading

1. Pandit JJ, Sathya-Krishna R, Gration P. Superficial or deep cervical plexus block for carotid endarterectomy: a systematic review of complications. *British Journal of Anaesthesia* 2007; 99: 159-69.

2. Chassot PG, Delabays A, Spahn DR. Preoperative evaluation of patients with, or at risk of, coronary artery disease undergoing non-cardiac surgery. *British Journal of Anaesthesia* 2002; 89: 747-59.
3. Bowyer MW, Zierold D, Loftus JP, *et al.* Carotid endarterectomy: a comparison of regional versus general anesthesia in 500 operations. *Annals of Vascular Surgery* 2000; 14: 145-51.
4. Sternbach Y, Illig KA, Zhang R, Shortell CK, Jeffrey M, Davies MG, Lyden SP, Green RM. Hemodynamic benefits of regional anesthesia for carotid endarterectomy. *Journal of Vascular Surgery* 2002; 35: 333-9.
5. GALA Trial Collaborative Group. General anaesthesia versus local anaesthesia for carotid surgery (GALA): a multicentre, randomised controlled trial. *The Lancet* 2008; 372: 2132-42.

Short case 7.2: Trifascicular heart block

A 68-year-old lady is scheduled for an extended right hemicolectomy. She is known to have hypertension, COAD and has had two previous episodes of myocardial infarction. Her regular medications are a salbutamol inhaler, aspirin, GTN spray and amlodipine.

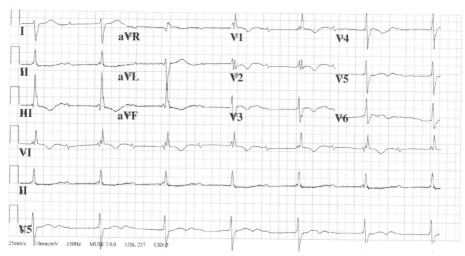

Figure 7.3 ECG.

Describe this ECG

This is a 12-lead ECG, calibrated at 1mV per cm and recorded at a speed of 25mm/sec. The heart rate is 42 per minute. There is a prolonged PR interval, right bundle branch block (RBBB), a wide QRS in V5 and V6 and right axis deviation (left posterior hemi-block), and T inversion in V1 to V6.

What information does the axis give in this situation?

♦ RBBB with left axis deviation is suggestive of left anterior hemi-block.
♦ RBBB with right axis deviation is suggestive of left posterior hemi-block.

Do you think this patient requires pacing before coming for surgery and why?

Yes, this patient will benefit from pacing prior to major surgery as there is a risk of complete heart block.

What are the different types of heart block?

Heart block can be classified according to the site of the block in the conduction system:

♦ Sinoatrial (SA) nodal block.
♦ Atrioventricular (AV) block.
♦ Bundle branch block.

In clinical practice AV block and bundle branch block are commonly encountered.

Atrioventricular (AV) block

AV block is due to a delay in conduction of the atrial impulse through the atrioventricular node and bundle of His. The impulse is either transmitted to the ventricles with certain delay or it may completely fail to reach the ventricles.

There are three types of AV blocks:

- First-degree AV block is characterised by a prolonged PR interval. All P waves are followed by a QRS complex. Causes of first-degree heart block include ischaemic heart disease, digoxin and beta-blockers.
- Second-degree AV block is characterised by intermittent absence of QRS complexes. In Mobitz type I AV block, the PR interval progressively increases and, finally, a QRS complex disappears. This is known as the Wenkebach phenomenon. In Mobitz type II AV block, there is a fixed drop in the QRS complex with a variable ratio of P wave to QRS complex (2:1, 3:2 or 3:1). This type of block is always pathological and can frequently progress to complete heart block.
- Third-degree AV block is characterised by complete block of all atrial impulses. Atrial and ventricular rhythms are independent and asynchronous. It is characterised by atrioventricular dissociation (P waves bear no relation to the QRS complexes), abnormal QRS complexes, and a slow ventricular rate.

Bundle branch block

This can either be block of the left bundle, right bundle or a combination of both. In left bundle branch block the left ventricle is activated from the right bundle branch which passes to the left side of the septum distal to the block. Block of the left anterior hemi-fascicle is characterised by left axis deviation in the absence of inferior myocardial infarction or other cause of left axis deviation. Block of the left posterior hemi-fascicle is characterised by right axis deviation. Bifascicular block is the combination of right bundle branch block and left anterior or posterior hemi-block.

Left bundle branch block is characterised by the following:

- Wide QRS of more than 0.1 second in leads V5 and V6.
- Wide notched R wave in leads 1, V5 and V6.
- Prominent, notched QS complex in lead V1.
- Absence of Q wave in leads V5 and V6.

In right bundle branch block, the right ventricle is activated by impulses from the left bundle branch through the septum, distal to the level of block. Right bundle branch block is characterised by:

- Wide QRS more than 0.1 second in leads V1 and V2.
- Secondary R wave in lead V1.
- Delayed S wave in lead 1.

Bifascicular block in association with first-degree heart block is known as trifascicular block.

What are the indications for cardiac pacing?

The following are indications for pacing:

- Sinus node: sick sinus syndrome, recurrent Stoke-Adams syndrome, sinus node dysfunction.
- Conduction system: complete heart block, symptomatic second-degree heart block, symptomatic bifascicular and trifascicular heart block.
- Chronic atrial fibrillation.
- Persistent and symptomatic second- or third-degree AV block associated with myocardial infarction.
- Atrio-biventricular pacing in moderate to severe heart failure.

Outline the pacemaker codes

The pacemaker type and function is described using a five letter code:

- The first letter describes the chamber paced.
- The second letter describes the chamber sensed.
- The third letter describes the response to sensing.
- The fourth letter describes the rate modulation or programmability.
- The fifth letter describes the anti-tachycardia function.

Table 7.3 Five letter pacemaker codes.

Chamber paced	Chamber sensed	Response to sensing	Rate modulation	Anti-tachycardia function
Atria (A)	Atria (A)	Triggered (T)	Rate modulated (R)	Pacing (P)
Ventricle (V)	Ventricle (V)	Inhibited (I)	No action (O)	Shocking (S)
Dual (D)	Dual (D)	Dual (D)		Dual (D)
No action (O)	No action (O)	No action (O)		No action (O)

What is the advantage of dual chamber pacing as opposed to sole ventricular pacing?

The advantage is its ability to maintain AV synchrony. The atria are responsible for 25-30% of ventricular filling. The loss of atrial kick can cause hypotension and decreased output in some patients.

What do you understand by the pacing threshold?

This is the threshold of the amount of energy needed to capture the atrium and/or ventricle. The level is determined by gradually decreasing the output in milliamperes until 1:1 capture is lost. The threshold should then be set at 2-3 times the current at which capture is lost.

What are rate-adaptive pacemakers?

These are pacemakers that have sensors that can increase the pacing rate with exercise and demand. They are identifiable by the letter R in the fourth position of the pacemaker code. They lead to subjective improvement in cardiac output and other haemodynamic variables.

Pre-operatively, how can you identify if the heart rate is completely pacemaker-dependent?

By performing a 12-lead ECG (there will be a pacemaker spike before every QRS complex).

Peri-operative management of patients with pacemakers

There are two important aspects of managing patients with a pacemaker during the peri-operative period:

- Ensuring that the pacemaker is functioning optimally.
- Ensuring that external electrical devices such as diathermy do not interfere with pacemaker function.

Pre-operatively

During pre-operative assessment there should be a detailed history including the indication for pacemaker insertion, hospital, date of insertion, type of pacemaker, model and serial number, along with the manufacturer and presence of any cardiovascular symptoms should be elicited. Most often these patients carry a registration card or passport with all the relevant details. Prior to surgery the implications of a pacemaker should be discussed with the surgeon. The pacemaker technician and the cardiologist should be informed. The pacemaker function and battery condition should have been checked within the last 3 months. During the intra-operative period, the pacemaker should be programmed so that inappropriate inhibition from electrical interference is minimised. A 12-lead ECG should be recorded to assess whether the patient is dependent on the pacemaker. It may also give additional information such as whether it is an atrial or ventricular pacemaker. A chest X-ray may be useful for checking the integrity of pacing leads.

Intra-operatively

Temporary external or transvenous pacing facilities should be available:

- Monitor cardiac rhythm and the peripheral pulse with a pulse oximeter and possibly intra-arterial monitoring.
- Bipolar diathermy is preferable to monopolar.
- If monopolar diathermy is unavoidable, limit its use to short bursts. Current strength and duration should be minimal.
- Place the earth plate as far away from the pacemaker to prevent electricity from crossing the generator-heart circuit.

- Ensure that diathermy cables are kept well way from the pacemaker site.

Care should be taken with central venous catheterisation, since it may dislodge the electrodes. Isoprenaline should be available to treat bradycardia associated with complete heart block in the event of pacemaker failure.

Postoperatively

Pacemaker function should be checked.

For emergency surgery the above procedure should be followed if possible. If it is not possible, the pacemaker should at least be checked before and after the procedure. The external defibrillator and cardiopulmonary resuscitation facility should be available.

For implantable cardioverter defibrillators, the shocking mode should be disabled, and defibrillator pads should be attached and connected to the defibrillator. The heart rhythm should be continuously monitored and if the rhythm changes to ventricular fibrillation (VF), the heart should be manually defibrillated using an external defibrillator.

Role of the magnet

A magnet placed over the pulse generator triggers the reed switch and converts the pulse generator into a non-sensing asynchronous mode. Switching to this asynchronous mode may trigger ventricular asynchrony in patients with myocardial ischaemia. The use of a magnet may be associated with the following problems:

- In the presence of electromagnetic interference (EMI) the magnet may alter the programmability of the pacemaker, resulting in malfunction.
- The response to application of the magnet varies from device to device.
- Its use is not indicated for programmable pacemakers.

(For further details on automated implantable cardioverter defibrillators please refer to section 2.4: Equipment, clinical measurement and monitoring in SOE2.)

Key points

♦ A symptomatic bifasicular or trifascicular block may require pacing prior to any major surgery.
♦ Diathermy can interfere with pacemaker function.
♦ It is important that in every patient with a pacemaker the appropriate precautions are taken in the peri-operative period.

Further reading

1. Saluke TV, Dob D, Sutton R. Pacemakers and defibrillators: anaesthetic implications. *British Journal of Anaesthesia* 2004: 93: 95-104.

2. Atlee JL, Bernstein AD. Cardiac rhythm management devices. Part I - indications, device selection and function. *Anesthesiology* 2001; 95: 1265-80.

3. Atlee JL, Bernstein AD. Cardiac rhythm management devices. Part II - perioperative management. *Anesthesiology* 2001; 95: 1492-506.

4. Guidelines for perioperative management of patients with implantable pacemakers or implantable cardioverter defibrillators, where the use of surgical diathermy/electrocautery is anticipated. http://www.mhra. gov.uk/Safetyinformation/Generalsafetyinformationandadvice.

Short case 7.3: Burns

A 30-year-old man is brought into the emergency department. He has been rescued from a house fire. He has burns to his face, arms and trunk.

How would you manage this patient?

This patient should be managed according to ATLS® guidelines. Both assessment and management should be carried out simultaneously.

Primary survey

Assessment and management of airway, control of cervical spine and administration of 100% oxygen.

If there are features of direct burns to the face, or inhalational injury, the airway may be compromised rapidly. Even if the airway is patent at that point in time there should be a very low threshold for early intubation. The features of inhalational injury include singeing of nasal hair, carbonaeceous soot in the sputum, and a hoarse voice. Succinylcholine can be used safely within the first 24 hours. Endotracheal tubes of various sizes should be available. Because of the airway oedema, intubation with a normal sized endotracheal tube may not be possible. In the presence of signs of upper airway obstruction (hoarseness, stridor, change of voice or a swollen uvula), muscle relaxants should be avoided and the patient should be anaesthetised using an inhalational technique.

Breathing

Breathing should be assessed clinically and one should bear in mind that pulse oximetry may over-read the oxygen saturation in the presence of carbon monoxide poisoning. Full-thickness burns around the chest can cause limited chest movements and escharotomy should be considered to improve ventilation.

Circulation and control of bleeding

Two large intravenous cannulae should be sited as soon as possible preferably through unburned skin, and a rapid assessment of the circulatory status should be made. Blood samples should be sent for a full blood count, urea and electrolytes, group and save/cross-match, and arterial blood gases along with carboxyhaemoblobin level. Patients may have potentially co-existing injury which may compromise the circulation. Warmed crystalloids should be administered.

The Parkland formula is often used to calculate the fluid requirement during the first 24 hours. The fluid required in the first 24 hours (from the time of burn) is 4ml/kg/% of total body surface area (TBSA) burned. Half of the calculated volume is given in the first 8 hours (from the time of burn) and the rest of the fluid is given over the next 16 hours. The normal maintenance fluid of 1-2ml/kg body weight should also be administered.

Fluid requirement in the first 24 hours = 4ml x weight in kg x % of burn.

Disability

Neurological assessment should be performed with the AVPU scale or Glasgow Coma Scale and assessing size and reactivity of the pupils. (AVPU = alert, vocalising, responding to pain, unconscious.)

Exposure

The patient should be completely exposed, and the degree of burn assessed. Burns patients can lose heat very rapidly so they should be kept warm.

Monitoring during resuscitation should include continuous peripheral oxygen saturation, ECG, blood pressure, fluid balance (input/output chart), hourly urine output and temperature.

Secondary survey

Close examination of the burn and assessment of the depth and degree of burn.

What problems might you encounter when monitoring burns patients?

- ECG. The ordinary gel electrodes may not pick up the signal through the damaged skin and the operating field may need to be avoided while placing the electrodes. Subcutaneous needle electrodes can be used.
- Pulse oximetry. It may over-read in the presence of carboxyhaemoglobin. Peripheral burns and vasoconstriction may lead to a poor trace and inaccurate values.
- . Blood pressure. It may be difficult to place the cuff if the arms are burned. The waveform of invasive blood pressure monitoring will provide extra information, and access to blood sampling is an additional benefit.
- Central venous pressure. Access may be difficult and there is an increased risk of infection from the entry site. Peripherally inserted long lines may be useful.

How would you classify a burn according to its depth?

- First-degree burn (superficial): limited to the epidermis and characterised by erythema, white plaque and minor pain.
- Second-degree burn (partial thickness): characterised by erythema and blistering. It may be very painful depending on the level of nerve involvement.
- Third-degree burn (full thickness): characterised by charring and extensive damage of the dermis.

How would you estimate the total body surface area involved in burns?

The total body surface area is estimated using the 'rule of nine', where each upper limb is 9%, each lower limb is 18%, the front of the trunk 18%, back of the trunk 18%, head 9% and neck 1%.

In children it is slightly modified; the relatively larger surface area of the head accounts for 18%. According to the age of the child the surface area of the body parts changes. Specific burn charts based on age of the child are available.

When will you refer a burns patient to a burns unit?

According to the British Burns Association the criteria for referral to a burns unit are:

- Total body surface area burnt: >10% TBSA in adults or >5% TBSA in children with dermal or full-thickness burns.
- Age: <5 years or >60 years of age.
- Areas involved: burns to hands, face, feet, genitals, perineum, major joints.
- Type of injury: inhalational injuries, chemical burns involving >5% TBSA, electrical burns.
- Special circumstances: burns with associated trauma, burns in patients with pre-existing diseases which may compromise the care and recovery of the patient, and pregnancy.

What would make you suspect an inhalation injury?

- History: burns in an enclosed space, inhalation and intoxication by toxic fumes (plastic).
- On examination:
  - facial burns;
  - singeing of hair in nostrils and eyebrows and eyelashes;
  - soot on face and in the sputum;
  - hoarseness or change of voice;
  - stridor.

How would you treat this patient's pain in the emergency department?

Cooling the patient's skin with tepid or cold water will terminate the burning process and reduce pain.

Small burns can be treated with paracetamol and NSAIDs and in more severe burns the mainstay is IV morphine titrated in small boluses until the patient is comfortable. Care should be given in shocked and elderly patients whilst administering opioids.

The other options available are:

- Patient-controlled analgesia.
- Ketamine.
- Inhalation of entonox: this is commonly used for changing dressings.

Two weeks later this patient presents for a skin graft for a wound on the chest. How would you anaesthetise this patient?

Pre-operative assessment

Pre-operative assessment includes a full history (any associated injury, history of epilepsy) and clinical examination. In addition to regular analgesia, the patient may require temazepam as an anxiolytic. The pre-operative haemoglobin should be checked and blood should be available for intra-operative transfusion.

Intra-operative monitoring

Intra-operative monitoring includes ECG, SpO_2, $ETCO_2$, NIBP, core temperature and urine output.

Induction of anaesthesia

Following pre-oxygenation, anaesthesia is induced with propofol or thiopentone. Muscle relaxation and tracheal intubation can be facilitated by a non-depolarising muscle relaxant such as vecuronium or atracurium. Succinylcholine should be avoided as a hyperkalaemic response is elicited from extrajunctional acetylcholine receptors. To avoid hypothermia, a warming mattress and warm intravenous fluids should be used. The wound debridement may involve significant fluid and blood loss. Burns patients have increased loss of fluid from evaporation.

It is important to also provide analgesia for the donor site. Local anaesthetic gel (e.g. 0.5% bupivacaine mixed with an equal quantity of aqueous gel) can be applied under the dressing.

Postoperatively

During the postoperative period analgesia should be provided using paracetamol, NSAIDs and opioids. PCA morphine has been found to be effective. Tolerance to opioids may develop and the patient may require large doses. An adjuvant such as ketamine may be useful.

Fluid management in burns

Adult patients with a burn greater than 15% of the total body surface area, and children with a burn greater than 10% require intravenous fluid resuscitation. There are various formulae available to calculate fluid requirement. These formulae are for guidance only and the actual fluid management should be determined by the clinical situation and frequent assessment of hydration status with parameters such as urine output.

The Parkland formula is widely used in the UK, and estimates total fluid requirement for the first 24 hours. A urinary catheter should be inserted to monitor the hourly urine output. There is a tendency for generalised capillary leaking and increased third space fluid loss. Crystalloids, usually Hartmann's (lactated Ringer's) solution, are generally used. Hourly urine output should be aimed at greater than 0.5ml/kg in adults and 1ml/kg in children.

Anaesthesia for dressing changes

Burns patient may require frequent change of dressings. A large burns dressing may take 1-2 hours to change. The anaesthetic options available are:

- General anaesthesia.
- Entonox supplemented with opioid analgesia.
- Intravenous sedation with benzodiazepines or propofol or a volatile anaesthetic agent.
- Intravenous ketamine.

Key points

- The initial assessment of a burns patient should be based on ATLS® trauma guidelines.
- In a burns patient with inhalational injury there should be a very low threshold for early intubation. The airway in these patients can become compromised very rapidly.
- Fluid management and analgesia are important components in the management of a burns patient.

Further reading

1. Referral criteria to burns centre. British Burns Association. http://www.britishburnsassociation.co.uk/.
2. Hilton PJ, Hepp M, The immediate care of the burned patient. *British Journal of Anaesthesia, CEPD Review* 2001; 1: 113-6.
3. Fenlon S, Nene S. Burns in children. *British Journal of Anaesthesia CEACCP* 2007; 7: 76-80.

4. Black RG, Kinsella J. Anaesthetic management for burns patients. *British Journal of Anaesthesia, CEPD Review* 2001; 1: 177-80.
5. Norman AT, Judkins KC. Pain in the patient with burns. *British Journal of Anaesthesia CEACCP* 2004; 4: 57-60.

Applied anatomy 7.1: Anatomy of the nose

Clinical Science

A 40-year-old female patient is scheduled for laparoscopic cholecystectomy. Her mouth opening is limited to 2cm due to ankylosis of the temporomandibular joint.

What is your preferred option for tracheal intubation in this patient?

Awake fibreoptic intubation via the nasal route is the preferred option.

You have chosen to do an awake nasal fibreoptic intubation. Describe the anatomical structures in the nose that you need to identify while inserting the fibreoptic scope

The important structures that should be identified during anterior rhinoscopy are the septum of the nose, the inferior turbinate and the floor of the nose. The intention is to advance the fibreoptic scope into the airspace between the floor of the nose and inferior turbinate.

Describe the anatomy of the nose in more detail

The nose is a pyramidal-shaped structure made up of bone and cartilage. A midline nasal septum divides the nose into two nasal cavities. The vestibule is the entrance to the nose which is lined with skin. The nasal cavity opens anteriorly onto the face via the nares and communicates posteriorly with the nasopharynx via the choane.

The roof of the nose is tent-shaped. The anterior third slopes downward and forward to the tip of the nose, the middle third is horizontal, and the posterior third slopes downward and backward. The anterior part is formed by the nasal cartilages and nasal bones. The middle third is formed by the cribriform plate of the ethmoid bone. The olfactory nerves perforate the cribriform plate and gain access to the olfactory bulb in the anterior cranial fossa. The posterior third of the roof is formed by the body of the sphenoid.

The floor is formed by the horizontal plate of the palatine bone and palatine process of the maxilla.

In the medial wall the anterior part of the nasal septum is formed by the septal cartilage. The posterior part is formed by the perpendicular plate of the ethmoid bone and vomer bone.

The lateral wall contains three turbinates or conche (superior, middle and inferior). They are covered by a highly vascular mucous membrane. The bony framework of the lateral wall is made up of the nasal aspect of the ethmoidal labyrinth (above), nasal surface of the maxilla (below) and perpendicular plate of the palatine bone (behind). The lateral wall lies medial to the orbit, ethmoid and maxillary sinuses and pterygopalatine fossa.

Table 7.4 Boundaries of the nose.

Part of the nose	Bones and components
Roof	Nasal cartilages, nasal bones, cribriform plate and body of the sphenoid
Floor	Horizontal plate of the palatine bone and palatine process of the maxilla
Medial wall	Septal cartilage, ethmoid and vomer
Lateral wall	Maxilla, lacrimal bone, ethmoid and palatine bone

What is the blood supply to the nose?

The arterial supply of the external nose is derived from the lateral branches of the facial, dorsal branch of the ophthalmic artery and infra-orbital branch of the maxillary artery. The sphenopalatine artery (a branch of the maxillary artery) provides blood supply to the anterior part of the inner aspect of the nose. The maxillary artery is a branch arising from the external carotid artery. The anterior and posterior ethmoidal branches of the ophthalmic artery supply the roof of the nose and nasal sinuses.

The ophthalmic artery is a branch arising from the internal carotid artery, and the labial and palatine from the facial artery.

Venous drainage is via a submucous plexus which drains into the facial, sphenopalatine and ophthalmic veins.

Table 7.5 Blood supply to the nose.		
Region of the nose	**Blood supply**	
	Main artery	**Branches**
External nose	Internal carotid	Ophthalmic artery
	External carotid	Facial and maxillary artery
Internal aspect of nose		
Anterior part	External carotid	Facial and maxillary artery
Roof of the nose	Internal carotid	Ophthalmic artery
Nasal sinuses	Internal carotid	Ophthalmic artery

What is Little's area?

This is the most common site for epistaxis. It is the area on the antero-inferior part of the nasal septum where the sphenopalatine branch of the maxillary artery anastomoses with the septal branch of the superior labial artery.

What is the nerve supply to the nose?

The trigeminal nerve divides into three divisions: the ophthalmic, maxillary and the mandibular. The ophthalmic and maxillary divisions provide sensory supply to the nose.

The anterior ethmoidal and nasociliary nerves (branches of the ophthalmic division of the trigeminal) provide sensory innervation to the bridge and tip of the nose.

The vestibule of the nose is supplied by the external nasal branches of the ophthalmic division and the infra-orbital branch of the maxillary division.

Septum

- Anterior and superior region: anterior ethmoidal branch of the ophthalmic division.
- Posterior and inferior region: nasopalatine branch of the maxillary division.

Lateral wall and floor

- Anterior and superior region of the lateral wall: anterior ethmoidal branch of the ophthalmic division.
- Anterior and inferior region: superior alveolar branch of the maxillary division.
- Posterior and superior region: posterior and inferior nasal branches of the maxillary division via the pterygopalatine ganglion.
- Posterior and inferior region: the greater palatine nerves of the maxillary division via the pterygopalatine ganglion.

Table 7.6 Nerve supply to the nose.

Part of the nose	Region	Division of trigeminal nerve	Branches
External nose	Vestibule and bridge of the nose	Ophthalmic	Anterior ethmoidal and nasociliary
Septum	Anterior and superior	Ophthalmic	Anterior ethmoidal
	Posterior and inferior	Maxillary	Nasopalatine
Lateral wall and floor	Anterior and superior	Ophthalmic	Anterior ethmoidal
	Anterior and inferior	Maxillary	Superior alveolar
	Posterior and superior	Maxillary	Nasal branches
	Posterior and inferior	Maxillary	Greater palatine

What is the function of the nose?

Its primary function is to provide a passage for entry of air into the respiratory system where it is warmed and humidified as it passes through. It provides a sense of smell. It also helps in the control of infection in the airway.

Describe the technique of awake fibreoptic intubation

Even though it is described as awake fibreoptic intubation, conscious sedation is often used combined with local anaesthesia to the airway. The procedure along with the benefits and complications such as nasal bleeding and coughing should be explained to the patient.

Premedication

An antisialogogue (e.g. glycopyrrolate 200-300µg IM or hyoscine hydrobromide 200-400µg SC) should be given about 30 minutes before the procedure.

Preparation

The intubating fibreoptic scope, video-camera system, appropriate endotracheal tubes, drugs for local anaesthesia, sedation and general anaesthesia should be checked and prepared.

Patient positioning

The sitting-up position at 45° with the operator facing the patient is preferred.

Monitoring

Peripheral oxygen saturation, ECG and NIBP should be monitored during the procedure.

Oxygen is administered via nasal prongs or through the working channel of the fibreoptic scope.

Airway preparation

The selected nostril, nasopharynx, tongue, oropharynx and larynx are anaesthetised using local anaesthetic. The nose and nasopharynx are anaesthetised by spraying the nose with 2.5ml of 5% lidocaine with 0.5% phenylephrine. The tongue and oropharynx is anaesthetised by gargling about 4-5ml of 4% lidocaine.

A combination of fentanyl 25µg and midazolam 1-2mg is used for providing conscious sedation. Alternatively, target controlled infusion of propofol (0.5-1.5µg/ml) or remifentanil (1-2ng/ml) can be used. Continuous verbal contact with the patient should be maintained throughout the procedure. The anti-tussive effect of opioids is beneficial in reducing coughing episodes during the procedure.

(For further details on remifentanil refer to Applied pharmacology 5.3 in SOE5 and for conscious sedation refer to Applied pharmacology 10.3 in SOE10.)

Once the upper airway is adequately anaesthetised the fibreoptic scope is preloaded with an endotracheal tube (ETT) and advanced through the air space between the inferior turbinate and the floor of the nose, and through the choana into the nasopharynx and oropharynx until the larynx is visualised. The lower airway is then anaesthetised by a 'spray as you go' technique. 2ml of 4% lidocaine is sprayed onto the epiglottis and around the vocal cords. Then the fibreoptic scope is advanced further and another 1-2ml of local anaesthetic is sprayed through the vocal cords to the trachea.

Once the lower airway is anaesthetised the fibreoptic scope is advanced into the trachea, and positioned just above the carina where the ETT is advanced. The ETT position is confirmed with the fibreoptic scope and capnography. The ETT is secured in place and general anaesthesia induced once correct placement is confirmed.

Awake fibreoptic intubation

The following are indications for awake fibreoptic intubation:

- Previous history of difficult intubation.
- Previous history of difficult mask ventilation.
- Predicted difficult intubation by airway assessment and clinical examination.
- Anticipate difficult mask ventilation.
- Suspected cervical spinal cord injury or unstable neck.

(For further details on predicting difficult intubation refer to the short case 1.2 in SOE1.)

Technique of airway anaesthesia

There are many ways by which one can provide local anaesthesia for awake fibreoptic intubation:

- Topical application.
- Nebulisation.
- Nerve blocks.

The nose and nasopharynx can be anaesthetised by direct application of local anaesthetic to the mucosa by spray or packing the nasal cavity with ribbon gauze soaked in 4% lidocaine. Cocaine paste can also be applied to the nasal cavity.

The nose, oropharynx and larynx can also be anaesthetised by using nebulised lidocaine 2%.

The glossopharyngeal nerve (9th cranial nerve) innervates the tonsillar areas, posterior one third of the tongue and the oropharynx. The lingual nerve, a branch of the mandibular division of the trigeminal nerve, innervates the anterior two thirds of the tongue.

The internal branch of the superior laryngeal nerve innervates the mucosa of the larynx above the level of the vocal cords and the recurrent laryngeal nerve innervates the mucosa of the larynx below the level of the vocal cords. The trachea is innervated from the tracheal branches of the vagus.

Lidocaine 4% can be applied to the nose and oropharynx as a 'jet' through a 20G venflon connected to the oxygen flow of 2L/min. Anaesthesia to the oropharyx can be supplemented by 4% or 10% lidocaine spray.

The larynx and trachea are usually anaesthetised by a 'spray as you go' technique (SAYGO).

Superior laryngeal nerve block

The internal laryngeal nerve (the branch of the superior laryngeal nerve) provides sensory innervation to the larynx above the level of the vocal cords. It can be blocked either by an internal or external approach.

Externally, the superior laryngeal nerve can be blocked by walking a 25G needle inferiorly off the greater horn of the hyoid bone and injecting 2ml of 2% lidocaine. Accidental arterial injection is a possible complication.

Internally, the nerve can also be blocked by applying a cotton wool ball soaked in 2% lidocaine, using Krause's forceps.

Transtracheal anaesthesia

The patient lies supine with their neck extended, and the skin over the cricothyroid membrane is infiltrated with local anaesthetic. A 22G or 20G cannula attached to a syringe containing 4% lidocaine is inserted through the cricothyroid membrane, and should be directed backwards and caudad to avoid trauma to the vocal cords. Correct placement is confirmed by aspiration of air via the needle. 2-3ml of 4% lidocaine should be injected at the end of expiration. During the process the patient will cough and anaesthesia should spread both above and below the cords. Complications such as haematoma, a broken needle and infection have been reported but they are very rare.

The total dose of lidocaine used varies between 6-8mg/kg. Some of the local anaesthetic may be spat out or swallowed by the patient. Because lidocaine has a high first-pass metabolism very little of the swallowed dose reaches the systemic circulation. In clinical practice a dose up to 9.3mg/kg has been used without systemic toxicity.

Table 7.7 Commonly used techniques of anaesthetising the airway for awake intubation.

Part of airway	Local anaesthetic (LA) technique	Nerve supply
Nose	5% lidocaine + 0.5% phenylephrine spray	Ophthalmic and maxillary division of trigeminal nerve
Nasopharynx	4% lidocaine spray	Maxillary division of trigeminal nerve
Tongue and oropharnx	4% lidocaine gargle	Glossopharyngeal nerve
Larynx	SAYGO technique or transtracheal injection	Superior laryngeal nerve
Trachea	SAYGO technique or transtracheal injection	Recurrent laryngeal nerve

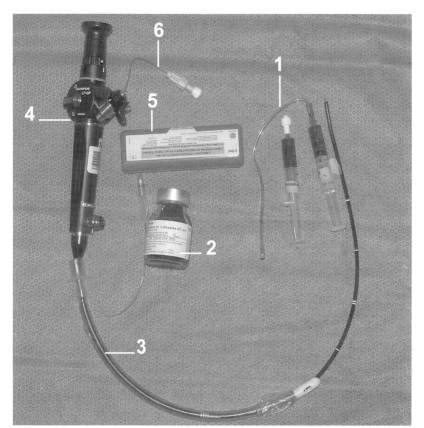

Figure 7.4 Drugs and equipment used for awake fibreoptic equipment.
1. Mucosal atomisation device; 2. 4% lidocaine; 3. Tracheal tube loaded on the fibreoptic scope; 4. Fibreoptic scope; 5. 5% lidocaine with 0.5% phenylephrine; 6. Epidural catheter.

Key points

- In an anticipated difficult airway awake fibreoptic intubation is a safe option.
- The nose is a pyramidal-shaped structure made up of bone and cartilage.
- The arterial blood supply is derived mainly from the branches of the ophthalmic, maxillary and facial arteries.
- The branches from the ophthalmic and maxillary divisions of the trigeminal nerve provide sensory innervation to the nose.

Further reading

1. Ellis H, Feldman S, Harrop-Griffiths W. *Anatomy for anaesthetists*, 8th ed. Oxford: Blackwell Science Ltd, 2004.
2. Popat M. *Practical fibreoptic intubation.* Butterworth-Heinemann, 2001.

Applied physiology 7.2: Haemorrhagic shock

A 29-year-old motor cyclist driving at 60 miles per hour has had a head on collision with a car. He was found lying on the road conscious and anxious by the paramedics. He has been brought to the resuscitation room in the emergency department. He is complaining of pain and swelling in his left thigh and abdomen.

On clinical examination, he is conscious and talking sensibly but is very anxious. His BP is 80/40 mmHg, HR is 120 bpm and RR is 25 breaths/minute.

What would be your initial management of this patient?

As this is a patient involved in a road traffic accident, the ATLS® protocol should be followed, assessing and ensuring patency of the airway, administration of 100% oxygen and protection of the cervical spine. Adequacy of breathing should be ensured and the circulatory system should be assessed. Measures are taken to resuscitate the patient and control the haemorrhage.

What is the most likely cause of haemodynamic instability in this patient?

As he has had a significant trauma, is hypotensive and tachycardic, and is complaining of pain and swelling in his left thigh and abdomen, the most likely cause is blood loss.

How would you classify hypovolaemic shock?

Hypovolaemia can be categorised according to the amount of blood loss into four classes.

Table 7.8 Classes of hypovolaemia.

	Class I	Class II	Class III	Class IV
Blood loss (ml)	750	750-1500	1500-2000	>2000
Blood loss (%)	<15	15-30	30-40	>40
Systolic BP	Normal	Normal	Reduced	Very low
Diastolic BP	Normal	Raised	Reduced	Unrecordable
Pulse (beats/minute)	<100	100-120	120-140	>140 and very thready
Capillary refill (seconds)	Normal	Slow >2 sec	Slow >2 sec	Undetectable
Respiratory rate	14-20	20-30	30-40	>40
Urine output (ml/hr)	>30	20-30	10-20	<10
Mental state	Slightly anxious	Mildly anxious	Anxious and confused	Confused and drowsy

What happens to the blood pressure in response to fluid resuscitation?

After fluid resuscitation (1-2L of fluids) in a trauma patient there may be any one of three responses:

- Responders: BP improves and is maintained (indicates adequate fluid resuscitation).
- Partial responders: BP improves initially and then falls again (indicates ongoing losses and partial fluid resuscitation).
- Non-responders: BP remains low despite fluid resuscitation (indicates massive ongoing losses and the need for emergency surgery to stop bleeding).

Describe the compensatory responses to one litre blood loss

Haemorrhage decreases the mean systemic filling pressure of the circulation and consequently reduces venous return resulting in a fall in cardiac output. The physiological effects of haemorrhage depend on the rate and degree of blood loss. Multiple compensatory mechanisms are activated, and these are important in modulating vascular resistance in the various tissues, bringing about the redistribution of the cardiac output. The blood flow to the brain and the myocardium is preserved as a result of these compensatory processes. The compensatory mechanisms can be classified under the following headings.

Immediate neuronal responses

As a result of a decrease in blood volume there is a decrease in arterial blood pressure which activates baroreceptors and low pressure vascular stretch receptors. This results in increased sympathetic activity and causes:

- Constriction of arterioles in most parts of the body, producing an increased total peripheral resistance.
- Constriction of the venous reservoirs which maintains venous return despite reduced blood volume.
- Increased heart rate and myocardial activity.

Progressive hypotension and inadequate tissue perfusion leads to increased anaerobic glycolysis and lactic acidosis which causes depression of the myocardium and reduces the peripheral vascular responses to catecholamine.

Baroreceptors are stretch receptors located in the carotid sinus and aortic arch. These receptors are progressively stimulated above a mean arterial pressure of 60mmHg with a maximum effect at 180mmHg. Afferent impulses are transmitted through branches of the glossopharyngeal nerve (carotid sinus nerve) and vagus nerve (from the aortic arch) to the centre in the medulla (which has the vasomotor centre and cardio-inhibitory centre). A rise in BP increases the firing rate and causes reflex inhibition of the vasomotor centre and excitation of the cardio-inhibitory centre resulting in lowering of the blood pressure. Hypotension reduces the stretch and firing rate, and results in less inhibition of the vasomotor centre and inhibition of the cardio-inhibitory centre.

Hormonal responses

As a result of decreased venous return the stretch of the right atrium is diminished. This results in a decrease in atrial natriuretic peptide (ANP) release and stimulates the release of anti-diuretic hormone (ADH).

Renal vasoconstriction causes renin secretion from the macula densa, which activates the renin-angiotensin pathway, enhancing the release of aldosterone from the adrenal cortex.

ADH and aldosterone promote water and sodium re-absorption in the kidney. Increased sympathetic activity also causes the release of cortisol and catecholamines from the adrenal gland.

Haematological responses

Absorption of interstitial fluid results in dilutional anaemia. Increased erythropoietin production by the kidneys stimulates bone marrow to produce red blood cells.

Fluid resuscitation in hypovolaemic shock

Warmed isotonic electrolyte solution is used for initial resuscitation. Hartmann's or Ringer's lactate is the initial fluid of choice. An initial fluid bolus is given as rapidly as possible. The usual adult dose is 1-2L and 20ml/kg for a child. The patient's response is observed and this will dictate further fluid management.

The amount of fluid and blood required for resuscitation is difficult to predict initially. Roughly, for each unit of blood lost three units of crystalloids are required. This is known as the 3-for-1 rule. Crystalloids, being isotonic, tend to distribute within the extracellular fluid (ECF) compartment. Intravascular (plasma) volume is about 25% of the ECF volume. When, therefore, a litre of crystalloid is administered, only about 250ml of the administered volume will eventually remain in the circulation. Blood, on the other hand, tends to stay within the intravascular compartment, so resuscitation with blood should be volume for volume. 5% dextrose should not be used for fluid resuscitation as it is rapidly lost from the intravascular compartment. The glucose component is metabolised leaving 1000ml of water. This distributes equally into the total body water (TBW). ECF being a third of TBW, only about 333ml remains in the ECF. Of this 333ml, only a quarter remains in the intravascular compartment, which is about 84ml.

It is important to measure the patient's response to fluid resuscitation. This is usually done clinically by observing the response of fluid resuscitation on heart rate, blood pressure, urine output, level of consciousness and peripheral perfusion.

Over the past few years many blood substitutes have being explored. These are either haemoglobin-based or perfluorocarbons:

◆ Haemoglobin(Hb)-based fluids, or stroma-free haemoglobin may contain free Hb that is liposome-encapsulated or modified. The aim of modification is to limit renal excretion and toxicity. Some advantages include the fact that the antigen-bearing RBC membrane is not present (stroma-free haemoglobin), so these substances do not require cross-matching. They can also be stored for more than a year, providing a more stable source than banked blood.
◆ Perfluorocarbons are IV carbon-fluorine emulsions that carry large amounts of O_2 without having a specific binding site. They have not, however, been proven to increase survival and cannot be given in amounts sufficient to compensate for critical RBC losses.

Key points

◆ Hypotension in trauma patients is often a late sign of severe hypovolaemic shock.
◆ The vast majority of shock in trauma is due to hypovolaemia (haemorrhagic shock).
◆ There are complex neural and humoral compensatory mechanisms which play an important role in both blood loss and fluid overload.

Further reading

1. ATLS Student Course Manual, 7th ed. American College of Surgeons Committee on Trauma, 2004; Chapter 3: 69-102.

Applied pharmacology 7.3: Alpha-adrenergic blockers

A 52-year-old male patient is scheduled for septoplasty. During the pre-operative visit it is revealed that he has a history of hypertension and has been suffering from intermittent headaches for the past 6 months. Subsequent 24-hour urine testing reveals an elevated metanephrine and vanillyl mandelic acid level.

What is the most likely cause of hypertension?

The most likely diagnosis is phaeochromocytoma, a tumour which originates from the adrenal medulla, or in the chromaffin tissues lying along the paravertebral sympathetic chain.

What substances does it secrete?

It secretes catecholamines, mainly norepinephrine and epinephrine and, rarely, dopamine.

Describe the structure of a catecholamine

The basic structure of a catecholamine includes a benzene ring with hydroxyl groups at the third and fourth position, and an amine side chain.

What are the mechanisms of action of epinephrine and norepinephrine?

Epinephrine and norepinephrine exert their effects by acting on ß-adrenergic and α-adrenergic receptors. They act as first messenger neurotransmitters at these receptors.

The effects of ß-receptor stimulation are largely mediated by activation of the enzyme adenyl cyclase on the inside of the cell membrane, which in turn results in production and activation of cyclic adenosine monophosphate (cAMP). Cyclic AMP acts as a second messenger. It activates the protein kinase which results in phosphorylation of proteins leading to altered ionic permeability of cell membranes.

Activation of $\alpha 1$ receptors leads to activation of the enzyme, phospholipase C, which hydrolyses phosphatidylinositol biphosphate (PIP2) to inositol triphosphate (IP3). IP3 increases the calcium influx into the cells.

The stimulation of α2 receptors causes activation of G inhibitory protein and inhibition of adenylate cyclase, leading to reduced cAMP.

On the other hand, activation of ß receptors causes activation of G stimulatory proteins, which in turn activate adenylate cyclase, increasing cAMP.

Table 7.9 Clinical effects of adrenergic receptor activation.

Organ	Receptor type	Effect
Eye	α1	Mydriasis
Arterioles	α1	Constriction
Pregnant uterus	α1	Contraction
Bladder sphincter	α1	Contraction
Intestinal smooth muscle	α1 and ß	Relaxation
Heart	ß1 and ß2	Increased rate, increased velocity on conducting tissue and increased contractility
Arterioles	ß2	Relaxation
Bronchioles	ß2	Relaxation
Uterus	ß2	Relaxation
Metabolic effects	ß2	Hypokalaemia, hepatic glycogenolysis and lipolysis

α2 receptors on the nerve endings (pre-synaptic) mediate negative feedback which inhibits norepinephrine release

α1 receptor stimulation produces vasoconstriction, relaxation of smooth muscle of the gut, increased secretion of saliva and hepatic glycogenolysis.

α2 receptor stimulation inhibits the release of autonomic neurotransmitters (mediates negative feedback which inhibits release of norepinephrine). It stimulates platelet aggregation.

β1 receptor stimulation causes an increased heart rate, increased myocardial contractility, relaxation of smooth muscle of the gut, and lipolysis.

β2 receptor stimulation results in vasodilatation, bronchodilatation, visceral smooth muscle relaxation and hepatic glycogenolysis.

Table 7.10 Action of catecholamines on adrenergic receptors.

	α1	α2	β1	β2
Epinephrine	+ +	+ +	+ + +	+ + +
Norepinephrine	+ + +	+ + +	+ +	+
Dopamine	+	0	++	+ +
+ = agonist activity				

How would you pharmacologically prepare a patient with a phaeochromocytoma for surgery?

The major goal is to partially block the responses to catecholamines thus avoiding the pressor effects of catecholamines.

Administration of α-adrenergic blockers has been the cornerstone of management. The most commonly used drugs are phenoxybenzamine, prazosin, doxazocin and phentolamine. During pre-operative preparation of phaechromocytoma:

♦ α-blockade with phenoxybenzamine should be started first, which results in volume expansion.

- A beta-blocker should be started only after adequate α-blockade.
- Both α- and beta-blockers should be continued until the night before the surgery.

Once α-blockade is established, the resultant tachycardia can be controlled by the cautious addition of a beta-blocker, such as propranolol. Beta-blockade should not be commenced until adequate α-blockade is achieved. Otherwise unopposed stimulation may precipitate a hypertensive crisis and cardiac failure. Pre-operative α-receptor blockade for at least 2 weeks before surgery is recommended.

Other drugs used are:

- Calcium channel blockers such as nicardipine. They act by inhibiting norepinephrine-mediated calcium influx.
- Labetalol has both α- and ß-blocking effects. The ß-block is 8-10 times greater than the α-block.
- α-methylparatyrosine inhibits tyrosine hydroxylase. This may decrease the catecholamine synthesis by 40-80% but it is not widely used.
- Magnesium sulphate blocks catecholamine release and acts as a direct vasodilator.

The following indicate adequate sympathetic blockade:

- 24-hour ambulatory blood pressure monitoring should record a BP of less than 140/90mm Hg.
- Presence of postural hypotension.
- Absence of ST-T changes in the ECG.
- Nasal congestion.

Can you tell me more about α-blockers?

These block α receptors and thus prevent their sympathetic actions. α-blockers can act on α1 or α2 receptors:

- Non-selective α-receptor blockers:
    - phentolamine;
    - phenoxybenzamine.

◆ Selective α-receptor blockers:
- α1 receptor blocker - prazosin, doxazosin;
- α2 receptor blocker - yohimbine.

Phenoxybenzamine

Phenoxybenzamine is a long-acting non-selective α-blocker, causing irreversible blockade of both α1 and α2 receptors. It is available as a capsule (10mg) and a 2ml ampoule containing 50mg of phenoxybenzamine per ml.

The oral dose is started at 10mg daily and increased by 10mg daily. The usual dose is 1-2mg/kg daily in two divided doses. Intravenously it is given as an infusion 1mg/kg over 2 hours.

Pharmacodynamics
◆ Cardiovascular system: it causes hypotension and may cause reflex tachycardia.
◆ Central nervous system: it can cause marked sedation.

Pharmacokinetics
Bioavailability after oral dose is 25%. It is metabolised in the liver and excreted in urine and bile.

Phentolamine

Phentolamine is a non-selective α-blocker, having more affinity for α1 than α2 receptors. It is available as a 1ml ampoule containing 10mg/ml. It is mainly used during the peri-operative period to control paroxysmal hypertension and particularly during operative handling of the tumour. The dose is 2-5mg IV, repeated if necessary.

Pharmacodynamics
◆ Cardiovascular system: it produces hypotension and reflex tachycardia. It has a direct vasodilatation effect and reduces systemic vascular resistance.
◆ Respiratory system: it can cause acute bronchospasm in asthmatics due to sulphites in the ampoule.

Pharmacokinetics

It is 50% protein bound, extensively metabolised and 10% excreted unchanged in urine. It has an elimination half-life of 20 minutes with a rapid onset of action with a peak effect at 2 minutes.

Doxazosin

Doxazosin is a selective α1 receptor antagonist, which inhibits the postsynaptic α-adrenergic receptors, resulting in vasodilatation of arterioles and veins. It is available as tablets of 1-2mg or as a modified release tablet of 4mg. The dosage is started at 1mg per day, increased weekly up to a maximum of 8mg/day.

Prazosin

Prazosin is a selective α1 receptor antagonist, which inhibits the postsynaptic α-adrenergic receptors, resulting in vasodilatation of arterioles and veins. It is available as tablets of 500μg to 5mg. The dosage is started at 500μg 2-3 times a day orally for a week and then increased to 1mg 2-3 times a day, up to a maximum of 20mg daily in divided doses.

What drugs should be avoided during the intra-operative period?

◆ All drugs releasing histamine (morphine, atracurium) should be avoided.
◆ Agents that cause an indirect increase in catecholamine levels (pancuronium, ketamine, and ephedrine) should be avoided.
◆ Droperidol and cocaine inhibit catecholamine reuptake and should be avoided.

How would you control the effects of catecholamine stimulation during the intra-operative period?

Drugs that can be used to control intra-operative hypertension include esmolol, labetalol, magnesium sulphate, sodium nitroprusside and phentolamine.

Phentolamine is a short-acting α-blocker, (2-5mg IV and repeated as necessary) and can be given as a continuous infusion to control blood pressure.

Sodium nitroprusside is a commonly used agent for controlling hypertension during surgery. It is started as an IV infusion at a dose of 0.3-0.5µg/kg/minute and titrated to control blood pressure. It is faster acting and has a shorter duration of action than phentolamine.

Magnesium sulphate is commonly used as an adjunct vasodilator.

Esmolol is a relatively cardio-selective beta-blocker and has a very rapid onset and offset. It can be given as bolus doses of 10mg and titrated according to the effect, or as an IV infusion at a dose of 50-200µg/kg/minute.

Labetalol is an α1 and non-selective beta-blocker. It is useful during the peri-operative period for control of blood pressure and heart rate. The dose is 5-20mg and titrated to effect up to a maximum of 200mg.

What postoperative measures should be considered after adrenalectomy?

- The patient should be managed in a critical care/high dependency unit.
- Steroid therapy may be required especially after bilateral adrenalectomy.
- Postoperatively the patient may be hypotensive and may require an epinephrine or norepinephrine infusion.
- The patient may have hypoglycaemic episodes.

Phaeochromocytoma

Phaeochromocytomas are catecholamine-secreting tumours of chromaffin tissue. They are usually located in the adrenal medullae or paravertebral sympathetic ganglion but may be found anywhere that chromaffin tissue exists. Although most phaeochromocytomas are found in the medullary portion of the adrenal gland, 10% of these tumours are located elsewhere.

Phaeochromocytomas account for only 0.1% of all cases of hypertension.

The 10% rule of phaeochromocytoma is:

◆ 10% are bilateral (adrenal involvement).
◆ 10% are extra-adrenal.
◆ 10% arise in childhood.
◆ 10% are malignant.
◆ 10% of patients may have hyperglycaemia.

Clinical features

The classic triad is severe headache, diaphoresis and palpitations. It may also be associated with perspiration, nausea, vomiting, anxiety, fever, paroxysmal hypertension, pallor, weight loss, elevated blood sugar, myocardial infarction, stroke or acute renal failure. The symptoms are usually paroxysmal in nature. These 'attacks' may last from a few moments to hours.

Phaeochromocytomas occur in both sexes, with a peak incidence in the third to fifth decades of life. It may occur as part of multiple endocrine neoplasia syndrome.

Table 7.11 Manifestations of multiple endocrine neoplasia (MEN).	
Type IIA (Sipples syndrome)	Parathyroid adenoma Medullary carcinoma - thyroid Phaeochromocytoma
Type IIB	Medullary carcinoma - thyroid Mucosal adenomas Marfanoid appearances Phaeochromocytoma
Von Hippel-Lindau syndrome	Haemangiomas of the retina, cerebellum Phaeochromocytoma

Investigations

Urine is collected over 24 hours and free catecholamines and the main metabolites, metanephrine and vanillyl mandelic acid (VMA), are measured. Elevated metanephrine is more sensitive than VMA.

About 90% of tumours are located in the adrenal glands, and 98% are within the abdomen.

An MRI scan is preferred to a CT scan, as MRI has a reported sensitivity of 100%. CT is less accurate for lesions smaller that 1cm.

An iodine[131] labelled meta-iodobenzyl guanidine (MIBG) isotope study is performed when phaeochromocytoma is suspected biochemically and the MRI scan is negative. Iodine[131] labelled MIBG resembles norepinephrine and is concentrated within the tumour.

Positron emission tomography has been shown to be useful in localising the tumour.

Synthesis of catecholamines

Catecholamines are formed by hydroxylation and decarboxylation of the amino acid, tyrosine. Most of the tyrosine is obtained from dietary intake and partly from phenylalanine. Tyrosine is transported into catecholamine-secreting neurons and the adrenal medulla. Tyrosine is converted into dopa in the adrenal medulla by the enzyme, tyrosine hydroxylase. Dopa is converted into dopamine by the enzyme, dopa dehydroxylase. The dopamine enters the granulated vesicles where it is converted to norepinephrine by the enzyme, dopamine beta-hydroxylase.

Norepinephrine is then converted into epinephrine by phenyl-ethanolamine-N-methyltransferase (PNMT).

Catabolism of catecholamines

Both epinephrine and norepinephrine are metabolised to inactive products by oxidation and methylation. The oxidation is catalysed by the enzyme, monoamino-oxidase (MAO). The methylation is catalysed by the enzyme, catechol-O-methyl transferase (COMT).

Norephinephrine is converted into normetanephrine by COMT, which is converted into 3-hydroxy 4-methoxy mandelic aldehyde and then to 3-methoxy, 4-hydroxy mandelic acid (VMA).

Key points

◆ Phaeochromocytomas are catecholamine-secreting tumours of chromaffin tissue.
◆ The major goal of pre-operative management is to partially block the responses to catecholamines and to avoid the pressor effects of catecholamines with an α-blocker.
◆ Beta-blockade should not be started until adequate α-blockade is achieved.

Further reading

1. Prys-Roberts C. Phaeochromocytoma - recent progress in its management. *British Journal of Anaesthesia* 2000; 85: 44-57.
2. Pace N, Buttigieg M. Phaechromocytoma. *British Journal of Anaesthesia CEPD review* 2003; 3: 20-3.

Equipment, clinical measurement and monitoring 7.4: Temperature measurement

An 85-year-old lady has had an elective laparotomy for a subtotal colectomy. She has been in the recovery room for the past 20 minutes. She is shivering, and her recorded temperature is 35.6°C.

What is the cause of her shivering?

Hypothermia.

What is hypothermia?

Hypothermia is a condition in which the temperature drops below that required for normal metabolism and bodily functions. In the peri-operative period hypothermia can be a result of deliberate induction or can arise inadvertently. It is defined as a core body temperature below 36°C.

How can you grade the severity of inadvertent peri-operative hypothermia?

According to NICE guidelines inadvertent hypothermia can be graded into:

◆ Mild hypothermia: 35°C to 35.9°C.
◆ Moderate hypothermia: 34°C to 34.9°C.
◆ Severe hypothermia: ≤33.9°C.

What are the risk factors for inadvertent peri-operative hypothermia?

◆ ASA grades II to V (the higher the grade, the greater the risk).
◆ Pre-operative temperature below 36°C.
◆ Combined regional and general anaesthesia.
◆ Major or intermediate surgery.
◆ Unwarmed intravenous fluids, irrigation fluids and blood.
◆ Lower theatre temperature.

How may temperature be measured?

Temperature can be measured by different methods and can be classified as non-electrical and electrical.

Non-electrical:

◆ Mercury thermometer.
◆ Alcohol thermometer.

- Bimetallic strip.
- Bourdon gauge thermometer.
- Infrared thermometry.

Electrical:

- Resistance thermometer.
- Thermistor.
- Thermocouple.

Electrical methods are commonly used for measuring temperature in the peri-operative period. The electrical probes have a shorter response time of 1-15 seconds, and a greater selection of sites for measurement is available.

The principle of the resistance thermometer involves a linear increase in the resistance of a metal with increasing temperature. It can either be a simple resistance thermometer or can be incorporated into the Wheatstone bridge circuit to improve accuracy.

A thermistor has a small bead of semiconductor (metal oxide) with a resistance that falls exponentially as temperature increases. The advantage is that it is convenient to use in theatres because of its compactness and fast response. It undergoes a greater change in resistance over the clinical range of temperature than the resistance thermometer. A major disadvantage of the thermistor is its calibration. It is liable to change over time ('drift') or if subjected to extremes of temperature as in sterilisation.

The thermocouple is made up of two dissimilar metals. At the junction of two dissimilar metals a voltage develops, the magnitude of which depends upon the temperature at the junction. This is called the Seebeck effect. Metals such as copper and constantan are commonly used. There is a reference junction kept at a constant temperature and a measuring junction that acts as a probe.

How does an infrared thermometer measure temperature?

Temperature measurement using an infrared thermometer is based on the principle of black box radiation. Objects (of a temperature greater than -273°C) emit radiant energy in an amount proportional to the fourth power of their temperature. Emissivity is a measure of the ratio of thermal radiation emitted by a surface to that of a black body at the same temperature. Measurement of infrared radiation emitted by a surface and the emissivity helps to calculate the temperature of the surface. This principle is used to measure temperature by infrared tympanometry, where infrared energy emitted by a tympanic membrane is detected and the temperature calculated.

What are the sites available for temperature measurement?

◆ Nasopharynx (approximates brain temperature).
◆ Ear: tympanic membrane.
◆ Lower oesophagus.
◆ Pulmonary artery.
◆ Rectum (usually 0.5°C-1.0°C higher than core temperature, because of bacterial fermentation).
◆ Urinary bladder.
◆ Skin (peripheral-core temperature gradient may give a useful index of adequacy of peripheral perfusion).

What steps can be taken to prevent inadvertent peri-operative hypothermia?

According to NICE guidelines on inadvertent peri-operative hypothermia, the following steps may help to prevent hypothermia.

Pre-operative phase

◆ Each patient should be assessed for their risk of inadvertent peri-operative hypothermia.
◆ Patients should be kept warm while waiting for surgery.
◆ Special care should be taken to keep patients comfortably warm when they are given premedication.
◆ The patient's temperature should be measured and documented.

- If it is below 36°C, forced air warming should be started pre-operatively.
- On transfer to the theatre suite the patient should be kept comfortably warm.

Intra-operative phase

- The patient's temperature should be measured and documented before induction of anaesthesia and then every 30 minutes until the end of surgery.
- Induction of anaesthesia should not begin unless the patient's temperature is 36°C or above (unless there is a need to expedite surgery because of clinical urgency).
- In the theatre suite the ambient temperature should be at least 21°C while the patient is exposed.
- The patient should be adequately covered throughout the intra-operative phase to conserve heat, and exposed only during surgical preparation.
- Intravenous fluids and blood products should be warmed to 37°C using a fluid warming device.
- Patients who are at higher risk should be warmed intra-operatively using a forced air warming device.
- All patients who are having anaesthesia for longer than 30 minutes should be warmed intra-operatively from induction of anaesthesia using a forced air warming device.
- All irrigation fluids used intra-operatively should be warmed.

Postoperative phase

- The patient's temperature should be measured and documented on admission to the recovery room and then every 15 minutes.
- Ward transfer should not be arranged unless the patient's temperature is 36°C or above.
- If the patient's temperature is below 36°C, they should be actively warmed using forced air warming.
- Patients should be kept comfortably warm when back on the ward.
- Their temperature should be measured and documented on arrival at the ward and every 4 hours.

Peri-operative hypothermia

Patients undergoing surgery under general anaesthesia are at risk of developing hypothermia due to several mechanisms. The cellular enzyme function is optimal within a narrow range of temperature (36.5°C-37.5°C).

The operating room temperature varies between 20-22°C, increasing the gradient between skin and room temperature. This increases the heat loss by mechanisms such as conduction, convection and radiation. General anaesthesia depresses the thermoregulatory centre and causes vasodilatation. Vasodilatation increases the blood flow to skin and increases heat loss from the skin. Other factors associated with heat loss include evaporation from the exposed body cavities, irrigation of the surgical site, body cavities with cold fluid and failure to warm intravenous fluids.

Adverse effects of mild to moderate hypothermia

Immediate effects:

◆ Increased intra-operative blood loss and need for allogenic blood transfusion.
◆ Increased oxygen requirement during recovery period.
◆ Increased incidence of myocardial ischaemia and arrhythmias.
◆ Prolonged duration of neuromuscular block.
◆ Increased duration of post-anaesthetic recovery.

Delayed effects:

◆ Increased risk of surgical wound infection.
◆ Prolonged hospital stay.

Key points

◆ Inadvertent peri-operative hypothermia is a common complication and is associated with a poor outcome for patients.
◆ Every effort should be made in the pre-operative, intra-operative and postoperative stages to prevent hypothermia.

◆ Electrical methods are commonly used for measuring temperature in the peri-operative period.

Further reading

1. Management of inadvertent hypothermia. London: NICE clinical guideline. http://www.nice.org.uk/CG65.
2. Kirkbride DA, Buggy DJ. Thermoregulation and mild peri-operative hypothermia. *British Journal of Anaesthesia CEPD review* 2003; 3: 24-8.

Structured oral examination 8

Long case 8

Information for the candidate

History

You are called to see a 28-year-old lady (Gravida 4 Para 3), who had an elective Caesarean section 7 hours ago at 38 weeks of gestation and delivered a male baby weighing 4.5kg. Intra-operative blood loss was 1.2L. Since the operation she has been continuously bleeding, and has passed large amounts of blood clots vaginally. She is pale, sweaty and drowsy. Her obstetric history includes an emergency Caesarean section under general anaesthesia 8 years ago for foetal distress. She had two subsequent elective Caesarean sections under spinal anaesthesia. She has been reviewed by the consultant obstetrician who wishes to perform an emergency laparotomy. She has received a transfusion of two units of cross-matched blood and a litre of Hartmann's solution. An intravenous infusion of oxytocin was commenced 4 hours ago.

Clinical examination

Table 8.1 Clinical examination.

Weight	69kg
Height	170cm
Respiratory rate	24 per minute
Heart rate	140 bpm
Blood pressure	70/40mmHg
Temperature	36.7°C
SpO_2	94%

She is breathing 60% oxygen via a face mask. On auscultation of her chest she has bilateral equal air entry.

She has been written up for the following drugs:

- Enoxaparin 40mg o.d.
- Co-amoxiclav 625mg t.d.s.
- Paracetamol 1g q.d.s.
- Diclofenac sodium 50mg t.d.s.

Investigations

Table 8.2 Haematology on the day before Caesarean section.

		Normal values
Hb	11.8g/dL	11-16g/dL
Haematocrit	0.42	0.4-0.5 males, 0.37-0.47 females
RBC	4.7×10^{12}/L	$3.8\text{-}4.8 \times 10^{12}$/L
WBC	6.2×10^9/L	$4\text{-}11 \times 10^9$/L
Platelets	240×10^9/L	$150\text{-}450 \times 10^9$/L
INR	1.1	0.9-1.2
PT	12 seconds	11-15 seconds
APTT ratio	1.0	0.8-1.2

Table 8.3 Haematology 6 hours post-Caesarean section.

		Normal values
Hb	3.2g/dl	11-16g/dl
Haematocrit	0.18	0.4-0.5 males, 0.37-0.47 females
RBC	3.7×10^{12}/L	$3.8\text{-}4.8 \times 10^{12}$/L
WBC	5.2×10^9/L	$4\text{-}11 \times 10^9$/L
Platelets	80×10^9/L	$150\text{-}450 \times 10^9$/L
INR	1.8	0.9-1.2
PT	18 seconds	11-15 seconds
APTT ratio	2.2	0.8-1.2
Fibrinogen	1.3g/L	1.5-4g/L
Fibrin degradation products	6mg/L	<5mg/L

Table 8.4 Biochemistry.		
		Normal values
Sodium	141mmol/L	135-145mmol/L
Potassium	4.4mmol/L	3.5-5.0mmol/L
Urea	10.5mmol/L	2.2-8.3mmol/L
Creatinine	123µmol/L	44-80µmol/L
Blood glucose	5.5mmol/L	3.0-6.0mmol/L

Examiner's questions

Please summarise the case

This is a young patient who has had an elective Caesarean section and is now scheduled for an emergency laparotomy to control the bleeding. She is in Class 4 haemorrhagic shock and has deranged clotting and abnormal renal function.

Comment on the blood results

The post-Caesarean section full blood count shows severe anaemia, a low platelet count, a prolonged INR, low fibrinogen level, and elevated fibrin degradation products.

What are the causes of primary post partum haemorrhage (PPH)?

There are four main causes in primary PPH:

◆ Tone: this is the most common cause, usually due to uterine atonia, often occurring after a prolonged labour and failure to progress. Other risk factors for uterine atonia include Caesarean section under general anaesthesia and multiparity.
◆ Tissue: retained products (placenta).
◆ Thrombin: low thrombin secondary to DIC due to massive blood transfusion.
◆ Trauma: there could be unrecognised trauma to abdominal structures, including major blood vessels, during Caesarean section. During vaginal delivery trauma can occur to the uterus, cervix and vagina.

(Remember the mnemonic: 4 Ts.)

How would you manage PPH?

The management of PPH involves immediate resuscitation, followed by an urgent assessment to establish the cause of bleeding. Simple measures such as manual massage of the uterus to stimulate contraction, and bimanual compression, may be useful at the initial stages. Other methods for bleeding control can be classified as pharmacological, radiological and surgical methods.

Pharmacological methods

- Oxytocin infusion. Five units of oxytocin is given as a slow IV bolus followed by an infusion of 10 units per hour for 4 hours. Care should be taken as oxytocin can cause hypotension and circulatory collapse.
- Ergometrine. This is an ergot alkaloid which causes uterine and vascular smooth muscle contraction. The dose is 0.5mg given intramuscularly or 100µg as a slow IV, repeated as necessary. Side effects include hypertension, bradycardia and pulmonary oedema. It should be avoided in hypertension and pre-eclampsia. It should be administered as a slow IV infusion with caution in patients with cardiac disease.
- Carboprost (prostaglandin F2α analogue). This is used for bleeding which has not been responsive to oxytocin and ergometrine. It can be given intramuscularly or as an intra-myometrial injection of 250µg repeated every 15 minutes up to a maximum of 2mg. It should not be given IV as severe bronchospasm and pulmonary hypertension can develop. Other side effects include nausea, vomiting and flushing. Excessive dosage can cause uterine rupture.
- Recombinant activated Factor VII (rFVIIa). This can be very effective in cases of refractory haemorrhage. It can be given at doses up to 100µg/kg IV. The indications for its use are: patients who are unresponsive to conventional treatment, unavailability of radiological facilities to control bleeding, and when emergency hysterectomy is the only other option.
- Antifibrinolytics such as tranexamic acid. This can be given at a dose of 0.5-1g as a slow IV.
- Blood and blood products. The haemoglobin concentration should be checked regularly and maintained above 7g/dL. Transfusion of blood

products should be guided by the coagulation studies and advice from a consultant haematologist.

Radiological methods

- Interventional radiological techniques may be available for selectively embolising the pelvic vessels, but not all centres have this facility.

Surgical methods

- Manual removal of the placenta and retained products.
- B-Lynch uterine suture. This is a relatively new technique for patients who have responded well to bimanual uterine compression. It involves placing a continuous suture through the uterus to provide compression.
- Internal iliac or uterine artery ligation.
- Uterine packing.
- Hysterectomy should be performed as a last resort when other methods to control the haemorrhage have failed.

What is meant by the term massive blood transfusion?

Massive blood transfusion is defined as replacement of a patient's total blood volume within 24 hours or acute transfusion of more than 50% of the patient's estimated blood volume per hour.

What are the complications of massive blood transfusion?

- Hypothermia. Blood is stored at 4°C. Infusion of cold blood results in hypothermia. Hypothermia reduces the metabolism of lactate and citrate which may contribute to acidosis and citrate toxicity. Hypothermia causes platelet dysfunction and increases bleeding. It shifts the oxygen-dissociation curve to the left, increasing the affinity of haemoglobin for oxygen. Core temperature should be monitored during massive blood transfusion.
- Coagulopathy. This occurs due to depletion of platelets and clotting factors. Packed red cell concentrates are deficient in clotting factors. During resuscitation, clotting factors are diluted by crystalloids and colloids.

- Hypocalcaemia. Stored blood contains citrate which is normally metabolised by the liver. If the rate of transfusion is greater than one unit every 5 minutes, or if liver function is impaired, citrate accumulates. Citrate binds to calcium and reduces free plasma calcium levels.
- Hyperkalaemia. Breakdown of RBCs in the stored blood releases K^+; the concentration of K^+ can be as high as 30mmol/L.
- Metabolic acidosis. Stored blood contains a high concentration of H^+ ions in the form of lactic acid generated in red cells during storage and from citric acid (an anticoagulant).
- Transfusion-related acute lung injury (TRALI). This is likely to be caused by donor leukocyte antibodies and micro-aggregates. It is characterised by respiratory distress, hypoxia and pulmonary infiltrates soon after transfusion. It is self-limiting with clinical improvement occurring in 2-4 days. The clinical diagnosis is based on a high degree of suspicion in the absence of other causes of respiratory distress. The management is mainly supportive and ventilatory support may be required.

What clotting tests would you perform during massive blood transfusion?

- APTT ratio/INR: aim for <1.5 .
- Platelets count: aim for >50 × 10^9/L.
- Fibrinogen: aim for >1g/L.

In most cases, including massive transfusion, FFP will supply the necessary clotting factors. FFP also contains a small amount of fibrinogen. If the APTT ratio or INR is >1.5, an adult dose of FFP (4 units) should be requested.

A low platelet count is corrected by giving platelets.

Low fibrinogen levels are corrected by transfusing cryoprecipitate. One adult dose of cryoprecipitate contains 3.2-4g of fibrinogen in a volume of 150-200ml and is therefore more efficient at replacing fibrinogen than FFP, avoiding volume overload.

Cryoprecipitate also contains Factors VIII, XIII and von Willebrand factor.

How would you manage this patient?

She is haemodynamically unstable and requires immediate resuscitation and laparotomy to control the haemorrhage.

Pre-operative management

◆ This patient is in Class 4 haemorrhagic shock. Immediate resuscitation involves an airway, breathing and circulation approach along with haemorrhage control. 100% oxygen should be administered via a face mask if breathing is adequate; rapid replacement of intravascular volume with blood and blood products is essential. Intravenous access should be secured with at least two wide-bore peripheral cannulae. At least 4 units of blood in the form of packed red cells should be transfused rapidly. Further blood and blood products such as FFP and platelets should be requested and transfused as soon as possible. The patient should be transferred to the operating theatre once resuscitation is in progress.

◆ A consultant obstetrician and consultant anaesthetist should be involved early in the management of this patient, with advice from a consultant haematologist.

◆ Invasive monitoring (arterial line and CVP line) should be established during resuscitation.

◆ Aspiration prophylaxis should be performed with 30ml of 0.3M sodium citrate administered orally just before transferring to the operating theatre or prior to induction. An H_2 receptor antagonist such as ranitidine 50mg should be administered as a slow IV.

Intra-operative management

Monitoring
◆ Invasive arterial blood pressure, CVP, body temperature (nasopharyngeal), urine output, blood loss estimation and intermittent blood gas monitoring (Hb) should be continued during the intra-operative period.

Induction

◆ Induction should be performed in theatre once the surgical team is scrubbed and ready. Following pre-oxygenation, rapid sequence induction should be performed using thiopentone and succinylcholine. Ketamine could be considered as an alternative induction agent.

◆ Fluid resuscitation and transfusion of packed red cells and other blood products should be continued. Further transfusion of blood and blood products should be guided by the haemoglobin and coagulation studies. All IV fluids and blood should be warmed during infusion to avoid hypothermia.

◆ A forced air warming device should be used to prevent hypothermia, as hypothermia can worsen the coagulopathy.

◆ Use of intra-operative cell salvage may be helpful in conserving blood and reducing homologous blood transfusion.

Postoperative management

Postoperatively, this patient should be managed in a high dependency /critical care unit. Metabolic acidosis and coagulation abnormalities should be corrected. Renal function should be monitored. Postoperative pain can be managed using PCA (morphine) and regular paracetamol. Measures should be taken to prevent hypothermia.

This patient underwent hysterectomy as a last resort to control the bleeding. During the postoperative period she required ventilatory support. On the second day, she is noted to have high airway pressures, her PaO_2 is 10kPa with 70% oxygen and a chest X-ray has been performed. Comment on this chest X-ray.

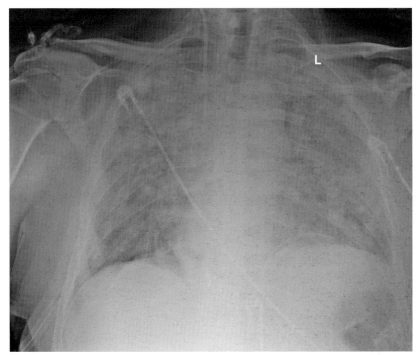

Figure 8.1 Chest X-ray.

This is an over-penetrated AP view; the central line inserted via the right internal jugular vein is correctly placed in the lower end of the superior vena cava. There are bilateral infiltrates over the lung fields.

What is the differential diagnosis?

The differential diagnosis includes:

- Cardiogenic pulmonary oedema.
- ARDS or non-cardiogenic pulmonary oedema.
- TRALI.

What is ARDS?

Acute respiratory distress syndrome (ARDS), also known as respiratory distress syndrome (RDS) or adult respiratory distress syndrome, is a serious reaction to various forms of injury to the lung. ARDS is associated with a high mortality, usually requiring mechanical ventilation and admission to an intensive care unit. A less severe form is called acute lung injury (ALI).

ARDS is characterised by:

- Acute onset.
- Bilateral infiltrates on a chest radiograph.
- Pulmonary artery wedge pressure <18mmHg or absence of clinical evidence for left ventricular failure.
- PaO_2/FiO_2 <300mmHg (~40kPa) suggests a diagnosis of ALI.
- If PaO_2/FiO_2 is <200mmHg (~27kPa) this suggests a diagnosis of ARDS.

Describe the ventilation strategies used when treating ARDS and any unconventional modes of ventilation

The overall goal is to maintain acceptable gas exchange and to minimise the adverse effects of ventilation. The following strategies are used:

- A tidal volume of 6ml/kg (compared to the traditional 12ml/kg) with permissive hypercarbia (ARDS Network).
- A plateau pressure less than 30cm H_2O is a secondary goal (ARDS Network).
- PEEP must be used in mechanically ventilated patients in order to oppose the tendency of affected alveoli to collapse.
- Prone position.
- Inverse ratio ventilation where the inspiratory time exceeds the expiratory time.

Complications of blood transfusion

Table 8.5 Complications of blood transfusion.

	Immunological	Non-immunological
Immediate		
	Haemolytic transfusion reactions	Hypothermia
	Febrile non-haemolytic transfusion reactions	Hypocalcaemia
	Anaphylaxis	Hyperkalaemia
	Urticaria	Metabolic acidosis
		Coagulopathy
Delayed		
	Delayed haemolytic transfusion reactions	Transmission of infections: viral: HIV, hepatitis C, hepatitis B, hepatitis A
	Delayed febrile reactions	bacterial: *Yersinia enterocolitica*,
	Transfusion-related acute lung injury (TRALI)	*Staphylococcus epidermidis* and *Klebsiella pneumoniae* parasites: malaria

Prone position for ARDS

Prone position ventilation is one of the ventilator strategies used in the management of ARDS. The main benefits of this mode of ventilation are:

◆ Better ventilation/perfusion matching.
◆ Recruitment of dependent alveoli.
◆ Improved respiratory mechanics.
◆ Facilitation of drainage of secretions.
◆ Reduction of ventilator-associated lung injury.

Oxygenation improves in approximately 70-80% of patients, but the beneficial effects of a prone position are short lived and reduce after a week of mechanical ventilation. Extreme care is necessary when this position is used; pressure sores are frequent and related to the number of pronations. Duration of stay in the ICU and hospital still remain high, as does mortality.

According to some recent research nitric oxide (NO) and almitrine when used in the prone position may help to improve outcome. NO inhalation improves gas exchange by inducing vasodilatation in ventilated areas and diverting blood flow away from atelectatic non-ventilated regions.

Almitrine is a piperazine derivative, a respiratory stimulant that augments hypoxic vasoconstriction, redirecting blood flow to well-ventilated alveoli. It may exacerbate severe pulmonary hypertension or right ventricular failure.

Key points

◆ Pharmacological and surgical methods should first be considered in managing PPH following Caesarean section before considering hysterectomy.
◆ Various ventilation strategies and unconventional modes of ventilation for ARDS can be used in the management of ARDS.

Further reading

1. Pelosi P, Brazzi L, Gattinoni L. Prone position in acute respiratory distress syndrome. *European Respiratory Journal* 2002; 20: 1017-28.
2. Donaldson MDJ, Seaman MJ, Park GR. Massive blood transfusion. *Journal of Anaesthesia* 1992; 69: 621-30.
3. Blood transfusion and anaesthetist - red cell transfusion. www.agbi.org. June 2008.
4. McLelland DBL. *Handbook of transfusion medicine*, 4th ed. United Kingdom Blood Services, 2007. http://www.transfusionguidelines.org.uk/docs/pdfs/htm_edition-4_all-pages.pdf.
5. Mechanical ventilation protocol summary in ARDS. ARDS Network, 2008 guideline. http://www.ardsnet.org/system/files/6mlcardsmall_2008 update_final_JULY2008.pdf.
6. Banks A, Norris A. Massive haemorrhage in pregnancy. *British Journal of Anaesthesia CEACCP* 2005; 6: 195-8.

Short case 8.1: Carcinoid syndrome

A 52-year-old male patient is scheduled for arthroplasty of his hip joint. He has been recently diagnosed with carcinoid syndrome.

What is carcinoid syndrome?

Carcinoid syndrome is the systemic manifestation of a carcinoid tumour. Carcinoid tumours are derived from argentaffin cells and cause production of peptides and amides. 75% occur in the gastrointestinal tract, usually in the terminal ileum; the rest are seen in the bronchus, pancreas and gonads.

They are usually benign and rarely malignant. The peptides and amides are mostly metabolised in the liver and do not reach the systemic circulation, so only tumours with hepatic metastasis or a primary tumour with non-portal venous drainage lead to the release of these mediators into the systemic circulation. The symptoms are usually due to secretion of 5-hydroxy tryptamine (5-HT), kinins, prostaglandins, histamine and substance P.

What are the clinical features?

Symptoms of carcinoid syndrome can be either due to the tumour itself or due to the release of vasoactive substances.

Symptoms due to the tumour

- Intestinal obstruction.
- Haemoptysis.

Symptoms due to vasoactive peptide release

- Flushing of head, neck and back.
- Diarrhoea.
- Bronchospasm and wheeze.
- Hypotension or hypertension.
- Tachycardia.
- Hyperglycaemia.
- Right heart failure secondary to endocardial fibrosis.

How would you confirm the diagnosis?

Measurement of 5-hydroxyindole acetic acid (metabolite of serotonin) in the urine is useful in confirming the diagnosis.

How would you control the symptoms due to carcinoid syndrome?

Various drugs have been used in the symptomatic treatment of carcinoid syndrome. The one that is most often used is a somatostatin analogue - octreotide. Other drugs that can also be used are 5-HT antagonists (e.g. ketanserin). Cyproheptadine is a non-specific anti-histamine which has also been used.

What is octreotide and what is its mechanism of action?

It is a somatostatin analogue.

Octreotide suppresses the secretion of pituitary growth hormone (GH) and thyrotropin, and decreases the release of a variety of pancreatic islet cell hormones including insulin, glucagon, and vasoactive intestinal peptide (VIP).

It causes reduction in:

- Splanchnic blood flow.
- Gastric acid secretion.
- GI motility.
- Pancreatic exocrine function.

The elimination half-life of IV octreotide is about 2 hours.

The standard initial therapy of octreotide acetate is 50-100µg subcutaneously every 8-12 hours, with titration based on clinical and biochemical effects.

Besides carcinoid syndrome it is used in acromegaly, VIP-secreting tumours and oesophageal varices.

Describe the anaesthetic management of a patient with carcinoid syndrome

Pre-operative

- Optimisation and symptomatic treatment with bronchodilators.
- Correction of dehydration and electrolyte imbalance.
- Octreotide 100µg SC, t.d.s. for 2 weeks prior to the surgery.
- Avoidance of factors which may trigger a carcinoid crisis, such as catecholamines, anxiety and histamine-releasing drugs such as morphine.
- Pre-medication should include anxiolytics (benzodiazepines) and octreotide 100µg SC 1 hour pre-operatively.

Intra-operative

- Invasive blood pressure and CVP monitoring.
- During induction of anaesthesia it is important to prevent the pressor response to intubation using opioids such as alfentanil or remifentanil.
- Succinylcholine is relatively contraindicated as it may increase mediator release due to increased intra-abdominal pressure associated with fasciculations.
- Anaesthesia can be maintained using either an inhalational agent or total intravenous anaesthesia. Atracurium is best avoided as it can cause histamine release. Vecuronium, rocuronium or cisatracurium are relatively safer.
- Hypotension should be treated initially with an IV bolus of 10-20µg of octreotide. Beta-blockers such as labetalol and esmolol can be used to treat hypertension.

Postoperatively

- Intensive care or high dependency care should be provided.
- Hypotensive episodes may occur requiring further IV boluses of octreotide 10-20µg.

5-HT receptors

5-hydroxytryptamine (5-HT) is an aminergic neurotransmitter found throughout the body. Other amine neurotransmitters include dopamine, norepinephrine and histamine. 99% of 5-HT is located peripherally, 1% is located in the central nervous system. There are about 14 sub-types of receptors which have been described. 5-HT is the most abundant in enterochromaffin cells in the wall of the stomach and gastrointestinal tract, platelets and mast cells.

5-HT is synthesised by the hydroxylation and decarboxylation of tryptophan and is metabolised by monoamine oxidase into 5-hydroxyindoleacetic acid (5HIAA) and melatonin. All the receptors besides 5-HT_3 are coupled to G proteins and 5-HT_3 is coupled to ligand gated ion (Na^+/K^+ ion) channels.

Systemic effects of 5-HT

Gastrointestinal system
- Increased gastric motility.
- Increased water and electrolyte secretion.
- Nausea and vomiting.

Central nervous system
- An inhibitory transmitter in the brain stem, descending spinal pathways, cortical, limbic and extrapyramidal systems.
- Affects mood, arousal and memory.

Cardiovascular system
- Increases vascular permeability.
- Increases platelet aggregation.
- Can cause both vasodilatation and vasoconstriction.

Respiratory system
- Bronchoconstriction.

Table 8.6 Drugs acting on the 5-HT (serotonin) receptors.

Receptor	Drug	Mechanism	Clinical use
5-HT$_{1A}$	Fluoxetine	Inhibition	Anti-depressant
5-HT$_{1A}$	Buspirone	Agonist	Anxiolytic
5-HT$_{1D}$	Sumatriptan	Agonist	Migraine
5-HT$_3$	Ondansetron	Antagonist	Anti-emetic
5-HT$_4$	Metoclopramide	Agonist	Pro-kinetic
5-HT$_{2A,2C}$	Methysergide	Antagonist	Refractory migraine

Key points

♦ Carcinoid syndrome is the clinical manifestation of a carcinoid tumour, mainly occurring when there is hepatic metastasis.
♦ Pre-operative optimisation and symptomatic treatment should be effective before surgery is attempted, if possible.
♦ For severe hypotension peri-operatively, octreotide should be used rather than catecholamines.

Further reading

1. Roy RC, Carter RF, Wright PD, Somatostatin, anaesthesia and the carcinoid syndrome. *Anaesthesia* 2007; 42: 627-32.
2. Caring for Carcinoid Foundation. http://www.caringforcarcinoid.org.
3. Chinniah S, French JLH, Levy DM. Serotonin and anaesthesia. *British Journal of Anaesthesia CEACCP* 2008; 8: 43-5.

Short case 8.2: Heart transplant

The first patient on your orthopaedic list is a 62-year-old male who is scheduled to have a total knee replacement. He underwent a cardiac transplant 6 years ago.

What are the implications of a transplanted heart to the anaesthetic management of this patient?

The anaesthetic implications of a transplanted heart are due to:

◆ Altered physiology of the transplanted heart.
◆ The effect of immunosuppressant drugs.

What are the physiological changes in a transplanted heart?

The transplanted heart is devoid of both sympathetic and parasympathetic innervation. There is absence of vagal tone on the sino-atrial node. The resting heart rate is usually around 100-110 bpm. There is poor tolerance of acute hypovalaemia because there is no reflex tachycardia. Normal autonomic system responses are lost. These include beat-to-beat variation in heart rate and response to the Valsalva manoeuvre. Atropine has no effect on the denervated heart.

How would these changes affect the anaesthetic management of the patient?

◆ There is no haemodynamic response to direct laryngoscopy.
◆ Haemodynamic response to light anaesthesia and pain will not occur.
◆ Intra-operative hypotension will require assessment of volume status and directly acting sympathomimetic agents should be considered.

What are the implications of immunosuppression?

Patients with a transplanted heart are on long-term immunosuppressant drugs. These are highly potent with significant side effects such as anaemia, thrombocytopenia, leucopenia and renal dysfunction. Patients are prone to infections, hence strict asepsis must be used with all invasive procedures. If they acquire an infection they will suffer higher morbidity and mortality. These patients may be on high doses of oral steroids, and may require supplemental steroids during the peri-operative period.

Can you name some immunosuppressant drugs this patient may be taking?

There are three classes of immunosupressants:

- ◆ Cyclosporin A, Tacrolimus (immunophilin binding drugs which cause prevention of cytokine-mediated T-cell activation and proliferation).
- ◆ Azathioprine (a nucleic acid synthesis inhibitor which causes blockage of lymphocyte proliferation).
- ◆ Steroids.

What are the implications of these drugs on the anaesthetic management?

- ◆ Chronic steroid treatment causes an abnormal stress response due to suppression of the hypothalamic-pituitary-adrenal axis.
- ◆ Azathioprine antagonises the action of non-depolarising neuromuscular blocking drugs, such that larger doses of muscle relaxants may be required.
- ◆ Due to the nephrotoxic effects of cyclosporin, it is best to avoid administration of drugs such as NSAIDs.

What would be your choice of anaesthetic?

Both regional and general anaesthesia have been safely used. Meticulous attention to blood pressure and fluid maintenance is essential.

What drugs would you use for treating intra-operative hypotension?

The volume status should be assessed and intravenous fluids should be administered as required. Directly acting sympathomimetic drugs such as norepinephrine, epinephrine, phenylephrine and dopamine are useful in treating intra-operative hypotension. Atropine has no effect on the denervated heart; the effect of ephedrine is reduced and unpredictable.

What are the indications for cardiac transplantation?

The indications for a cardiac transplant are:

- End-stage heart failure which is refractory to medical treatment.
- Cardiomyopathy (idiopathic or ischaemic dilated).
- Congenital defects.
- Valvular heart disease.

Nerve supply to the heart

The parasympathetic supply is provided by branches of the vagus; the sympathetic nerve supply arises from the first four thoracic segments (T1 to T4). The pre-ganglionic fibres ascend in the paravertebral sympathetic chain to synapse in the cervical and upper thoracic ganglia.

Branches from the sympathetic ganglia and vagus form the cardiac plexus which is divided into superficial and deep parts.

The superficial part is formed by the superior cardiac branch of the left sympathetic chain and superior cervical cardiac branch of the vagus.

The deep cardiac plexus is formed by cardiac branches of the cervical and upper thoracic sympathetic ganglia, and cardiac branches of the vagus and recurrent laryngeal nerves. The right and left coronary plexus are formed from the deep and superficial cardiac plexus; they accompany the coronary arteries and innervate the atria and ventricles.

Stimulation of the sympathetic system increases heart rate (positive chronotropy), increases myocardial contractility (positive inotropy), and increases conduction velocity (positive dromotropy). Conversely, parasympathetic stimulation reduces heart rate, reduces contractility and reduces conduction velocity.

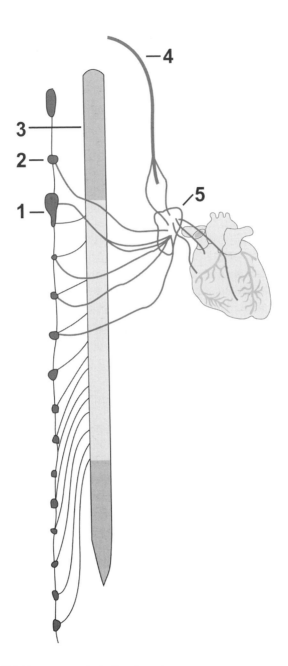

Figure 8.2 Nerve supply to the heart.

1. Stellate ganglion; 2. Middle cervical ganglion; 3. Spinal cord; 4. Vagus nerve; 5. Cardiac plexus.

Key points

♦ The transplanted heart is devoid of innervation.
♦ Atropine has no effect on the transplanted heart.
♦ Directly acting sympathomimetic agents should be used for treating hypotension.

Further reading

1. Cheng DC, Ong DD. Anaesthesia for non-cardiac surgery in heart transplanted patients. *Canadian Journal of Anesthesia* 1993; 40: 981-6.
2. Shaw IH, Kirk AJB, Conacher ID. Anaesthesia for paients with transplanted hearts and lungs undergoing non-cardiac surgery. *British Journal of Anaesthesia* 1991; 67: 772-8.
3. Lyons JB, Chambers FA, MacSullivan R, Moriarty DC. Anaesthesia for non-cardiac surgery in the post-cardiac transplant patient. *Irish Journal of Medical Science* 1995; 164: 132-5.

Short case 8.3: Postoperative confusion

You are called to assess a 50-year-old female patient in the recovery room who underwent total abdominal hysterectomy under general anaesthesia. The recovery nurse states that she is very confused and agitated.

How would you assess her?

♦ Airway, breathing and circulation (A, B, C) approach.
♦ Administer 100% oxygen.
♦ Check the vital parameters including oxygen saturation, pulse rate, and blood pressure.

What are the possible causes of postoperative confusion and agitation?

♦ Residual effects of drugs used in anaesthesia: inadequate recovery from muscle relaxants, intravenous/inhalational anaesthetic agents, opioids, etc. Hypothermia may contribute to impaired drug metabolism.

- Surgical causes: pain, acute abdomen, full urinary bladder, paralytic ileus, sepsis.
- Cardiovascular system: hypotension, hypovolaemia, acute coronary syndrome.
- Respiratory system: hypoxia, hypercapnia, pneumonia, aspiration
- Metabolic causes: electrolyte disturbances (especially hyponatraemia), hypoglycaemia, dehydration, hepatic and renal impairment.
- Neurological causes: cerebrovascular accident, convulsion, the post-ictal state, intracranial pathology.
- Infective causes: meningitis, respiratory infection, urinary tract infection, sepsis.
- Drug and alcohol abuse: withdrawal effects.
- Personality or behavioural disorder.

How would you investigate and treat?

Reviewing the anaesthetic chart to find the details, timing and dosage of drugs used will point to the possibility of a residual drug effect. Inspired and expired gas monitoring may identify residual inhalation agents.

If an opioid or a benzodiazepine overdose is suspected, specific antagonists such as naloxone or flumazenil should be administered.

Neuromuscular monitoring helps in assessing the degree of neuromuscular blockade. If residual paralysis is revealed, a further dose of neostigmine and glycopyrrolate can be given (the total dose of neostigmine should not be more than 5mg).

Blood glucose, serum electrolytes and temperature should be checked and the abnormalities corrected.

Monitoring the vital parameters is essential. Apart from heart rate, pulse and blood pressure, the ECG should be monitored for abnormal rhythms. When simple measures fail to identify any immediately correctable cause, arterial blood gas analysis of $PaCO_2$, PaO_2 and acid-base status can help to determine gas exchange and the metabolic status of the patient.

Comment on this ECG

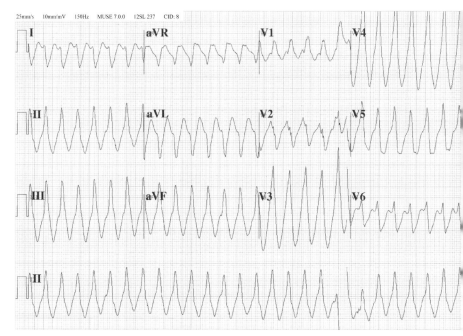

Figure 8.3 ECG.

The ECG shows regular broad complex tachycardia with a rate of approximately 175 bpm. It could be ventricular tachycardia or supraventricular tachycardia with conduction defects.

How would you treat this patient?

The management should follow the European Resuscitation Council guidelines.

As this patient has a heart rate of 175 bpm and impaired consciousness, she is considered to be unstable and will require urgent synchronized electrical cardioversion. This is commenced with a 120-150J biphasic shock (200J monophasic) and is increased in increments if this fails. She may require sedation.

In a stable patient, drug management such as amiodarone 300mg over 20-60 minutes followed by an infusion of 900mg over 24 hours should be considered.

Potentially reversible causes for the arrhythmia including electrolyte abnormalities (e.g. magnesium, potassium) should be identified and corrected.

The following adverse signs indicate that the patient is unstable:

- Signs of low cardiac output include pallor, sweating, cold, clammy extremities, impaired consciousness and hypotension.
- Heart rate >150 bpm reduces coronary perfusion.
- Blood pressure <90mm Hg.
- Presence of chest pain.
- Presence of cardiac failure.

What are the causes of irregular broad complex tachycardia?

This is most likely to be atrial fibrillation (AF) with bundle branch block, but a careful examination of a 12-lead ECG should enable precise identification of the rhythm. Other possible causes are AF with ventricular pre-excitation (in patients with Wolff-Parkinson-White [WPW] syndrome), or polymorphic VT (e.g. torsade de pointes).

How would you treat torsade de pointes?

All drugs known to prolong the QT interval should be stopped. Electrolyte abnormalities, especially hypokalaemia, should be corrected. Magnesium sulphate 2g intravenously over 10 minutes should be given. Expert help should be obtained, as other treatment (e.g. overdrive pacing) may be needed to prevent a relapse once the arrhythmia has been corrected. If adverse features develop, which is not uncommon, immediate synchronised cardioversion should be arranged.

Long QT syndrome

Long QT syndrome is characterised by a prolonged QT interval on the ECG with a tendency to develop ventricular tachyarrhythmias. The QT interval is measured from the beginning of the QRS complex to the end of the T wave. The normal QT interval corrected to the heart rate is less than 0.44 seconds. It represents the duration of ventricular activation and recovery.

A prolonged QT interval may lead to polymorphic ventricular tachycardia, which may lead to ventricular fibrillation and sudden cardiac death.

The causes of prolonged QT interval include hypocalcaemia, hypothermia, acute myocarditis, acute myocardial infarction and sympathetic stimulation. Drugs which may increase the risk of torsade de pointes include chloroquine, quinidine, amiodarone, erythromycin, methadone, thioridazine and procainamide.

Key points

◆ Immediate assessment and management of a severely confused patient involves an airway, breathing and circulation approach.
◆ Regular broad complex tachycardia compromising haemodynamic stability should be treated with cardioversion.

Further reading

1. European Resuscitation Council guidelines. http://www.erc.edu/index. php/guidelines_download_2005/en/.

Applied anatomy 8.1: Ankle block

A 55-year-old lady is on a day-case orthopaedic list for metatarsal osteotomy.

Clinical Science

What are the anaesthetic options for this patient?

The following are available options:

- General anaesthesia.
- Spinal/epidural anaesthesia.
- Ankle block.
- Combination of general anaesthesia and ankle block.

What is the nerve supply to the ankle?

The ankle is supplied by five different nerves:

- Saphenous nerve (terminal branch of femoral nerve).
- Tibial nerve (branch of sciatic nerve).
- Deep peroneal nerve (branch of sciatic nerve).
- Superficial peroneal nerve (branch of sciatic nerve).
- Sural nerve (branch of sciatic nerve).

Describe the course of these nerves

The sciatic nerve terminates at the apex of the popliteal fossa and divides into the common peroneal and tibial nerves. The tibial nerve leaves the popliteal fossa between the heads of gastrocnemius to run on the tibialis posterior, then passes medially, entering the foot behind the medial malleolus between the posterior tibial artery and flexor hallucis longus tendon. It terminates as the medial and lateral plantar branches which provide sensory supply to the sole of the foot. The tibial nerve provides sensory innervation over the calf, the heel, and the medial aspect of the plantar surface.

In the popliteal fossa, the tibial nerve gives off a sensory branch, the sural nerve, which passes downwards along the lateral aspect of the leg and then behind the lateral malleolus to provide sensory innervation of the postero-lateral aspect of the calf, the plantar surface of the heel, the lateral surface of the foot and the fifth toe.

The common peroneal nerve winds round the neck of the fibula and divides into the superficial peroneal and deep peroneal branches. It is at this location the nerve is vulnerable to pressure neuropathy. The superficial peroneal nerve provides sensory supply to the lower and outer aspect of the leg and dorsum of the foot. The deep peroneal nerve supplies the skin over the web space between the first and second toe.

The saphenous nerve is the largest sensory branch of the femoral nerve. It provides sensory innervation to the medial calf, medial malleolus, and a portion of the medial arch of the foot. It has a fairly superficial course and runs along the long saphenous vein.

What are the indications and contraindications for an ankle block?

Indications

Ankle bock can provide analgesia and anaesthesia for any operations on the foot and toes such as metatarsal osteotomy, Morton's neuroma excision, bunionectomy, incision and drainage of an abscess and amputation of the forefoot.

Absolute contraindications

◆ Patient refusal.
◆ Local infection.

Relative contraindications

◆ Coagulopathy.
◆ Systemic infection.

Describe the procedure

Ensure that IV access is secured and that SpO_2, ECG and NIBP are monitored during the procedure. The block should be performed under aseptic conditions, using 0.5% bupivacaine or levobupivacaine.

Tibial nerve

To block the tibial nerve, the area between the medial malleolus and the Achilles tendon is approached. The nerve lies in the posterior groove of the medial malleolus and is blocked by inserting a short bevelled needle anterior to the tibial artery pulsation, injecting 3-5ml of local anaesthetic.

Sural nerve

To block this nerve, the posterior groove behind the lateral malleolus is identified. The area between the lateral malleolus and Achilles tendon is approached. The nerve is blocked either by eliciting paraesthesia in the groove or by subcutaneous infiltration behind the lateral malleolus using 5ml of local anaesthetic.

Saphenous nerve

To block the nerve at the ankle, the tendon of external hallucis longus is identified. This tendon can be made more prominent by asking the patient to extend the big toe against resistance. A subcutaneous injection of 5ml of local anaesthetic is injected medial to the tendon towards the medial malleolus.

Deep peroneal nerve

To block this nerve, the external hallucis tendon is located as described earlier. The nerve is blocked between the external hallucis longus tendon and dorsalis pedis artery in the proximal portion of the first metatarsal space, using 3-5ml of local anaesthetic.

Superficial peroneal nerve

The nerve is blocked by subcutaneous infiltration of 5-10ml of local anaesthetic between the extensor hallucis longus tendon and the lateral malleolus.

What complications can occur as a result of an ankle block?

Immediate

- Vascular injury.
- Nerve injury.
- Local anaesthetic toxicity.
- Failure of block.

Delayed

◆ Haematoma.
◆ Infection.

Management of local anaesthetic toxicity

Local anaesthetic (LA) toxicity may occur sometime after the initial injection. Signs of severe toxicity include loss of consciousness, tonic-clonic convulsions, cardiovascular collapse, bradycardia, conduction blocks, asystole and ventricular tachyarrhythmias.

Management

◆ Stop injecting the LA.
◆ Call for help.
◆ Maintain the airway, administer 100% oxygen and assess breathing; if necessary, secure the airway with a tracheal tube and establish intravenous access with a wide-bore cannula.
◆ Control seizures with a benzodiazepine, thiopental or small incremental doses of propofol.
◆ If cardiac arrest occurs start cardiopulmonary resuscitation (CPR) using the advanced life support (ALS) protocol.
◆ Consider intravenous infusion of intralipid. Give an intravenous bolus injection of intralipid 20%, 1.5ml/kg over one minute (~100ml for an average adult) and start an IV infusion of intralipid 20% at 0.25ml/kg/minute (~100ml over 5 minutes for an average adult patient). The bolus injection can be repeated twice at 5-minute intervals if an adequate circulation has not been restored and the rate of infusion can be doubled.

Key points

◆ Five nerves supply the ankle and all need to be blocked for a complete ankle block.
◆ The saphenous nerve is a branch of the femoral nerve; all other nerves are branches of the sciatic nerve.

Further reading

1. Ankle block. New York Society of Regional Anaesthesia (NYSORA). www.nysora.com/techniques/ankle-block/.
2. Guidelines on management of severe local anaesthetic toxicity. Association of Anaesthetists of Great Britain and Ireland, 2007. http://www.aagbi.org/publications/guidelines/docs/latoxicity07.pd.

Applied physiology 8.2: Weaning from ventilation

A 66-year-old male patient has been ventilated for 6 days for type 2 respiratory failure secondary to acute exacerbation of COAD. Intravenous sedation and inotropic support has been gradually withdrawn so that the patient can be weaned off the ventilatory support.

What are the criteria used for weaning a patient off ventilator support?

- Cause of the respiratory failure should have been resolved.
- FiO_2 should be <0.5.
- PEEP should be <10cm H_2O.
- The patient should be able to initiate spontaneous breaths and be able to cough.
- The patient should be haemodynamically stable and inotrope requirement should be minimal.

What other indices are used to predict successful weaning from a ventilator?

- Minute ventilation <10L/min.
- Vital capacity >10ml/kg body weight.
- Respiratory rate <35 bpm.
- Tidal volume >5ml/kg body weight.
- Maximum inspiratory pressure <-25 cmH_2O.
- PaO_2/PAO_2 >0.35.
- Respiratory rate/tidal volume <100 litre^{-1}.
- PaO_2/FiO_2 >200mm Hg (>26kPa).

What do you mean by PEEP?

PEEP or positive end expiratory pressure is produced by maintaining a positive pressure during both inspiration and expiration. It helps to minimise airway and alveolar collapse and helps to increase functional residual capacity (FRC), helping to improve oxygenation.

Can you define FRC?

Functional residual capacity (FRC) is the sum of the residual volume and expiratory reserve volume. It is the volume of gas remaining in the lung at the end of normal expiration. It represents the equilibrium point where the tendency of the lungs is to collapse is balanced by the tendency of the thoracic cage to expand. The normal FRC is 2.5-3L.

Table 8.7 Factors affecting the FRC.

Increased FRC	Decreased FRC
Asthma	Supine position
Emphysema	General anaesthesia
Application of PEEP and CPAP	Obesity
	Pregnancy
	Pulmonary fibrosis

What do you understand by the Rapid Shallow Breathing Index (RSBI)?

The RSBI is used as a predictor of weaning from a ventilator and is the ratio of respiratory rate to tidal volume:

$$RSBI = respiratory\ rate/tidal\ volume$$

It is measured using a hand-held spirometer attached to the endotracheal tube with the patient breathing spontaneously for 1 minute. In patients who are likely to fail weaning, the frequency increases and tidal volume falls.

An RSBI of <80 means the patient is likely to succeed in weaning; an RSBI of >100 means the patient is likely to fail in weaning.

What is meant by the term spontaneous breathing trial (SBT)?

An SBT is a method by which a patient can be weaned off the ventilator, which is done by allowing the patient to breathe spontaneously using a T-piece, CPAP or a low level of pressure support. After 30 minutes the patient may be ready for extubation.

When would you terminate a SBT?

The SBT should be terminated if:

- Respiratory rate >35 bpm.
- SpO_2 <90%.
- Heart rate >140 bpm.
- Systolic blood pressure >180 or <90mmHg.
- The patient becomes agitated, or is sweating or very anxious.

What is the role of a tracheostomy in weaning from mechanical ventilation?

Tracheostomy facilitates weaning. It is better tolerated by the patient than an endotracheal tube and thereby reduces the need for sedation. It reduces airway resistance, and the work of breathing. It facilities tracheal suctioning and removal of secretions.

Are there any other advantages of a tracheostomy compared with an endotracheal tube?

When long-term ventilation is needed a tracheostomy is useful in reducing complications associated with prolonged tracheal intubation.

The benefits of tracheostomy include:

- Better patient comfort and compliance with the treatment.
- The patient is able to talk.
- The patient can have oral nutrition.

◆ Reduction in dead space.
◆ Easier nursing.
◆ Early tracheostomy may reduce the duration of mechanical ventilation, the incidence of pneumonia, duration of intensive care stay and overall mortality.

Measurement of FRC

FRC can be measured by three different methods:

◆ Helium dilution. The patient is made to breathe through a spirometer with a known initial volume of fresh gas (V_1) with a known initial concentration of helium (C_1). This is continued until a state of equilibrium is reached where helium is diluted to a final concentration (C_2) in the larger combined volume V_2 (which is V_1 + FRC). From the available values FRC can be derived using the equation $C_1V_1 = C_2 V_2$.
◆ Body plethysmography. The patient makes an inspiratory effort in a closed chamber and the pressure and volume changes before and after the inspiratory effort are measured by applying Boyle's gas law ($P_1V_1 = P_2V_2$).
◆ Nitrogen washout. At the end of expiration the patient breathes 100% oxygen for 7 minutes and the total volume of expired gas is analysed for nitrogen content using a nitrogen meter at the lips and by using the following formula:

$$V_1 \times 80 = (V_1 \times C_3) + (V_2 \times C_2)$$

where:

V_1 = FRC;
V_2 = total volume of gas exhaled at the end of 7 minutes;
80 = (C_1) concentration of nitrogen in the lungs before washout = 80%;
C_2 = concentration of nitrogen exhaled at the end of 7 minutes;
C_3 = concentration of nitrogen left in the lungs at the end of 7 minutes by sampling end expired gas with a nitrogen meter at the lip.

Tracheostomy

Tracheostomy can be performed using two different techniques:

◆ Surgical tracheostomy.
◆ Percutaneous tracheostomy.

Percutaneous tracheostomy

The procedure is usually performed on the intensive care unit under fibreoptic guidance. The proposed benefits of the technique compared with surgical tracheostomy include a reduced delay in performing the procedure, ease of performance at the bed side, a lower incidence of peristomal bleeding and reduced postoperative infection. Both techniques are, however, safe when conducted by experienced and skilled practitioners.

Pre-procedure preparation involves pre-oxygenation. Clotting tests should be normal.

Procedure
◆ Positioning: the neck should be extended by placing a sandbag under the shoulder.
◆ Full aseptic precautions are necessary (scrubbed, mask, gloves, gown).
◆ Local anaesthetic (lidocaine with epinephrine) is infiltrated at the junction of the first and second tracheal ring.
◆ After making a vertical incision in the space between the first and second tracheal ring, a syringe and needle with saline is used to locate the trachea.
◆ A fibreoptic scope is used to ensure the correct placement of the needle.
◆ A guidewire is inserted through the needle; the needle is removed with the guidewire left in place.
◆ Special dilators lubricated with sterile water are used to dilate the site of entry. Serial dilators are used from small to large.
◆ Finally, the tracheostomy tube is railroaded over the dilator and passed over the guidewire.
◆ A fibreoptic scope is used throughout to ensure correct placement.

+ The breathing system is connected to the tracheostomy tube and adequate ventilation of the lungs should be confirmed before completely removing the tracheal tube.
+ A chest X-ray is performed to ensure correct placement and to rule out pneumothorax.

Key points

+ A patient being weaned from a ventilator should be haemodynamically stable, the cause of the respiratory failure resolved and oxygen requirement should be minimal.
+ A spontaneous breathing trial will help in deciding which patients may be extubated.

Further reading

1. Trac-man. A randomised trial looking at the timing of tracheostomy management in adult intensive care patients. www.tracman.org.uk.
2. Jaber S, Chanques G, Matecki S, *et al*. Post-extubation stridor in intensive care patients. *Intensive Care Medicine* 2003; 29: 69-74.
3. Dries DJ, McGonigal MD, Malian MS. Bor BJ, Sullivan C. Protocol-driven ventilator weaning, use of mechanical ventilation, rate of early re-intubation, and ventilator-associated pneumonia. *Journal of Trauma* 2004; 56: 943-51.

Applied pharmacology 8.3: Post-herpetic neuralgia

A 65-year-old male was admitted to hospital with a rash on his chest 4 months ago. He has been readmitted with a constant burning pain over his chest (where the rash was) which at times becomes sharp and stabbing, and comes and goes. The skin over the rash is very sensitive and even slight touch such as the rubbing of clothes on the affected area causes pain.

What do you think is the most likely diagnosis?

Post-herpetic neuralgia (PHN).

What is post-herpetic neuralgia (PHN)?

PHN is a painful condition associated with reactivation of the *Varicella zoster* virus in a particular dermatome(s). Pain that persists for longer than 1-3 months after resolution of the rash is a strong indicator of PHN.

What is the pathophysiology of PHN?

During primary infection, the virus gains entry to the sensory root ganglia. The virus remains dormant for decades due to *Varicella zoster* virus-specific cell-mediated immunity acquired during the primary infection. Following a decrease in virus-specific cell-mediated immunity, reactivation of the virus can occur. The reactivated virus travels down the sensory nerve and causes the dermatomal distribution of pain and the skin lesions.

Is there any age group particularly predisposed to developing PHN?

It is usually seen in adults over 50 and more likely to be severe in people aged over 60. About one in four people aged over 60 who have had shingles develop PHN that lasts more than 30 days.

What are the clinical features of PHN?

The prodromal phase consists of hyperaesthesia, paraesthesia, burning dysaesthesia or pruritus along the affected dermatomes.

A characteristic skin lesion follows the prodromal phase with a maculopapular rash in the affected dermatomes. The vesicles become haemorrhagic or turbid and then crust over within 7-10 days.

Ocular complications include:

- Mucopurulent conjunctivitis.
- Episcleritis.
- Keratitis.

- Anterior uveitis.
- Extraocular motility which may be affected, due to the effect on the 3rd, 4th and 6th cranial nerves.

What are the features of pain suffered in PHN?

Pain in PHN is described as constant, burning, gnawing, lancinating and unrelenting. At times, the patient complains of sharp or stabbing pain which comes and goes. The affected skin is very sensitive. Even slight touch such as rubbing of clothes or a draught of air may cause pain.

Which dermatomes and cranial nerves are commonly affected?

It commonly affects the thoracic dermatomes (T5/T6) and also the ophthalmic division of the trigeminal nerve.

What is the natural progression of PHN?

PHN is generally a self-limiting condition but can last indefinitely. Treatment is directed at pain control whilst waiting for the condition to resolve.

What are the various treatment modalities available to treat PHN?

General measures

Loose fitting cotton clothes may reduce irritation of the affected area of the skin. Pain may be eased by cooling the affected area with ice cubes (wrapped in a plastic bag), or by having a cool bath.

Topical measures

- Lidocaine 5% patch.
- Capsaicin cream.

Systemic analgesics

Paracetamol, codeine, tramadol or anti-inflammatory drugs such as ibuprofen may give some relief. Strong painkillers such as morphine and oxycodone may be needed in some cases.

Antidepressant drugs

Tricyclic antidepressants are used commonly as a treatment for PHN, as they ease neuralgia (nerve pain). Amitriptyline is a drug commonly used. Pain ceases, or is greatly eased, in up to 8 in 10 cases of PHN treated with amitriptyline. Imipramine and nortriptyline are other tricyclic antidepressants that are occasionally used to treat PHN.

Anticonvulsant drugs

These are an alternative to antidepressants. Gabapentin and pregabalin are commonly used for PHN.

Other methods

- Infiltration with local anaesthetics.
- Sympathetic blockade.
- Nerve blocks.
- Extradural steroid injection.
- Transcutaneous electrical nerve stimulation (TENS).
- Behavioural therapy.

Which topical medications are used to treat PHN?

Topical lidocaine

Lidocaine may block the pain signals coming from the nerve. Patches need to be worn for 12 hours per day. It can be applied over unbroken skin. It is chosen when the pain is localised, when other neuropathic pain medicines are ineffective or not tolerated.

Capsaicin cream

Capsaicin is the active 'burning' component of chilli peppers. It causes release of substance P from pain fibres, causing a burning sensation. Analgesia occurs when substance P is depleted from the nerve fibres. Capsaicin cream should be applied 3-4 times a day.

What is the role of tricyclic antidepressants (TCAs) in PHN?

These are effective adjuncts in the reduction of neuropathic pain of PHN. The commonly used TCAs in PHN are amitriptyline, nortriptyline, desipramine and imipramine. Their onset of action is slow. A tricyclic antidepressant will often ease the pain within a few days, but it may take 2-3 weeks, and it can take several weeks before achieving maximum benefit. The onset may be enhanced by commencing the treatment early in the course of *Herpes zoster* infection in conjunction with antiviral agents. The side effects include sedation, dry mouth, postural hypotension, blurred vision and urinary retention. Occasionally, TCAs can cause cardiac conduction abnormalities or liver toxicity (more likely in elderly patients with cardiac or liver disease).

What is the role of anticonvulsants in the treatment of PHN?

Anticonvulsants such as phenytoin, carbamazepine, gabapentin and pregabalin have been shown to be effective in treating the pain of PHN. Lack of response to one of these medications does not necessarily predict a poor response to another.

The role of antiviral drugs in the treatment of PHN

Famciclovir is an antiviral drug used for the treatment of Herpes virus infection. It is a pro-drug of peciclovir with better oral bioavailability. If administered within 72 hours of the onset of the vesicles of shingles, the damage to peripheral nerves can be minimised and the subsequent pain of PHN is attenuated. The dose is 500mg tablets orally, three times a day for 1 week.

Key points

- PHN is a painful condition associated with reactivation of the *Varicella zoster* virus.
- It usually affects the T5/T6 dermatomes and the ophthalmic division of the trigeminal nerve.

Further reading

1. Dworkin RH, Boon RJ, Griffin DRG, DePhung. Post-herpetic neuralgia: impact of famciclovir, age, rash, severity and acute pain in a *Herpes zoster* patient. *The Journal of Infectious Diseases* 1998; 178: S76-80.
2. Johnson RW, Dworkin RH. Treatment of *Herpes zoster* and post-herpetic neuralgia. *British Medical Journal* 2003; 326: 748-50.
3. Stankus SJ, Dlugopolski M, Packer D. Management of *Herpes zoster* (shingles) and post-herpetic neuralgia. *Journal of American Family Physician* 2000; 61: 2437-44.

Equipment, clinical measurement and monitoring 3.4: Measurement of blood gases

A 38-year-old known asthmatic is admitted to the emergency department with acute exacerbation of asthma. He is short of breath and not able to speak in sentences.

On clinical examination, his BP is 135/80mmHg, HR is 110 bpm, RR is 26/minute and SpO_2 is 92%. He is receiving oxygen via a face mask at 12L/min. On auscultation, he has extensive bilateral expiratory wheezes.

What blood tests are useful in the further management of this patient?

- Full blood count.
- Urea and electrolytes.
- Arterial blood gas analysis.

What are the various parameters that can be measured by blood gas analysis?

Basic parameters

- Hydrogen ion concentration (pH).
- Carbon dioxide tension ($PaCO_2$).
- Oxygen tension (PaO_2).

- Base excess.
- Bicarbonate and standard bicarbonate concentration.

Additional/optional parameters

- Na^+, K^+, Ca^{2+} concentrations.
- Lactate.
- Haemoglobin.
- Carboxyhaemoglobin and other abnormal haemoglobins.

What do you understand by the term pH?

pH is the negative logarithm to the base 10 of the hydrogen ion concentration:

$$pH = - \log [H^+]$$

The normal pH of an arterial blood gas sample is 7.35-7.45. It is basic/alkaline if pH >7.45 and acidic if the pH <7.35. The higher the concentration of hydrogen ions, the lower will be the pH:

- pH 7.0 = 100nmol/L i.e., 10^{-7}mol/L.
- pH 8.0 = 10nmol/L.
- pH 6.0 = 1000nmol/L.

Hydrogen ions are produced daily by the reaction of carbon dioxide and water. For normal cellular functioning, the acid base balance needs to be within normal limits. The normal hydrogen ion concentration is 35-45nmol/L which corresponds to a pH of 7.35-7.45.

How does a blood gas analyser measure the hydrogen ion concentration and pH in a blood sample?

The blood gas analyser directly measures pH using a pH electrode. It consists of two separate electrodes: a pH measuring electrode and a reference electrode.

The pH measuring electrode is a glass electrode (silver/silver chloride) incorporating a bulb made of pH(hydrogen ion)-sensitive glass holding a buffer solution of constant pH.

The reference electrode is calomel (mercury/mercury chloride) or a silver/silver chloride electrode which contains potassium chloride as an electrolyte solution. The arterial blood sample comes into contact with the potassium chloride solution via a membrane.

When a sample is passed through the pH-sensitive glass bulb, an electrical potential is developed due to the difference in H^+ ion concentration. The potential difference across the two electrodes is measured and converted to a direct reading of H^+ or pH.

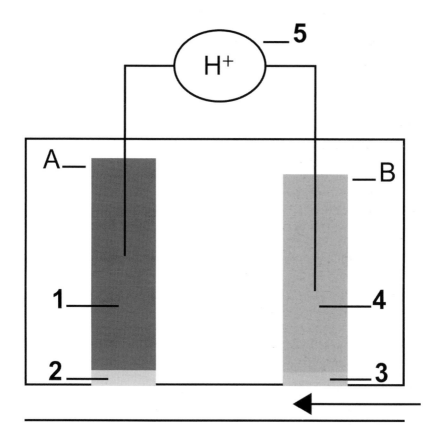

Figure 8.4 pH electrode. A) Measuring electrode; B) Reference electrode; 1. Buffer; 2. pH-sensitive glass; 3. Leaky membrane; 4. Potassium chloride solution; 5. pH display.

Is temperature control important when measuring pH?

Yes. The electrodes are surrounded by a thermal control system to maintain a constant temperature at around 37°C. The pH decreases by 0.015 units for each degree Celsius rise in temperature.

How would you measure carbon dioxide tension ($PaCO_2$) in arterial blood?

$PaCO_2$ is measured using the Severinghaus CO_2 electrode. This consists of a H^+-sensitive glass electrode and a silver/silver chloride reference electrode. The electrode is surrounded by nylon mesh containing sodium bicarbonate (electrolyte) solution and a Teflon membrane permeable to CO_2. Carbon dioxide reacts with the water present in the electrolyte solution producing hydrogen (H^+) ions, resulting in a change in pH:

$$CO_2 + H_2O \longrightarrow H^+ + HCO_3^-$$

The numbers of H^+ ions produced are in proportion to the partial pressure of CO_2 (0.01 pH units for every 0.1kPa CO_2).

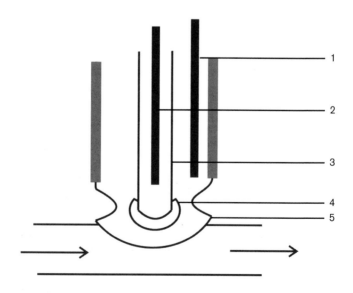

Figure 8.5 Severinghaus CO_2 electrode.
1. Reference electrode; 2. H^+ sensitive glass electrode; 3. H^+ sensitive glass; 4. Bicarbonate-containing nylon mesh; 5. CO_2 permeable membrane.

As with a pH electrode, the CO_2 electrode needs to be maintained at 37°C and is calibrated with known mixtures of CO_2 and O_2.

How would you measure oxygen tension in arterial blood?

Oxygen tension in blood can be measured by the Clark electrode, also known as the polarographic electrode.

The Clark electrode has a platinum cathode and a silver/silver chloride anode in a potassium chloride solution. Electrons are produced at the anode by the reaction of silver and chloride ions. In the presence of oxygen, electrons are consumed at the cathode.

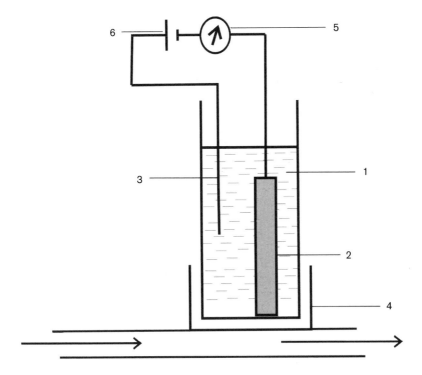

Figure 8.6 Clark electrode.

1. Electrolyte, buffered KOH, KCl or NaCl; 2. Platinum cathode; 3. Anode (silver/silver chloride); 4. Plastic membrane; 5. Galvanometer; 6. Battery.

A voltage of 0.7V is applied between the electrodes, and a small electric current flows. The current flow is measured. The greater the oxygen tension the greater the current flow.

What is meant by standard bicarbonate?

Standard bicarbonate is the plasma concentration of bicarbonate when haemoglobin is fully saturated, arterial PCO_2 is corrected to 5.3kPa and the temperature is 37°C. The normal value is 24-33mmol/L.

What is meant by a base excess or deficit?

This is the amount of base or acid that is required to restore 1L of blood to normal pH at a PCO_2 of 5.3kPa and at a temperature of 37°C.

Calibration

To assure appropriate functioning of the electrodes, calibration procedures are performed. The blood gas analyser automatically performs one-point and two-point calibrations at regular intervals. There is an option for the operator to perform a re-calibration at any time.

One-point calibration measures each parameter (PaO_2, $PaCO_2$ and pH) on one gas or solution of known concentration, giving one value per parameter.

Two-point calibration measures each parameter on two different solutions or gases of known concentration, giving two values per parameter. A 'low' concentration and a 'high' concentration are used at both ends of the physiological range to be measured.

Multiple-point calibration (three or more points) helps to assess whether the gas analyser response is linear or not.

PO_2 and PCO_2 electrodes are calibrated using calibration gas mixtures of known oxygen and carbon dioxide concentration. The pH electrode is calibrated using solutions of known hydrogen ion concentration.

Key points

◆ PCO_2, PO_2 and pH are measured directly; the other values are usually calculated.

◆ For normal cellular functioning, acid base balance needs to be within normal limits.

◆ To ensure appropriate functioning of the electrodes, calibration procedures need to be performed.

Further reading

1. Shapiro BA, Cane RD. Blood gas monitoring: yesterday, today, and tomorrow. *Critical Care Medicine* 1989; 17: 573-81.

2. Venkatesh B, Clutton Brock TH, Hendry SP. A multiparameter sensor for continuous intra-arterial blood gas monitoring: a prospective evaluation. *Critical Care Medicine* 1994; 22: 588-94.

3. Abraham E, Gallagher TJ, S. Fink S. Clinical evaluation of a multiparameter intra-arterial blood-gas sensor. *Intensive Care Medicine* 1996; 22: 507-13.

Structured oral examination 9

Long case 9

Information for the candidate

History

A 76-year-old lady is scheduled for an extended colectomy for confirmed adenocarcinoma of the colon. She has never had an operation in the past. Her past medical history includes hypertension and a myocardial infarction 5 years ago. A subsequent coronary angiogram showed an 80% stenosis of the left anterior descending artery and moderate mitral regurgitation.

She gave up smoking 3 months ago. Her current medication is bendroflumethiazide 5mg o.d., perindopril 4mg o.d. and aspirin 75mg o.d.

Clinical examination

Table 9.1 Clinical examination.	
Weight	72kg
Height	172cm
Heart rate	75 bpm
Respiratory rate	14/minute
Blood pressure	150/80mmHg
Temperature	37°C

Investigations

Table 9.2 Biochemistry.

		Normal values
Sodium	138mmol/L	135-145mmol/L
Potassium	4.1mmol/L	3.5-5.0mmol/L
Urea	10.5mmol/L	2.2-8.3mmol/L
Creatinine	103μmol/L	44-80μmol/L
Blood glucose	5.5mmol/L	3.0-6.0mmol/L

Table 9.3 Haematology.

		Normal values
Hb	9.8g/dL	11-16 g/dL
Haematocrit	0.34	0.4-0.5 males, 0.37-0.47 females
RBC	3.7×10^{12}/L	$3.8-4.8 \times 10^{12}$/L
WBC	4.2×10^9/L	$4-11 \times 10^9$/L
Platelets	220×10^9/L	$150-450 \times 10^9$/L
INR	1.0	0.9-1.2
PT	12.5 seconds	11-15 seconds
APTT ratio	1	0.8-1.2

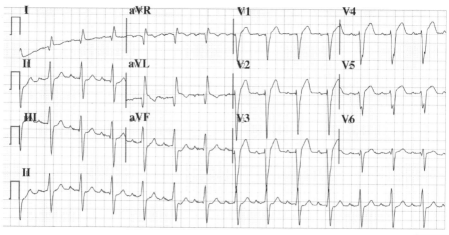

Figure 9.1 ECG.

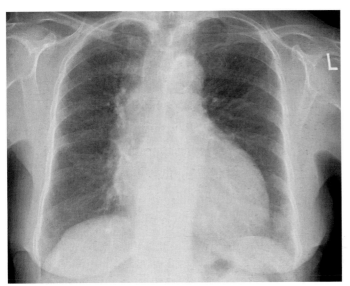

Figure 9.2 Chest X-ray.

Examiner's questions

Please summarise the case

An elderly lady with significant cardiovascular comorbidity and renal impairment is scheduled for major abdominal surgery.

Comment on the haematology results

The haemoglobin is low at 9.8g/dL.

What could be the reasons for the low haemoglobin?

These could be due to nutritional deficiency, decreased production or increased loss. In this lady the possible causes are:

- Iron deficiency due to poor appetite and poor intake.
- Deficiency of B12 and folate.
- Blood loss due to bleeding from the colonic cancer.
- Bone marrow depression from anticancer drugs or bone marrow infiltration by malignant cells.

Would you transfuse blood to this patient pre-operatively?

The usual pre-operative transfusion trigger in a healthy patient is approximately 7g/dL. The concerns in this patient are significant cardiac disease and major abdominal surgery with anticipated blood loss of 0.5 to 1 litre. This patient could benefit from a higher Hb to maintain adequate myocardial oxygen delivery. A slightly higher transfusion trigger of 8-9g/dL could be beneficial, but with her level there is no need to transfuse pre-operatively. The haemoglobin concentration should be monitored intra-operatively and blood should be available for transfusion.

Can you read this ECG in a systematic way?

This ECG is recorded at a speed of 25mm/sec and properly calibrated with a standardisation of 1mV =10mm.

Table 9.4 Systematic reading of ECG.	
Heart rate	75 beats per minute
Rhythm	Normal sinus rhythm
PR interval	0.24 second; this is prolonged and indicates first-degree heart block
P wave	Normal
QRS complex	Widened in V4, V5 and V6 suggesting left bundle branch block Abnormal Q waves in leads I, aVL and non-progression of R waves from V4-V6 indicating an old lateral/ anterior myocardial infarction
QT interval	Normal
ST segment	Normal

Q waves are pathological when wide (greater than 0.04 seconds) and deep (greater than 4mm).

Comment on the chest X-ray

This is a postero-anterior view of a chest X-ray of a female patient. It is an erect, centralised film with adequate exposure of the lung fields. The trachea is deviated to the right. There is cardiomegaly.

How would you stratify cardiac risks in a patient presenting for non-cardiac surgery?

A detailed pre-operative evaluation of cardiovascular status is performed in order to identify patients with severe ischaemic heart disease and to stratify the risks. The important decision that should be made is whether a revascularisation procedure and/or modification of medical therapy is required prior to the proposed surgery.

Based on the surgical procedure the cardiac risk can be stratified into high, intermediate and low.

High (mortality >5%):

- Emergency major operations especially in the elderly.
- Aortic and other major vascular surgery.
- Peripheral vascular surgery.
- Anticipated prolonged surgical procedures associated with large fluid shifts and blood loss.

Intermediate (mortality <5%):

- Carotid endarterectomy.
- Head and neck surgery.
- Intraperitoneal and intrathoracic surgery.
- Orthopaedic surgery.
- Prostate surgery.

Low (cardiac risk generally <1%):

- Endoscopic procedures.
- Superficial procedures.
- Cataract surgery.
- Breast surgery.

As this patient is scheduled for major abdominal surgery with anticipated large fluid shifts and blood loss, she has a high risk of cardiac mortality.

Cardiac risk stratification based on Goldman cardiac risk factors

In Goldman's cardiac risk evaluation there are nine independent factors which are evaluated on a point scale:

- Presence of third heart sound (S3) or elevated jugular venous pressure (11 points).
- Myocardial infarction in the past 6 months (10 points).
- ECG showing premature atrial contractions or any rhythm other than sinus (7 points).
- ECG showing >5 premature ventricular contractions per minute (7 points).
- Age >70 years (5 points).
- Emergency operation (4 points).
- Intrathoracic, intra-abdominal or aortic surgery (3 points).
- Poor medical condition, or bedridden (3 points).
- Significant aortic stenosis (3 points).

Patients with scores >25 points have a 56% incidence of death, and a 22% incidence of severe cardiovascular complications.

The Goldman risk index was modified by Detsky and further simplified by Lee *et al*. The predictors of adverse cardiac outcome include high risk surgery, ischaemic heart disease, cardiac failure, cerebrovascular disease, Type I diabetes mellitus and renal failure.

How would you classify the risk based on functional status?

Functional capacity is a measure of exercise tolerance and it can be deduced from the ability to perform the activities of daily living. It is expressed in metabolic equivalent (MET) levels:

- 1 MET=3.5ml/kg per minute of oxygen consumption (oxygen consumption [VO_2] of a 70kg, 40-year-old man in a resting state).
- 4 METs are equivalent to climbing a flight of stairs.
- 6 METs are equivalent to a short run.

The functional capacity can be classified as:

- Excellent: exercise tolerance greater than 7 METS.
- Moderate: exercise tolerance between 4 and 7 METS.
- Poor: exercise tolerance less than 4 METS.

Patients with exercise tolerance 4 METs and above are considered to be at low risk of peri-operative morbidity; 4 METs or less increase the risk of peri-operative morbidity.

The New York Heart Association classifies patients into four groups depending on clinical symptoms (the symptoms include shortness of breath and angina on exertion):

- Class 1: no symptoms at ordinary physical activity.
- Class 2: mild symptoms and slight limitation of physical activity.
- Class 3: symptoms at minimal exertion and marked limitation of physical activity.
- Class 4: symptoms on minimal exertion or at rest.

Are there any other investigations which may be useful in assessing the severity of ischaemic heart disease?

Echocardiogrphy

This is useful in assessing the degree of the valvular lesion. Myocardial ischaemia leads to ventricular wall and septal motion abnormalities which can also be detected by echocardiography.

Dobutamine stress echocardiography

Dobutamine increases the heart rate and myocardial contractility, increasing myocardial oxygen demand. Echocardiography can identify regional wall motion abnormality produced by inadequate oxygen supply and also ischaemia within the distribution of affected vessels. This test is useful in patients in whom exercise testing is not possible.

Dipyridamole-thallium scintigraphy scanning

Dipyridamole causes coronary dilatation and increases blood flow in normal vessels. The coronary vessels distal to the significant stenosis are already dilated. It therefore increases blood flow to the region supplied by normal coronary arteries. Distribution of thallium in the myocardium is detected using a gamma camera. The diseased, under-perfused area of the myocardium will have less thallium distribution.

Is there any other objective test to evaluate cardiorespiratory function?

Cardiopulmonary exercise testing (CPET) is a more objective method of assessing cardiopulmonary function. CPET is a non-invasive test that involves submaximal and maximal exercise, either on a treadmill or a bicycle with respiratory gas analysis and continuous ECG monitoring. The respiratory analysis involves continuous spirometry, oxygen uptake and CO_2 output. It helps to simultaneously assess ventricular function, respiratory function and myocardial ischaemia, and a number of parameters such as maximal oxygen consumption (VO_2 max), anaerobic threshold (AT), peak heart rate and respiratory gas exchange ratio. The AT is the point at which the oxygen consumption of the exercising muscle outstrips the aerobic supply and the metabolism switches to anaerobic glycolysis. At this point there is a sudden increase in CO_2 production. If a patient is scheduled for major abdominal surgery and had an AT >11ml/kg/minute and a VO_2 max >15ml O_2/kg/minute, they would be regarded as fit to undergo surgery. An AT <11ml/kg/minute is associated with significantly increased peri-operative cardiorespiratory morbidity and a higher mortality rate. A VO_2 max of 15ml O_2/kg/ minute and an AT >11ml O_2/kg/minute is clinically equivalent to climbing two flights of stairs or walking 600m on level ground.

How would you optimise this patient prior to surgery?

As this patient has ischaemic heart disease with an 80% stenosis of the left anterior descending artery, she has a significant risk of peri-operative cardiac mortality. Although she may benefit from coronary revascularisation and optimisation, this may not be possible due to the urgency of surgery. If a patient undergoes coronary revascularisation with a bare-metal stent, surgery may not be possible for 4-6 weeks due to the required antiplatelet therapy and increased risk of myocardial events during that period. Surgery can be performed 2-4 weeks following balloon angioplasty.

A multidisciplinary team approach involving consultant surgeon, consultant anaesthetist and cardiologist is essential in the management of this patient. If time is available the patient should be referred to a cardiologist for evaluation of left ventricular function by stress testing and echocardiography. Use of drugs such as beta-blockers, calcium channel blockers and statins should be considered:

♦ Beta-blockers. Initial studies suggested survival benefits when patients were treated with a beta-blocker in the peri-operative period. The Peri-Operative ISchaemic Evaluation (POISE) trial, however, published in 2008, found an increased mortality with peri-operative beta-blockade. Clinically significant peri-operative hypotension and bradycardia were associated with increased mortality.
♦ Calcium channel blockers. Calcium channel blockers may offer cardio protection in the peri-operative period, but the results of meta-analysis are conflicting.
♦ α-2 adrenoceptor agonists. α-2 adrenoceptor agonists (clonidine) may improve cardiovascular morbidity and mortality following non-cardiac and cardiac surgery. They attenuate peri-operative haemodynamic instability and inhibit central sympathetic discharge.
♦ Statins. Statins reduce vascular inflammation, improving endothelial function and stabilising the atherosclerotic plaque. Peri-operative statin usage in patients undergoing major vascular surgery has been associated with reduced peri-operative mortality.

You have referred this patient to a cardiologist but before she is seen by the cardiologist she presents with abdominal pain and vomiting. On clinical examination her BP is 110/64 mmHg, HR is 110 beats per minute, and SpO$_2$ is 94%. Her abdomen is distended and tender on palpation. What is the likely cause for her sudden deterioration?

The most likely cause is due to bowel perforation.

How would you anaesthetise her for an emergency laparotomy?

Pre-operative management

She should be assessed and resuscitated in a critical care environment. Further investigations including a full blood count, urea, electrolytes, blood glucose, ECG and chest X-ray should be performed. Her hydration status should be assessed, and fluid and electrolyte imbalance should be corrected. Pre-operative resuscitation and management involves the following:

◆ Ensure her airway is patent, breathing is adequate and administer 100% oxygen.
◆ Secure the venous access with at least two large-bore intravenous cannulae and start fluid resuscitation with crystalloids.
◆ Blood should be grouped and two units of blood should be cross-matched.
◆ The stomach should be emptied by inserting a nasogastric tube, allowing free drainage.
◆ Hypotension should be treated with intravenous fluids and a titrated infusion of inotropic drugs. Vasopressor drugs should be used with caution.

Intra-operative management

Monitoring
Intra-operative monitoring should include invasive arterial blood pressure, central venous pressure, body temperature (nasopharyngeal), urine output, blood loss estimation and intermittent measurement of blood gases, haemoglobin and blood glucose.

Anaesthetic technique
A combination of general anaesthesia and epidural analgesia with a low concentration of local anaesthetic can be used. An epidural catheter at low thoracic level can be inserted prior to induction of general anaesthesia. Epidural anaesthesia can result in hypotension which may have deleterious effects on myocardial oxygen delivery. However, a titrated epidural infusion of a low concentration of local anaesthetic (0.1 to 0.125% bupivacaine or levobupivacaine) can provide analgesia without significant cardiovascular effects.

Induction

Prior to induction the nasogastric tube should be aspirated. Rapid sequence induction should be performed with a titrated dose of thiopentone and succinylcholine. Hypothermia is avoided by using a warm air blanket and by warming the intravenous fluids.

Cardiac output monitoring using transoesophageal Doppler or LiDCO (lithium indicator dilution cardiac output) monitoring is useful in optimising myocardial and tissue oxygen delivery. Inotropic drugs such as epinephrine, dobutamine and vasodilators such as glyceryl trinitrate may be required during the intra-operative period.

Postoperative management

This patient should be managed in the intensive care unit. Ventilator support may be needed based on the acid-base balance, inotropic support and oxygen requirement. Invasive monitoring should be continued during the postoperative period. The options for postoperative analgesia include epidural analgesia, morphine infusion or PCA with morphine. Supplemental oxygen should be administered for the first 3-4 days postoperatively.

What are the principles of haemodynamic management during anaesthesia in a patient with mitral regurgitation?

- Preload: a sudden increase in preload may cause pulmonary oedema. Adequate preload is essential to maintain stroke volume.
- Myocardial contractility: normal contractility should be maintained.
- Afterload: an increase in systemic vascular resistance reduces the forward flow from the left ventricle and increases the regurgitant flow from the left ventricle. Relatively low systemic vascular resistance facilitates forward flow and maintains stroke volume.
- Heart rate: bradycardia should be avoided as it increases the diastolic filling of the left ventricle, and may lead to further dilatation of the valve ring. Relative tachycardia is preferred as it maintains the cardiac output.

Antiplatelet therapy

Antiplatelet therapy is commonly used in patients with ischaemic heart disease, particularly following insertion of coronary stents. Aspirin and clopidogrel are two current drugs commonly used in cardiac patients. Aspirin irreversibly inactivates the cyclo-oxygenase enzyme, and by reducing the synthesis of thromboxane A_2, reduces platelet aggregation. Clopidogrel binds to the P2Y12 subtype of adenosine diphosphate (ADP) receptors on the platelet membrane and prevents the activation of the glycoprotein IIb/IIIa pathway. This inhibits platelet aggregation. The effect of both drugs lasts for the life-time of platelets (7-10 days).

Drug-eluting stents (DES) are designed to reduce the rate of restenosis. They are coated with either sirolimus or paclitaxel. As the action of these drugs will delay endothelialisation, there is an increased risk of thrombosis which is prevented by administering antiplatelet agents. Patients with bare metal stents require life-long aspirin and at least a month's treatment with clopidogrel.

Key points

- There are various methods of cardiac risk stratification based on the surgical procedure, Goldman's cardiac risk factors and CPET.
- Supplemental oxygen should be administered for the first 3-4 days following major surgery to reduce the incidence of postoperative MI.
- Postoperative anaemia, hypothermia and inadequate analgesia can result in an imbalance between myocardial oxygen demand and supply.

Further reading

1. Goldman L, Caldera DL, Nussbaum SR. Multifactorial index of cardiac risk in non-cardiac surgical procedures. *New England Journal of Medicine* 1977; 297: 845-50.
2. Priebe HJ. Perioperative myocardial infarction - aetiology and prevention. *British Journal of Anaesthesia* 2005; 95: 3-19.
3. Allman KG, Wilson IH. Ischaemic heart disease. In: *Oxford handbook of anaesthesia*, 2nd ed. Oxford: Oxford University Press, 2006: 20-3.

Short case 9.1: Ulcerative colitis

A 45-year-old female patient known to have ulcerative colitis has presented with toxic megacolon and is scheduled for an urgent laparotomy. Her regular medication includes prednisolone 10mg o.d. and mesalazine 800mg b.d.

What is toxic megacolon?

Toxic megacolon is a life-threatening complication of severe fulminant ulcerative colitis. Usually the transverse colon acutely dilates and may perforate. Patients may present with fever, tachycardia, abdominal pain and distension, dehydration, electrolyte imbalance, hypotension and possible sepsis.

What are the aims of treating toxic megacolon?

The main aims are to:

◆ Reduce the risk of colonic perforation.
◆ Correct fluid-electrolyte imbalance.
◆ Treat toxaemia and precipitating factors.

What are the implications for anaesthesia in a patient with ulcerative colitis?

Ulcerative colitis may have associated systemic manifestations involving the joints, liver, haematological and renal systems. These patients are usually on a wide range of medications such as steroids, aminosalicylates and immuno-modulatory drugs. Patients may present with the following systemic effects:

◆ Fragile skin due to both the disease process and also long-term steroid use.
◆ Limited joint mobility due to arthritis can cause difficulty in neck positioning for tracheal intubation. Rarely, it can affect the temporomandibular joint and restrict mouth opening.

◆ Ulcerative colitis can cause renal and hepatic impairment which may affect drug metabolism and excretion.
◆ In severe disease there may be multiple episodes of diarrhoea which can cause dehydration and electrolyte imbalance.
◆ Patients may be anaemic which may require blood transfusion.
◆ In fulminant cases patients may be systemically very unwell and haemodynamically unstable.

This patient is on mesalazine. What is it?

Mesalazine or 5-aminosalicylic acid (5-ASA) is a bowel-specific aminosalicylate. It is used to treat ulcerative colitis and mild to moderate Crohn's disease. It is mainly metabolised in the gut. It is available as a tablet, rectal suppository, suspension or enema.

The dosage in an acute episode is 2.4g daily in divided doses. For maintenance, 1.2-2.4g per day in divided doses is used. To treat an acute episode affecting the rectosigmoid region, one metered application can be used as a foam enema (mesalazine 1g) into the rectum daily for 4-6 weeks; for an acute episode affecting the descending colon, two metered applications (mesalazine 2g) can be used once daily for 4-6 weeks. It can also be administered as a suppository, 0.5 to 1.5g/day in divided doses, both for an acute episode and for maintenance.

Side effects include diarrhoea, nausea, vomiting, abdominal pain, exacerbation of symptoms of colitis, headache and hypersensitivity reactions (including rash and urticaria). Rare side effects can include pancreatitis, hepatitis, myocarditis, peripheral neuropathy and blood disorders (agranulocytosis, aplastic anaemia and thrombocytopaenia).

What are the side effects of corticosteroids?

These can be classified as general side effects, those due to mineralocorticoid effects, and those due to glucocorticoid effects. They can be minimised by using the lowest effective dose for the shortest period possible.

Mineralocorticoid effects

The most marked effects are seen with fludrocortisone and hydrocortisone:

◆ Sodium and water retention.
◆ Hypertension.
◆ Electrolyte imbalance such as hypokalaemia and hypocalcaemia (particularly with fludrocortisone use).

Glucocorticoid effects

◆ Diabetes.
◆ Osteoporosis which may cause fractures.
◆ Avascular necrosis of the femoral head.
◆ Muscle wasting (proximal myopathy).
◆ Peptic ulceration and perforation.
◆ Cushing's syndrome (moon face, striae, and acne).

General side effects

Gastrointestinal system
◆ Dyspepsia and abdominal distension.
◆ Acute pancreatitis.
◆ Ulceration.

Musculoskeletal system
◆ Muscle weakness.
◆ Osteoporosis causing vertebral and long bone fractures.

Endocrine system
◆ Menstrual irregularities.
◆ Weight gain.
◆ Tendency to catch infections.

Effects on the eye

◆ Glaucoma.

◆ Cataracts (posterior subcapsular).

Effects on the skin

◆ Impaired healing.

◆ Petechiae and ecchymoses.

Complications of acute therapy include hyperglycaemia, peptic ulceration, fluid retention, hypokalaemia, delayed wound healing, psychosis and myopathy.

How does steroid therapy affect the stress response in a surgical patient?

The stress response is the name given to the hormonal and metabolic changes which follow injury or trauma. It encompasses a wide range of endocrinological, immunological and haematological effects. The endocrinological effect is characterised by increased secretion of pituitary hormones and activation of the sympathetic nervous system. There is increased secretion of ACTH from the anterior pituitary with a resultant increase in the release of glucocorticoids from the adrenal cortex. The renin-angiotensin system increases the release of aldosterone from the adrenal cortex leading to water and sodium retention.

The normal cortisol production is about 25-30mg per day. During the stress response this may increase up to 75-100mg per day, and may remain elevated for up to 3 days following surgery.

Patients on long-term steroid therapy, however, with a dose >10mg per day of prednisolone (or the equivalent of other steroids) are likely to have a suppressed hypothalamic-pituitary adrenal (HPA) axis. These patients are unable to produce a normal stress response to surgery. This may be manifested as hypotension, hyponatraemia and hypoglycaemia during the peri-operative period.

How would you test the function of the hypothalamic-pituitary adrenal (HPA) axis?

The HPA axis can be tested using the short synacthen test. It involves intravenous administration of 250µg of synacthen (synthetic corticotrophin) and measurement of serum cortisol levels. A low cortisol level indicates suppression of the HPA axis. In equivocal cases the insulin tolerance test can be used. The insulin tolerance test involves intravenous administration of 0.1u/kg of insulin and measurement of serum glucose and cortisol levels. A low cortisol level and hypoglycaemia suggests the need for peri-operative glucocorticoid treatment. As hypoglyacaemia can occur during the test, the availability of 50% glucose should be ensured before starting the test.

Describe the steroid replacement regime

Patients on long-term steroid therapy equivalent to >10mg per day of prednisolone within the previous 3 months need peri-operative supplemental steroid therapy. The dose and duration of supplemental hydrocortisone needed depends on the type of surgery.

Table 9.5 Steroid replacement regimes.

Minor surgery (cataract)	25mg hydrocortisone IV at induction
Moderate surgery (hysterectomy)	Usual pre-op steroids + 25mg hydrocortisone IV at induction + 100mg hydrocortisone per day
Major surgery (laparotomy, nephrectomy)	Usual pre-op steroids + 25mg hydrocortisone IV at induction + 100mg hydrocortisone per day for 2-3 days Resume normal oral therapy when gastrointestinal function has returned

You have a patient who is on 6mg per day of dexamethasone. What is the equivalent dose of prednisolone?

6mg of dexamethasone is equivalent to 40mg of prednisolone.

Table 9.6 Equivalent dose of prednisolone.	
	Betamethasone 750µg
	Cortisone acetate 25mg
Prednisolone 5mg =	Dexamethasone 750µg
	Hydrocortisone 20mg
	Methylprednisolone 4mg

Ulcerative colitis

Ulcerative colitis is a form of inflammatory bowel disease (IBD). It causes inflammation of the large bowel. The colon become inflamed, and in severe cases, ulcers may form on the lining of the colon. These ulcers can bleed and produce mucus and pus.

There are periods of exacerbations of symptoms, and periods of quiescence. Symptoms can be related to the gastrointestinal tract or may be extra-intestinal and vary according to the severity of the disease. Gastrointestinal features include intermittent watery diarrhoea, and may be associated with blood or mucus, cramping abdominal pain, nausea and loss of appetite. Extra-intestinal features include fatigue, weight loss, low grade fever and anaemia which are seen during exacerbations of the disease. There may be multi-system involvement which can affect any organ but usually these are the eye, joints, skin and soft tissues.

Eye

- Iritis.
- Uveitis.
- Episcleritis.

Joints

◆ Sero-negative arthritis.
◆ Ankylosing spondylitis.

Skin and soft tissues

◆ Erythema nodosum.
◆ Pyoderma gangrenosum.

Key points

◆ Ulcerative colitis may have multi-system involvement and as well as affecting the gastrointestinal tract, it can also affect the eyes, joints and skin.
◆ Patients on long-term steroid therapy may have a suppressed HPA axis and need steroid replacement during the peri-operative period.

Further reading

1. Baumgart DC, Sandborn WJ. Inflammatory bowel disease: clinical aspects and established and evolving therapies. *The Lancet* 2007; 369: 1641-57.
2. Podolsky DK. Inflammatory bowel disease. *New England Journal of Medicine* 2002; 347: 417-29.
3. Nicholson G, Burrin JM, Hall GM. Peri-operative steroid supplementation. *Anaesthesia* 1998; 53: 1091-104.

Short case 9.2: Intravenous drug abuse

A 29-year-old male patient is scheduled for an emergency appendicectomy. He is known to have been an intravenous drug abuser in the past. He is currently on methadone 20mg three times a day.

Summarise the problems that may be encountered when anaesthetising this patient

The problems are those related to intravenous drug abuse. These include:

- An incomplete history as the patient may not want to reveal the issues surrounding drug abuse.
- He may be agitated and unco-operative at induction if a dose of methadone has been omitted during the concurrent illness.
- Difficult venous access, as the veins may be thrombosed due to repeated venepuncture.
- Postoperative pain relief, as the patient may be tolerant to opioids.
- Coexisting infective diseases such as hepatitis B and C, and HIV infection.

What is methadone?

Methadone is a long-acting μ-receptor agonist with pharmacological properties similar to morphine. It differs from other opioids in having a relatively low first-pass metabolism, high oral bioavailability (75%) and long plasma half-life. After oral administration it is absorbed within 30 minutes and peak plasma concentration is achieved within 4 hours. It can also be administered intravenously and intramuscularly.

It is less sedative than morphine, and tolerance develops more slowly. Other effects on the respiratory system, gastrointestinal tract and biliary tract are similar to morphine.

It is 90% protein bound and extensively metabolised in the liver by N-demethylation and cyclization to form pyrrolidines and pyrrolines which are excreted in the urine and bile.

Name the commonly abused drugs

These are classified into four different classes:

- Cannabis.
- Opioids (morphine, heroin, opium).
- Stimulants (amphetamine, ecstasy).
- Hallucinogens (LSD, ketamine).

What precautions would you take when anaesthetising this patient?

Precautions should be taken to ensure personal safety, staff safety and patient safety as follows:

- Appropriate communication with other theatre staff is essential.
- Anaesthetising the patient in theatre rather than the anaesthetic room can help to minimise any possible contamination.
- All sharps should be disposed of safely.
- Single-use breathing equipment should be used where possible.
- Any reusable equipment should be sterilised after use.
- Universal precautions should be strictly followed. They are designed to protect workers from exposure. All patients should be assumed to be carriers of blood-borne diseases such as HIV and hepatitis B.

How would you manage postoperative pain in this patient?

A regular dose of methadone should be continued during the peri-operative period. Analgesics with opioid-sparing effects such as paracetamol and NSAIDs drugs should be administered at regular intervals. Infiltration of local anaesthetic to the surgical wound can provide supplementary analgesia. If this patient requires morphine this may be best administered as PCA.

What advice would you give to a theatre nurse who sustains an accidental needlestick injury to the finger during this patient's operation?

- Encourage bleeding by squeezing the finger.
- Wash the wound thoroughly with soap and water.
- Report the accident to the department manager and seek advice from the occupational health department.
- Complete a critical incident form.
- Perform a risk assessment of the incident.
- When the patient is awake and orientated he will need to be counselled and give informed consent for blood to be tested for Hepatitis B and C, and HIV.
- Passive immunisation with hepatitis B immunoglobulin, antiviral drugs, antibiotics and anti-tetanus immunisation should be considered.

How would you conduct a risk assessment of a needlestick injury?

It is important to identify the cases which are at higher risk so that post-exposure prophylaxis (PEP) can be started as soon as possible after the injury. Three factors need to be considered: assessment of the wound, patient and staff.

Assessment of the wound

High risk features:

◆ Injury caused by the blade.
◆ Injury caused by a hollow needle.

Low risk features:

◆ Blood on solid skin.
◆ Injury caused by suture needle.

Assessment of the patient

High risk group patients:

◆ History of IV drug abuse.
◆ Sexual history: homosexuality, multiple partners.
◆ Patients who are from sub-Saharan Africa.
◆ History of blood transfusions.

Assessment of staff

◆ Hepatitis B immunisation status.

What PEP regimes do you know of?

PEP is used when the risk assessment indicates a high risk of contracting infections as a result of the needlestick injury.

HIV PEP

◆ Usually a three-drug prophylaxis is used.

- They are classified into two groups:
  - nucleoside reverse transcriptase inhibitors (NRTI): zidovudine, lamuvidine;
  - protease inhibitors (PI): nelfinavir, ritonavir.

A combination of two NRTIs and a PI is usually used.

Hepatitis B PEP

- A booster dose of hepatitis B vaccine if the person is immunised and has good titre levels.
- The person who is not immunised will need a hepatitis B immunisation course.

Universal precautions

Universal precautions are those which a health care worker should take for all patients regardless of their infection status. These must be used when there is a possibility of contact with blood, any body fluids, non-intact skin and mucous membrane. The key principles of universal precautions are:

- Hands must be washed with soap and water at the beginning of every session and case, and whenever they are soiled. If the hands are not soiled, antimicrobial hand rub should be used in between every patient contact. Any cuts or abrasions should be covered with waterproof dressings.
- Gloves must be worn when contact with body fluids and blood is anticipated. They should be worn before each activity and removed soon after the activity.
- Gown, apron, and goggles or eye shields must be worn when spillage of blood or body fluids is expected.
- Sharps must be disposed appropriately after use. Needles should not be re-sheathed.

Key points

◆ IV drug abuser patients should be given alternatives to opioids whenever possible to provide postoperative pain relief, but should not be denied them should they be required.

◆ Risk assessment of a needlestick injury is important in order to identify cases in which post-exposure prophylaxis (PEP) should be started as soon as possible after the injury.

◆ Universal precautions should be followed when dealing with any patient.

Further reading

1. Mitra S, Sinatra RS. Perioperative management of acute pain in the opioid-dependent patient. *Anesthesiology* 2004; 101: 212-27.

2. Wood PR, Soni N. Anaesthesia and substance abuse. *Anaesthesia* 2007; 44: 672- 80.

3. Moller A. Substance abuse and anaesthesia: the substance abusing patient. Euroanaesthesia 2005. http://www.euroanesthesia.org/ Education/~/media/Files/Publications/RefresherCourse/rc2005 vienna/1rc3.ashx.

Short case 9.3: Ruptured abdominal aortic aneurysm (AAA)

A 75-year-old man is brought into the accident and emergency department with sudden onset abdominal pain radiating to the back. In the past he has been investigated for an abdominal aortic aneurysm (AAA). He has been reviewed by a vascular surgeon who suspects a ruptured AAA and wants to take the patient to the operating theatre immediately for an AAA repair. You are the senior resident on-call anaesthetist.

How would you manage this patient?

A ruptured AAA is a surgical emergency. The initial approach should be to maintain the airway, breathing and circulation. High flow oxygen should be administered via a face mask. Intravenous access should be secured with at least two wide-bore peripheral cannulae. Blood samples should be collected for full blood count, serum urea and electrolytes, coagulation screen, blood group and cross-match. The diagnosis and management plan should be discussed with the surgeon.

The emergency theatre team and blood bank should be alerted. A relevant history should be elicited and a clinical examination performed. This patient is likely to be in hypovolaemic shock due to blood loss. A litre of warm Hartmann's solution should be administered rapidly and further fluid resuscitation continued to maintain the systolic blood pressure at 90-100mm Hg.

The patient may be in severe pain; small incremental doses of morphine (1mg of morphine every 5 minutes) can be administered.

Blood should be available for immediate transfusion. In the absence of cross-matched blood, O negative or group-specific blood should be made available.

While you are resuscitating this patient, a year 1 specialist trainee is available to help you in the theatre. What instructions would you give him regarding preparation in theatre?

Intra-operative management of ruptured AAA requires additional assistance for the anaesthetist in the operating theatre. Appropriate roles must be delegated to all available theatre staff and anaesthetic assistants. The on-call consultant anaesthetist should be informed. The preparation in theatre involves the following:

◆ Anaesthetic drugs including induction agents (thiopentone, ketamine), muscle relaxants, inotropic drugs (epinephrine, norepinephrine) and vasopressors (metaraminol) should be prepared.
◆ A transducer system for invasive arterial blood pressure monitoring and central venous pressure monitoring should be set up.
◆ Passive warming devices such as a fluid warmer and a forced air warming device should be prepared.
◆ A rapid IV fluid infusion device should be set up.
◆ A cell salvage system, if available, should be set up and kept on stand by for use during the intra-operative period.

This patient has now been transferred to the operating theatre. What would you do next?

Monitoring

Invasive arterial blood pressure, central venous pressure, body temperature (nasopharyngeal), urine output, blood loss estimation and intermittent blood gas monitoring including haemoglobin should be monitored. Invasive blood pressure monitoring should ideally be established prior to induction. Central venous access can be established after induction of anaesthesia.

Induction

Induction of general anaesthesia should take place in the operating theatre once the surgical team is scrubbed and ready. A rapid sequence induction should be performed using a titrated dose of thiopentone followed by succinylcholine. Ketamine can be used in the absence of significant ischaemic heart disease. Opioids such as fentanyl and alfentanil may be administered at induction to reduce the dose of induction agent. Blood should be available.

Maintenance

Anaesthesia should be maintained using a volatile agent, fentanyl and a non-depolarising neuromuscular blocking agent. All IV fluids and blood should be warmed during infusion to avoid hypothermia. Hypotension should be treated with fluids and judicious use of vasoactive drugs.

Once the aorta is cross-clamped, there is an increase in systemic vascular resistance which may cause hypertension proximal to the clamp. This can be managed by increasing the depth of anaesthesia and with intravenous infusion of glyceryl trinitrate.

During release of cross-clamp there is a sudden decrease in afterload which may be associated with severe hypotension, lactic acidosis, myocardial ischaemia and cardiovascular collapse. This can be minimised by maintaining an adequate circulating volume, by giving IV fluids (to maintain the CVP 5mm Hg above the baseline). Inotropic support and vasoconstrictors are usually required at this stage to maintain the mean arterial pressure.

How would you manage him postoperatively?

This patient should be managed in a critical care unit. Most patients require ventilatory support for the first 24 hours. Metabolic acidosis and coagulation abnormalities should be corrected. Renal function should be monitored. Postoperative pain during the immediate postoperative period can be managed using intravenous paracetamol, and a morphine or alfentanil infusion. Associated cardiovascular instability and coagulopathy may contraindicate the use of epidural analgesia. Active warming should be continued to prevent hypothermia. Tracheal extubation can be planned once the patient is normothermic, haemodynamically stable and any acidosis resolved.

There is a high mortality (about 50%) associated with emergency repair of AAA. The main problems in the postoperative period are hypothermia, bleeding, acidosis, coagulopathy, renal failure, abdominal compartment syndrome and spinal cord ischaemia.

What would you do to ensure renal protection?

One of the risks of AAA repair is renal failure due to inadequate blood supply to the kidneys from hypovolaemia, hypotension and suprarenal aortic cross-clamping.

Renal impairment can be minimised by maintaining mean arterial pressure using adequate fluid resuscitation and inotropic support. Mannitol 0.5g/kg administered during the cross-clamp time has been used. It acts as a free radical scavenger and an osmotic diuretic. There is, however, no convincing evidence for the use of mannitol, furosemide or dopamine in preventing renal failure.

Endovascular aneurysm repair (EVAR)

During an EVAR, an aortic stent graft is passed via the femoral arteries through the aortic lumen to fit tightly above and below the aneurysm. The aim is to exclude the aneurysm sac from the systemic circulation. This procedure is usually carried out by a radiologist and a vascular surgeon working together. The procedure can be performed under general anaesthesia or regional anaesthesia (spinal, epidural or combined spinal epidural). In 1994, the EUROSTAR registry (European collaborators on stent graft techniques for abdominal aortic aneurysm repair) was established for the purpose of collection and analysis of data on patients who undergo EVAR. Data from nearly 3000 procedures performed between 1994 and 2000 showed that the incidence of device-related complications decreased from 21.7 to 7.3%.

Key points

♦ A ruptured AAA is an anaesthetic and surgical emergency.
♦ Initial management includes an airway, breathing and circulation approach with emphasis on fluid resuscitation.
♦ Severe hypotension and cardiovascular collapse may be seen at induction of general anaesthesia and during release of the cross-clamp.
♦ Abdominal compartment syndrome and renal failure are common postoperative problems.

Further reading

1. Nataraj V, Mortimer AJ. Endovascular abdominal aortic aneurysm repair. *British Journal of Anaesthesia CEACCP* 2004; 4: 91- 4.
2. Leonard A, Thompson J. Anaesthesia for ruptured abdominal aortic aneurysm. *British Journal of Anaesthesia CEACCP* 2008; 8: 11-5.

Applied anatomy 9.1: Brachial plexus block

Describe the sensory nerve supply to the hand

The ulnar nerve supplies the ulnar (medial) half of the dorsum of the hand and the medial two and half fingers. The radial nerve supplies the lateral half of the dorsum of the hand and lateral two and half fingers as far as the

Clinical Science

distal interphalangeal joints. The medial side of the palm and medial one and half fingers including the finger tips and nail beds are supplied by the ulnar nerve. The lateral side of the palm and the palmar aspect of the lateral three and half fingers including finger tips and nail beds are supplied by the median nerve.

What is the origin of the median nerve?

The median nerve is formed from the terminal branches of the lateral and medial cords of the brachial plexus along the lower part of the axillary artery. The fibres of the median nerve are derived from the 6th, 7th, and 8th cervical and first thoracic nerves (C6-T1).

Describe the anatomy of the brachial plexus

The brachial plexus is formed by the union of the anterior primary rami of the lower four cervical nerves and the anterior primary rami of the first thoracic nerve (C5-T1). The brachial plexus provides cutaneous and muscular innervation to the entire upper limb, except for the trapezius muscle which is innervated by the spinal accessory nerve, and the skin over the medial aspect of the axilla which is innervated by the intercostobrachialis nerve.

One can remember the order of brachial plexus elements by using the mnemonic, Read The Damn Cadaver Book (Roots, Trunks, Divisions, Cords, Branches):

- ◆ Roots: the roots emerge from the intervertebral foramina of the cervical vertebrae immediately posterior to the vertebral artery and enter the interscalene groove formed by scalenus anterior and scalanus medius.
- ◆ Trunks: the roots of the 5th and 6th cervical nerves unite to form the upper trunk. The root of the 7th cervical nerve continues as the middle trunk. The roots of the 8th cervical nerve and 1st thoracic nerve roots unite to form the lower trunk.
- ◆ Divisions: each trunk divides into anterior and posterior divisions. In total there are six divisions from three trunks; three anterior and three posterior.

- Cords: these six divisions regroup to become the three cords. Cords are named according to their relationship to the second part of the axillary artery behind the pectoralis minor muscle. The posterior cord is formed from the three posterior divisions of the trunks (C5-T1). The lateral cord is formed from the anterior divisions from the upper and middle trunks (C5-C7). The medial cord is simply a continuation of the anterior division of the lower trunk (C8-T1).
- Branches: most branches arise from the cords, but a few branches arise from the roots and trunks as well.

In the neck the roots and trunks lie in the posterior triangle, covered by skin, platysma and deep fascia. Superficially the plexus is crossed by the external jugular vein and the supraclavicular nerves. The trunks emerge from the space between the scalenus anterior and scalenus medius muscles. This space becomes wider in the anteroposterior plane as the muscles approach their insertion on the first rib. The plexus leaves the neck by crossing the clavicle near its midpoint.

Table 9.7 Branches arising from the cords.

Cords	Branches
Lateral cord	Lateral pectoral nerve, musculocutaneous nerve, lateral root of the median nerve
Medial cord	Medial pectoral nerve, medial cutaneous nerve of the arm, medial cutaneous nerve of the forearm, medial root of the median nerve and ulnar nerve
Posterior cord	Upper subscapular nerve, lower subscapular nerve, thoracodorsal nerve, axillary nerve and radial nerve

What are the causes of brachial plexus injury during anaesthesia and surgery?

The commonest cause is stretching of the brachial plexus. This occurs during excessive rotation or extension of the neck, abduction, or external rotation of the arm. During surgery around the head and neck region the plexus may be compressed by surgical retractors. Prolonged application of a tourniquet on the upper limb can cause ischaemia to the major nerves. The ulnar nerve can be damaged due to direct pressure behind the elbow whilst the arm is resting on a hard surface.

During regional anaesthesia, the nerve can be damaged by direct injury from the needle.

What precautions would you take to minimise nerve injury?

Optimum care should be taken whilst positioning the patient to avoid stretching and compression of the plexus and nerves. Pressure points should be appropriately padded. The abduction of the arm should be limited to 90° or less.

During regional anaesthesia, purpose made regional anaesthesia needles should be used. A sound knowledge of anatomy is essential in order to avoid multiple needle passes. When injecting local anaesthetic high pressures should be avoided; if there is excessive resistance, the needle should be re-positioned. Many peripheral nerve blocks are performed with the patient awake, so that any injection or further advancement of the needle can be stopped if the patient complains of severe pain. Ultrasound is now increasingly used for regional anaesthesia. The needle and injection of local anaesthetic can be performed under direct vision, which may reduce the incidence of nerve injury.

Describe the supraclavicular approach to the brachial plexus block

Preparation

The benefits and complications of the procedure should be explained to the patient. The availability of drugs and equipment should be checked.

ECG, peripheral oxygen saturation and NIBP should be monitored. Venous access should be secured.

Patient positioning

The block is usually performed awake or sedated with the patient in a semi-sitting position and the head rotated to the opposite side. The semi-sitting position is more comfortable than the supine position both for the patient and the operator. The patient is asked to lower the shoulder and flex the elbow, so the forearm rests on his/her lap. The wrist is supinated so the palm of the hand faces the patient's face. This manoeuvre allows for the detection of any subtle finger movement produced by nerve stimulation.

Point of needle entry

The posterior border of the sternocleidomastoid (SCM) muscle is identified and followed distally to the point where it meets the clavicle. The needle entry point is 1.5cm lateral and 1.5cm above the clavicle from the point where the SCM muscle meets the clavicle.

Either a peripheral nerve stimulator or ultrasound should be used to locate the nerve.

The skin at the point of needle entry is infiltrated with 1ml of 1% lidocaine. An insulated nerve stimulator needle should be inserted perpendicular to the skin. Using a nerve stimulator (1.5mA and 2Hz), contraction of the forearm muscles should be elicited. Once the muscle contractions occur at a current less than 0.5mA, 30-40ml of local anaesthetic is injected, following a careful negative aspiration.

What are the complications of a supraclavicular brachial plexus block?

Common:

♦ Phrenic nerve palsy.
♦ Horner's syndrome.
♦ Failed block.

Uncommon:

+ Pneumothorax.
+ Nerve damage.
+ Intravascular injection of local anaesthetic.
+ Infection.

What are the contraindications to a supraclavicular nerve block?

General contraindications include patient refusal, allergy to local anaesthetics, bleeding disorders and infection at the site.

Relative contraindications are a short and stiff neck, large goitre, previous radiotherapy to the neck, previous radical neck surgery, recurrent laryngeal nerve palsy, and pneumothorax in the opposite side.

What other approaches may be used to block the brachial plexus?

The brachial plexus can be blocked using the interscalene, infraclavicular and axillary approaches.

Interscalene block

This block should be considered for shoulder and upper arm surgery.

Patient positioning
The patient should lie supine with the head turned slightly away from the side to be blocked.

Point of needle entry
The interscalene groove lies between scalenus anterior and medius at the level of C6 (cricoid cartilage). An awake patient should be asked to lift their head off the pillow to make the groove more prominent. In the majority of patients the external jugular vein crosses the groove at the level of C6. The needle is passed perpendicular to the skin in all planes in a slightly caudad direction.

Muscle contractions in the anterior shoulder and arm muscles are used to assess the endpoint for this block.

Infraclavicular block (sub-coracoid approach)

This block is used for surgery on the elbow, forearm, wrist and hand.

Patient positioning
The patient should lie supine with the head turned away from the side to be blocked.

Point of needle entry
2cm medial and 2cm caudad to the coracoid process.

A flexion or extension response of the fingers (median or radial nerve) is used as an endpoint.

Deltoid contraction indicates stimulation of the axillary nerve; biceps contraction is due to stimulation of the musculocutaneous nerve. Both are branches from the plexus at a higher level.

Axillary block

This block is suitable for surgery on the hand and forearm. The musculocutaneous nerve is usually missed when this block is performed.

Patient positioning
The patient should lie supine with their arm abducted to 90° and elbow flexed.

Point of needle entry
The axillary artery pulsation is traced towards the apex of the axilla to the level of the lateral border of pectoralis major. The needle is inserted above (for median nerve) and below (for ulnar and radial nerves) the axillary artery pulsation.

Ultrasound guidance for regional nerve blocks

In January 2009, NICE published guidelines on ultrasound-guided regional nerve block, in which use of ultrasound enables visualisation of the nerve and helps in accurate placement of the needle tip adjacent to the nerve. Satisfactory spread of local anaesthetic solution around the nerve can be visualised. It improves the success rate of nerve block and may reduce the incidence of complications. The onset of block appears to be faster and the volume of local anaesthetic required to produce block is smaller with ultrasound guidance compared with a landmark technique.

Key points

♦ The brachial plexus is formed by the union of the anterior primary rami of the lower four cervical nerves and the anterior primary rami of the first thoracic nerve (C5-T1).

♦ Stretching of the plexus due to excessive neck rotation or hyperabduction of the arm can result in nerve injury.

♦ The cords are named according to their relationship to the second part of the axillary artery.

♦ The use of ultrasound guidance for regional nerve block can improve the success rate and can reduce the incidence of complications.

Further reading

1. Fischer HBJ. Upper limb blocks. In: *Principles and practice of regional anaesthesia,* 3rd ed. Wildsmith JAW, Armitage EN, McClure JH, Eds. Elsevier Science Limited, 2003: 193-211.
2. Ultrasound-guided regional nerve block: guidance 285. http://www.nice.org.uk/nicemedia/pdf/IPG285Guidance.pdf.

Applied physiology 9.2: Coagulation cascade

A 56-year-old, morbidly obese female patient sustained an ankle fracture 2 days ago. Her past medical history includes carcinoma of the left breast treated with surgery and chemotherapy 3 years ago. On admission to the orthopaedic ward she is complaining of chest pain, and an ECG is recorded.

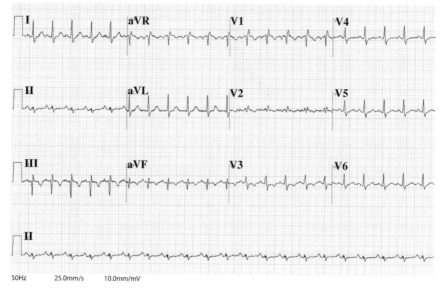

Figure 9.3 ECG.

What are the abnormal findings in this ECG?

The ECG shows sinus tachycardia with a heart rate of approximately 150 per minute. QRS complexes are widened in V1 and V2 with an rSR pattern. There are S waves in lead 1, Q waves in lead III, and inverted T waves in leads III, V1 to V3. Along with clinical history, this ECG is suggestive of pulmonary embolism.

What are the risk factors for deep vein thrombosis (DVT) in this patient?

This patient has a history of malignancy, she is obese and she has sustained an ankle fracture which will give her restricted mobility.

How does immobility contribute to DVT?

Immobility leads to venous stasis in the lower limbs. This forms one of the components of Virchow's triad. This consists of three broad factors that are thought to contribute to thrombosis:

- Alteration in the normal blood flow, e.g. stasis.
- Injuries to the vascular endothelium.
- Alteration in the constitution of blood (hypercoagulability).

Describe the initial phase of the formation of a clot

Formation of a clot following a vessel injury can be explained by a revised coagulation cascade. With the disruption of the vessel walls, tissue factor (TF) from the endothelium is exposed and brought into contact with circulating Factor VII. This produces an activated factor VII-TF complex. This in turn triggers coagulation by activating Factors IX and X; Factor X binds very rapidly with Factor II to produce thrombin. This is the initiation phase.

What occurs following this initial phase?

The following three phases then contribute to the formation of clot:

- Amplification phase. The amount of thrombin produced by the initial phase is too small to activate fibrinogen. Thrombin initiates several feedback mechanisms by activating Factors V, VIII and XI to increase the production of thrombin.
- Propagation phase. Ongoing generation of activated Factor X by Factors IXa and VIIIa maintains continuous thrombin production. This ensures the formation of a large clot.
- Stabilisation phase. Maximum thrombin generation occurs only after the formation of fibrin monomers. Thrombin then activates Factor XIII, which cross-links the fibrin monomers to a stable fibrin meshwork.

What is 'tissue factor'?

Tissue factor (TF) is a trans-membrane glycoprotein receptor, and consists of an extracellular domain, a trans-membrane segment and a cytoplasmic tail. It is found in the cell membrane of blood vessels, macrophages, monocytes, fibroblasts, the adventitia of blood vessels, organ capsules and the epithelium of skin. There is also circulating TF present in whole blood and serum.

What non-homeostatic functions does TF have?

TF is involved in the pathophysiology of systemic inflammatory disorders, coagulopathies, atherosclerotic disease, tumour angiogenesis and metastasis.

What is fibrinolysis?

It is the process whereby a fibrin clot is broken down by plasmin into fragments which are then cleared by proteases or excreted by the liver and the kidney. Inactive plasminogen is incorporated into the fibrin mesh during the clot formation and is activated by tissue plasminogen activator and urokinase. The activated plasmin, a protease, then breaks down the clot into soluble fibrin degradation products.

What is a D-dimer test?

It is a measurement of a specific fibrin degradation product, the D-dimer. D-dimer is increased in DVT. It is a sensitive but not specific test for DVT and pulmonary embolism.

If a 42-year-old lady is scheduled for a vaginal hysterectomy on a gynaecology list, would you implement DVT prophylaxis?

It is advisable to implement mechanical prophylaxis for this patient. The pharmacological prophylaxis would depend on whether the patient had any other risk factors (one or more) for developing a DVT (NICE guidelines).

What are the risk factors which would lead to the implementation of pharmacological prophylaxis?

These are classified into surgical and patient factors.

Surgical factors

◆ High risk surgery for the development of DVT includes cardiothoracic, major orthopaedic and vascular surgery followed by major abdominal general surgical procedures.

Patient factors

- Age >60 years.
- Obesity.
- Past history of DVT.
- Inherited thrombophilia, e.g. Factor V Leiden mutation, protein C and S deficiency.
- Acquired thrombophilia, e.g. antiphospholipid antibody syndrome.
- Malignancy.
- Dehydration.
- Chemotherapy.
- Varicose veins.
- Oral contraception and hormone replacement therapy.
- Active cardiac and respiratory failure.
- Nephrotic syndrome.
- Myeloproliferative syndrome.
- Immobility.

Which pharmacological agent would you use?

- Low-molecular-weight heparins (LMWH) are considered the gold standard.
- Unfractionated heparin.
- Oral anticoagulants (warfarin) are associated with a high risk of peri-operative haemorrhage.
- Newer agents: danaparoid, fondaparinux and melagatran.

What types of mechanical prophylaxis do you know of?

- Graduated compression stockings.
- Intermittent pneumatic compression devices.
- Foot impulse devices.

What is the mechanism of action of graduated compression stockings?

They exert a graded circumferential pressure from the distal to proximal regions of the leg thereby increasing blood velocity and promoting venous return.

What are the contraindications for the use of graduated compression stockings?

◆ Peripheral arterial disease.
◆ Arteriosclerosis.
◆ Severe peripheral neuropathy.
◆ Massive leg oedema or pulmonary oedema.
◆ Oedema secondary to congestive cardiac failure.
◆ Local skin/soft tissue diseases such as local dermatitis, or a recent skin graft.
◆ Extreme deformity of the leg.
◆ Gangrenous limb.
◆ Doppler pressure index (Ankle Brachial Pressure Index) <0.8.
◆ Gross limb cellulitis.

How does the foot impulse device (FID) work?

The FID mimics the action of normal walking of the sole of the foot. By compressing the sole of the foot artificially it stimulates the action of walking on the sole of the foot causing compression and thereby emptying the venous plexus of the sole into the deep veins. This produces a pulsatile flow which reduces stasis and thrombus formation.

Tissue factor pathway inhibitor

Tissue factor pathway inhibitor (TFPI) acts on the activated Factor VII-TF complex and is the main regulator of the tissue factor pathway. It occurs in two main forms: TFPI-1 and TFPI-2. TFPI is stored in endothelial cells and is released by platelet activation and heparin. Binding of TFPI with activated Factor X deactivates activated Factor X. TFPI binds with the activated Factor VII-TF complex and prevents further activation of Factor X. The properties of TFPI lead to the revised coagulation cascade.

Heparin may exert its antithrombotic effect through the TFPI pathway, by inducing TFPI synthesis and increasing secretion of TFPI by endothelial cells.

Key points

◆ The old concept of a two-pathway coagulation cascade has been replaced by a revised coagulation cascade.
◆ A risk assessment for DVT should be performed for all patients undergoing surgical procedures.
◆ Tissue factor pathway inhibitor is the main regulator of the coagulation cascade.

Further reading

1. Price GC, Thompson SA, Kam PCA. Tissue factor and the tissue factor pathway inhibitor. *Anaesthesia* 2004; 59: 483-93.
2. Bombeli T, Spahn DR. Updates in perioperative coagulation: physiology and management of thromboembolism and haemorrhage. *British Journal of Anaesthesia* 2004; 93: 275-87.
3. Venous thromboembolism: reducing the risk in surgical inpatients. NICE guidance CG46, April 2007. http://www.nice.org.uk/CG046.

Applied pharmacology 9.3: Insulin and hypo-glycaemic drugs

A 25-year-old female patient who suffers with known Type 1 diabetes presents to the emergency department. She has been generally unwell for 2 weeks. On clinical examination she is drowsy and appears dehydrated. Her pulse rate is 110 beats per minute. Her blood glucose is 25mmol/L.

What is Type 1 diabetes?

Type 1 diabetes is due to an absolute deficiency of insulin and is also known as insulin-dependent diabetes mellitus (IDDM). Patients with Type 1 diabetes are most likely to develop diabetic ketoacidosis when insulin is omitted because of missed meals during intercurrent illness. Patients become rapidly dehydrated and acidotic. Tachypnoea or Kussmaul breathing is prominent, with the smell of ketones on the breath. Acidosis with increased hydrogen ions results in a reduced level of consciousness. Type 2 diabetes, also known as non-insulin dependent diabetes mellitus (NIDDM), is caused by a relative deficiency of insulin. This may be either due to reduced insulin secretion from the ß cells in the islets of Langerhans or due to peripheral resistance of insulin.

How would you manage this patient?

This patient is likely to have diabetic ketoacidosis, and needs assessment and resuscitation in a critical care environment. Airway, breathing and circulation should be assessed and supplemental oxygen should be administered. The aim is to control the blood glucose and correct dehydration and electrolyte and acid-base imbalance.

Monitoring should include continuous ECG, pulse oximetry, invasive arterial blood pressure, central venous pressure, urine output and temperature. Further investigations such as urine analysis for ketone bodies, arterial blood gas for pH, serum electrolytes (K^+), a full blood count, and urine and blood cultures should also be performed.

Control of blood glucose should be done using a short-acting insulin (Actrapid) infusion on a sliding scale regimen. There are several locally agreed regimens for insulin infusion. Commonly, 50 IU of insulin is diluted in 50ml of 0.9% sodium chloride (1 IU/mL). In this patient, an insulin infusion can be commenced at a rate of 6 IU/hour and then titrated according to the blood glucose. The aim is to maintain the blood glucose between 4-8mmol/L. Once the blood glucose is less than 12mmol/L, a 5% dextrose infusion should be started at a rate of 125ml/hour to prevent hypoglycaemia.

Serum potassium should be monitored two-hourly; it should be maintained between 4-5mmol/L. The following regimen can be used for intravenous infusion of potassium chloride through a central venous line.

Table 9.8 Potassium chloride infusion regimen.

Serum K^+ mmol/L	KCl (mmol/hour)
<3	40
3-4	30
4-5	20
5-6	10

Correction of dehydration should be based on clinical signs of dehydration; 1L of 0.9% sodium chloride should be administered intravenously over the initial 30 minutes. Further administration of normal saline should be guided by clinical signs, CVP and urine output.

What is insulin?

Insulin is a hormone secreted by the islet of Langerhans cells in the pancreas. It is a polypeptide containing 51 amino acids arranged in two chains. These are A and B chains linked by disulphide bridges. It has anabolic effects including increased glucose and amino acid uptake, an increase in glycogenesis, lipogenesis and protein synthesis. It also has anti-catabolic effects such as the inhibition of lipolysis and protein breakdown. The plasma half-life after endogenous secretion from cells is about 4-6 minutes.

What are the actions of insulin?

The most immediate effect of insulin is hypoglycaemia. It also modifies fat and protein metabolism and has effects on electrolyte transport.

Hypoglycaemic effects

◆ Liver. It inhibits hepatic glucose production by decreased gluconeogenesis. It stimulates glucose uptake and storage in the liver as glycogen. In the absence of insulin, glycogen synthesis in the liver ceases and glycogen breakdown is stimulated. Absence of insulin and glucagon both will facilitate glycogen breakdown.
◆ Muscle. It facilitates glucose uptake in the muscles.
◆ Adipose tissue. It facilitates glucose uptake and stimulates glucose storage as triglycerides.

Fat metabolism

◆ Liver. Insulin promotes the synthesis of fatty acids in the liver. Insulin is stimulatory to synthesis of glycogen in the liver. However, when glycogen accumulates to produce high levels (roughly 5% of liver mass), further synthesis is strongly suppressed. When the liver is saturated with glycogen, any additional glucose taken up by hepatocytes is shunted into pathways leading to synthesis of fatty acids, which are exported from the liver as lipoproteins.

◆ Adipose tissue. Insulin inhibits breakdown of fat in adipose tissue by inhibiting the intracellular lipase that hydrolyzes triglycerides to release fatty acids. Insulin facilitates entry of glucose into the fat cells and within these cells, glucose can be used to synthesize glycerol. This glycerol, along with the fatty acids delivered from the liver, is used to synthesize triglyceride within the fat cells. By these mechanisms, insulin is involved in further accumulation of triglycerides in fat cells.

Protein metabolism

Insulin stimulates protein synthesis and inhibits protein degradation. It stimulates the uptake of amino acids and contributes to its overall anabolic effect. When insulin levels are low, as in the fasting state, the balance is pushed toward intracellular protein degradation.

Electrolyte transport

Insulin increases the activity of sodium-potassium ATPase in the cell membranes, causing a flux of potassium into the cells. It also increases the permeability of cells to magnesium and phosphate ions.

Describe the mechanism of action of insulin

The receptors for insulin are embedded in the plasma membrane. They are membrane spanning glycoproteins composed of two alpha subunits and two beta subunits linked by disulphide bonds. The α chains are entirely extracellular and house insulin binding domains, while the linked ß chains penetrate through the plasma membrane. Insulin initially binds to the α subunit. This causes ß subunits to phosphorylate themselves (autophosphorylation) and activate the catalytic activity of the receptor. The activated receptor then phosphorylates a number of intracellular proteins which in turn alter their activity and generate a biological response.

What insulin preparations are available?

Insulin preparations can be classified according to their species of origin and to their duration of action. Insulin has been prepared from porcine or beef pancreas. With the advent of recombinant DNA technology, a human insulin preparation is more commonly used. Human insulin differs from porcine by one amino acid. It contains threonine instead of alanine at the carboxyl terminal of the ß chain. Human insulin is more soluble than porcine insulin in aqueous solution.

Insulin preparations are classified based on the onset and duration of action into rapid, short, intermediate and long-acting:

- Rapid-acting: onset within 15 minutes; duration up to 3 to 4 hours.
- Short-acting: onset 30 minutes to 1 hour; duration up to 3 to 6 hours.
- Intermediate-acting: onset 1 to 2 hours; duration up to 12 to 18 hours.
- Long-acting: onset 2-4 hours; duration up to 24 hours.

Table 9.9 Insulin products.

Type of insulin	Generic name	Brand name
Rapid-acting	Insulin lispro	Humalog
	Insulin aspart	Novolog
Short-acting	Insulin regular	Humulin R
	Insulin regular	Novolin R
Intermediate-acting	NPH	Humulin N
	NPH	Novolin N
Long-acting	Insulin detemir	Levemir
	Insulin glargine	Lantus

Insulin pens

Insulin is available as both disposable and re-usable pen devices. The patient-specific dose can be programmed into these. This is beneficial for patients as it allows self-administration resulting in improved compliance and better outcome.

Describe the oral hypoglycaemic drugs

They can be classified as:

◆ Sulphonylureas: tolbutamide, glibenclamide, glimepiride, gliclazide.
◆ Biguanides: metformin.
◆ Thiazolidinediones: pioglitazone, rosiglitazone.
◆ Meglitinide analogues: nateglinide, repaglinide.
◆ α-glucosidase inhibitors: acarbose.

Sulphonylureas

These act by increasing the endogenous insulin secretion from the cells in the pancreas. They block the ATP-dependent potassium channel and depolarise the membrane of the cells. As a result calcium influx increases which in turn increases the insulin secretion. They therefore require functioning cells to exert their effect.

These drugs are metabolised in the liver to active metabolites and are eventually excreted in urine. Sulphonylureas are extensively bound to plasma proteins and hence concurrent administration of other highly protein-bound drugs such as aspirin can increase the freely available sulphonylurea in the plasma. They can cause prolonged and severe hypoglycaemia.

Biguanides

Unlike sulphonylureas biguanides have no effect on insulin secretion. They act more peripherally by increasing the sensitivity of the tissues to insulin. They increase the glucose utilisation in the skeletal muscles and reduce hepatic gluconeogenesis. They can cause lactic acidosis. This may possibly be due to inhibition of oxidative phosphorylation at the cellular level.

Thiazolidinediones

These reduce peripheral insulin resistance. They can be used in combination with insulin and other oral hypoglycaemic drugs. They bind to the peroxisone proliferator-activated receptor-γ (PPAR-γ) which activates insulin-responsive genes regulating carbohydrate and lipid metabolism. Thiazolidinediones also increase the glucose transport into the muscle and fat by enhancing the synthesis of specific forms of glucose transporters. Both pioglitazone and rosiglitazone are administered as a once daily dose; it may take about 6-12 weeks before any clinical effect is observed. They have been shown to lower the haemoglobin A1C levels in patients with Type 2 diabetes.

Meglitinides

The mechanism of action is similar to sulphonylureas, increasing the insulin secretion from the cells. The onset of action is more rapid and duration of action is shorter as compared with sulphonylureas. They are useful in controlling postprandial hyperglycaemia in patients with Type 2 diabetes.

α-glucosidase inhibitors

These inhibit the action of α-glucosidases on the intestinal brush border and reduce the absorption of starch and disaccharides. They are usually used in combination with other oral hypoglycaemic drugs and insulin. Like thiazolidinediones, they also lower the haemoglobin A1C levels.

Pathophysioloy of diabetic ketoacidosis

Due to the lack of insulin, glucose cannot enter into cells, and the carbohydrate-based metabolism is changed over to fat oxidation. This is an extension of normal physiological mechanisms that compensate for starvation. Free fatty acids are produced in fat cells and transported to the liver. In the liver, they are broken down into acetate, then to ketoacids (acetoacetate and beta-hydroxybutyrate). The ketoacids are then exported from the liver to peripheral tissues (notably brain and muscle) where they can be oxidised.

Both the absence of insulin and excess glucagon results in inhibition of glycolysis. Such inhibition not only raises glucose levels, but stimulates ketone formation. Insulin deficiency and other stress hormones also promote increased glucose production via glycogen breakdown. The combination of reduced cellular uptake of glucose and gluconeogenesis increases plasma glucose. Hyperglycaemia promotes osmotic diuresis with loss of water, sodium, potassium and phosphate. Further associated nausea and vomiting exacerbate dehydration.

The main causes of death in diabetic ketoacidosis include severe hyperkalaemia, hypokalaemia, aspiration of gastric contents and cerebral oedema. Poor prognostic features include an impaired conscious level, acidosis with a pH <7.0, oliguria and hypokalaemia.

Key points

- ◆ Insulin-dependent (Type 1) diabetes is due to an absolute deficiency of insulin.
- ◆ Insulin increases the activity of sodium-potassium ATPase in the cell membrane and shifts potassium into cells.
- ◆ Sulphonylureas increase the secretion of endogenous insulin secretion.
- ◆ Biguanides act peripherally by increasing the sensitivity of tissues to insulin.
- ◆ α-glucosidase inhibitors such as acarbose reduce the absorption of carbohydrates.

Further reading

1. Robinson S, Smith M. Insulin. In: *Anaesthetic pharmacology - physiologic principles and clinical practice.* Evers AS, Maze M, Eds. Philadelphia: Churchill Livingstone, 2004: 835-52.
2. The endocrine pancreas and the control of blood glucose. In: *Pharmacology.* Rang HP, Dale M, Ritter JM, Eds. Churchill Livingstone; 2001: 385-98.
3. Ferrari LR. New insulin analogues and insulin delivery devices for the peri-operative management of diabetic patients. *Current Opinion in Anaesthesiology* 2008; 21: 401-5.

Equipment, clinical measurement and monitoring 9.4: Fibreoptic bronchoscope and sterilisation

What are the components of an intubating fibreoptic bronchoscope?

It consists of three main parts: the body, insertion cord and a light source or light cable. The body houses a lever which controls the movement of the tip of the scope, eyepiece, dioptre ring and working channel. The eyepiece can be connected to a video camera. The dioptre ring allows focusing of the image. The working channel port incorporates the suction connector. The working channel can be used for suction, delivering oxygen and administration of local anaesthetics.

The insertion cord is about 55-60cm in length, allowing railroading of the tracheal tube to facilitate intubation. The insertion cord consists of a light transmission bundle, image transmission bundle, working channel and control wires which connect the tip of the scope to the control lever.

Most of the newer fibreoptic scopes have the option to use a battery-operated light source as well as a light cable connected to a halogen light.

What are the physical principles involved in the fibreoptic scope?

Light transmission bundles in the fibreoptic scope carry light to the tip of the scope which illuminates the object. Light from the object is reflected onto the objective lens at the tip of the scope. The lens focuses the light onto the image transmission bundle which carries the image to the eyepiece where the image is reconstructed.

What is the principle of transmission of light in a fibreoptic scope?

The light transmission bundle consists of thousands of optical fibres of 6-10 microns in diameter arranged in bundles. Each optical fibre consists of a thin glass centre where the light travels (core), an outer optical material surrounding the core (cladding) and a plastic coating (buffer coating) which protects the fibre from damage and moisture.

The light is transmitted via total internal reflection. The light travels in the fibreoptic core by constantly bouncing off the cladding. The cladding does not absorb any light from the core, so the light wave can travel great distances. Signal degradation occurs due to impurities in the glass; the extent depends on the purity of the glass and the wavelength of transmitted light.

What do you understand by total internal reflection?

When light travels through a glass fibre, part of it is absorbed, part of it is reflected and the rest is transmitted. At a certain angle of incidence (critical angle) all light falling on the glass surface is internally reflected with no transmission taking place. It is repeatedly reflected between the core and cladding until it emerges at the other end.

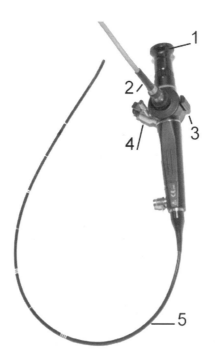

Figure 9.4 Intubating fibreoptic bronchoscope.
1. Eye piece; 2. Light cable; 3. Control lever; 4. Working channel; 5. Insertion cord.

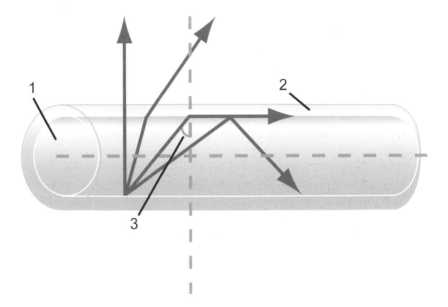

Figure 9.5 Total internal reflection in a glass fibre.
1. Core; 2. Cladding; 3. Critical angle.

In a fibreoptic scope, the fibreoptic relay system amplifies and decodes the transmission of light signal. The fibreoptic relay system consists of the following components:

◆ A transmitter: produces and encodes the light signals.
◆ An optical fibre: conducts the light signal over a distance.
◆ An optical regenerator: required to boost the light signal.
◆ An optical receiver: receives and decodes the light signals; the receiver uses a photodiode to detect the light.

How would you disinfect a fibreoptic scope after use?

It should be cleaned and disinfected as soon as possible after its use. The process of cleaning and sterilisation involves the following steps:

◆ Cleaning. A leakage test should be performed by pressurising the inside of the scope to ensure that there is no damage to the outer cover of the scope. A thorough manual cleaning and rinsing is done under running water to remove most of the micro-organisms. The fibreoptic scope has a blue ring around the control handle indicating that it is fully immersible in water. Any debris within the working channel should be removed by brushing and flushing the working channel.

◆ Chemical disinfection. Glutaraldehyde 2%, peracetic acid and chlorine dioxide are used for disinfecting the fibreoptic scope. Chemical disinfectants are capable of destroying gram-positive and gram-negative vegetative bacteria and enveloped viruses (also called lipophilic viruses). Glutaraldehyde is very effective but is an irritant to the skin, eyes and respiratory tract which exposes health care workers to an unacceptable risk. Peracetic acid is only irritant to the eyes. Chlorine dioxide is non-irritant. A 10-minute contact time with the disinfectant is sufficient to disinfect the scope. Both peracetic acid and chlorine dioxide have good microbiocidal activity against spores, mycobacteria, bacteria and viruses.

◆ Rinsing and drying. After 10 minutes of contact time the scope is rinsed with sterile water and dried with an alcohol swab.

◆ Transport and storage. After disinfecting, it should be stored in a clean sealed bag which has been appropriately labelled.

There are automated systems available which will perform all the above steps and produces a printout of a label with the time and date of disinfection.

Disposable sheaths are available as an alternative to disinfection. These can be used for a scope without a working channel.

What is the difference between sterilisation and disinfection?

Sterilisation is a process which renders the equipment free from viable micro-organisms including bacterial spores and viruses.

Disinfection is a process which reduces the number of viable micro-organisms to a safe level but does not necessarily include bacterial spores and viruses. Disinfection can be performed using pasteurisation, boiling or using chemical methods.

Pasteurisation involves heating the equipment to 70°C for 20 minutes or 80°C for 10 minutes. Bacterial spores are not killed by this method. Glutaraldehyde, 70% ethyl or isopropyl alcohol in water, chlorhexidine (0.5-5%), hydrogen peroxide, phenols and aldehydes are the various chemicals that are used for disinfection.

What is decontamination?

It is the combination of a process including cleaning and disinfection and/or sterilisation. This should ensure that the equipment is safe for re-use on the patient and safe to be handled by the staff.

How would you classify surgical and anaesthetic equipment based on the risk of infection?

They can be classified into critical, semi-critical and non-critical equipment.

Critical items

Critical items are introduced into tissue or the vascular system and pose a high risk of infection if contaminated. This category includes surgical instruments, cardiac and urinary catheters, central lines, implants and needles.

Semi-critical items

Semi-critical items contact the mucous membranes and non-intact skin but should not breach the blood barrier. Examples include breathing circuits, laryngoscopes, fibreoptic endoscopes and thermometers. Intact mucous membranes are generally resistant to infection by bacterial spores but susceptible to bacteria, bacilli and viruses, therefore these items require at least high-level disinfection.

Non-critical items

Non-critical items come into contact with healthy skin but not mucous membranes; examples include blood pressure cuffs and pulse oximeter probes. Skin is an effective barrier to most micro-organisms and non-critical items can be cleaned at the point of use as there is a low risk of transmitting infectious agents to patients with these items.

What is cleaning?

Cleaning is physical removal of infectious agents or organic matter. It involves washing with a solvent (water and detergent) which may be heated. The water temperature should not exceed 45°C as higher temperatures may lead to coagulation of proteinacious material forming a protective layer for micro-organisms. This process is usually performed at the sterile supplies department (SSD). Automated methods have largely replaced manual cleaning.

Steam sterilisation

Steam sterilisation is the most efficient and safest method for surgical instruments; it is a non-toxic, non-corrosive, rapid and fully automated process. Micro-organisms are killed at a lower temperature if moist (rather than dry) heat is used. Before sterilisation, items should be cleaned to reduce the population of viable infectious agents (bioburden) to the lowest possible level. The instruments are packaged to permit effective sterilisation and ensure sterility until the pack is opened. Temperatures >100°C are required to kill some micro-organisms and increasing the pressure in the autoclave allows these temperatures to be obtained. The efficacy of steam sterilisation is dependent upon the time and temperature of the cycle. The most common combinations are sterilisation temperatures of 115°C with a minimum holding time of 15 minutes or a temperature of 134°C with a minimum holding time of 3 minutes.

Chemical sterilisation

Chemical sterilisation is an alternative for items that cannot withstand steam sterilisation, e.g. endocsopes.

Ethylene oxide is used commonly for the sterilisation of heat- and moisture-sensitive devices. It is a colourless gas which is very flammable. Microbiocidal activity is thought to be due to the result of alkylation of protein, DNA and RNA. Temperatures of 29-65°C are used and each cycle can take 5-12 hours. After sterilisation, items are aerated to make them safe for personnel handling and patient use. Ethylene oxide is highly penetrative, effective and non-corrosive; it does not require high temperatures or pressures.

Immersion in glutaraldehyde 2% is a form of sterilisation and is used for optical instruments such as cytoscopes or fibreoptic scopes as it is non-corrosive and has no deleterious effects on the lens. Immersion must be for more than 10 hours to ensure effective sterilisation.

Gas plasma sterilisation is a relatively new technique which may in the future replace ethylene oxide sterilisation. Gas plasma is a highly ionized gas containing ions and free radicals capable of inactivating micro-organisms. These particles can diffuse through packaging materials in the chamber and sterilise their contents. Gas plasma provides non-toxic, dry, low-temperature sterilisation with a cycle time of only 75 minutes.

Prion disease

Variant Creutzfeldt-Jakob disease (vCJD) in humans and bovine spongiform encephalopathy (BSE) in cattle are caused by the same prion. A prion is an infectious protein. vCJD prions are found in the brain, spinal cord, posterior segment of the eye, lymph nodes, tonsils, and appendix.

None of the standard methods of sterilisation can prevent transmission of prion disease. Despite thorough cleaning and sterilisation, traces of tissue with prions remain on surgical instruments. After about ten decontamination cycles, infectivity becomes negligible. The only way of preventing transmission of prion disease is by the use of single-use equipment.

If a patient is definitely known to have vCJD, all equipment should be single-use or should not be re-used.

If a patient is suspected of having vCJD, all re-usable equipment should be quarantined. If at a later date the diagnosis is confirmed, the equipment should be destroyed.

Key points

♦ The insertion cord of the fibreoptic scope houses light transmission and image transmission bundles.

♦ Because of total internal reflection, the light is transmitted from one end to the other of a flexible scope.

♦ A fibreoptic scope can be cleaned and decontaminated using a chemical disinfectant such as glutaraldehyde or peracetic acid.

♦ None of the standard methods of sterilisation can prevent transmission of prion disease.

Further reading

1. Department of Health Medical Devices Agency. Sterilization, disinfection and cleaning medical devices and equipment: guidance on decontamination from the Microbiology Advisory Committee to Department of Health Medical Devices Agency, Part 1-3. London: Department of Health; 1996, 1999, 2000.

2. Sabir N, Ramachandra V. Decontamination of anaesthetic equipment. *British Journal of Anaesthesia CEACCP* 2004; 4: 103-6.

3. The Association of Anaesthetists of Great Britain and Ireland. Guidelines for infection control in anaesthesia. *Anaesthesia* 2008; 63: 1027-36.

Structured oral examination 10

Long case 10

Information for the candidate

History

A 72-year-old male patient is scheduled for a right total knee replacement. His past medical history includes chronic obstructive airway disease and osteoarthritis. He has smoked 10-15 cigarettes for the past 50 years, and has a chronic cough with occasional white sputum. His best exercise tolerance is about 200 yards on the level ground. He denies any chest pain, dizziness or ankle oedema.

His current medication includes a salbutamol inhaler 200µg b.d., a beclomethasone dipropionate inhaler 200µg b.d., prednisolone 5mg o.d., omeprazole 20mg o.d., paracetamol 1g q.d.s. and codeine phosphate 30mg q.d.s.

Clinical examination

Table 10.1 Clinical examination.

Weight	68kg
Height	176cm
Heart rate	76 bpm
Respiratory rate	18 per minute
Blood pressure	150/75mmHg
Temperature	37.1°C

Cardiovascular system

First and second heart sounds are heard, and no audible murmur.

Respiratory system

On auscultation scattered wheezes are heard over the lung fields.

Investigations

Table 10.2 Biochemistry.

		Normal values
Sodium	141mmol/L	135-145mmol/L
Potassium	4.4mmol/L	3.5-5.0mmol/L
Urea	5.7mmol/L	2.2-8.3mmol/L
Creatinine	68μmol/L	44-80μmol/L

Table 10.3 Haematology.

		Normal values
Hb	15.1g/dL	11-16g/dL
Haematocrit	0.52	0.4-0.5 males, 0.37-0.47 females
RBC	$4.85 \times 10^{12}/L$	$3.8\text{-}4.8 \times 10^{12}/L$
WBC	$8.5 \times 10^9/L$	$4\text{-}11 \times 10^9/L$
Platelets	$334 \times 10^9/L$	$150\text{-}450 \times 10^9/L$
MCV	86.4fL	80-100fL
MCHC	32.2g/dL	31.5-34.5g/dL
INR	1.0	0.9-1.2
PT	10.0 seconds	11-15 seconds
APTT ratio	0.9	0.8-1.2

Table 10.4 Lung function tests.

		Predicted value	Observed value Pre	% predicted	Observed value Post	% predicted
FVC	L	4.2	3.6	86	3.6	86
FEV1	L	3.2	1.8	56	1.9	61
FEV1/FVC %		73	50		53	
FEF 25-75 L/s		2.8	1.2	43		
PEFR	L/s	7.5	3.5	47	3.8	51
Lung volumes						
FRC	L	3.4	4.2	123%		
VC	L	3.9	3.5	89%		
RV	L	2.1	3.2	152%		
TLC	L	7.3	7.7	106%		

Pre=prior to bronchodilator therapy; Post=after bronchodilator therapy

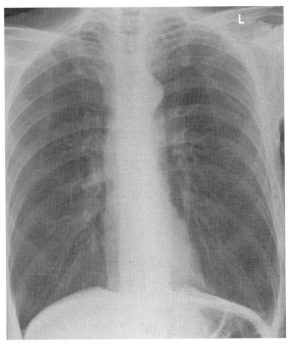

Figure 10.1 Chest X-ray.

Examiner's questions

Please summarise the case

An elderly man with significant respiratory illness and reduced exercise tolerance presents for an elective orthopaedic operation. He needs further optimisation of his respiratory function before surgery is performed.

What are the abnormal findings in the haematology and biochemistry results?

The haemoglobin and haematocrit are on the higher side of normal, probably because of his smoking habit.

What are the abnormalities in the pulmonary function tests?

FEV1 and PEFR are markedly reduced by about 50%. The ratio of FEV1 and FVC is also reduced by 50% indicating severe obstructive airway disease.

Describe the chest X-ray in a systematic way

This is a postero-anterior view of a chest X-ray of a male patient. It is an erect, centralised film with adequate exposure of lung fields and adequate penetration.

The chest X-ray can be described as follows using an ABCDEFGH approach:

- ◆ A = airway: trachea in midline.
- ◆ B = bones: no obvious bony defects seen.
- ◆ C = cardiac silhouette: heart shadow is tubular in shape.
- ◆ D = diaphragm: contour of the diaphragm is flattened and the costophrenic angles are obtuse.
- ◆ E = effusion/empty space: costophrenic angles are clear, no pneumothorax.
- ◆ F = fields (lungs): lung fields are hyper-translucent with increased vascular markings in both lung fields with widening of lower intercostal spaces.
- ◆ G = gastric air bubble: this is present indicating that the X-ray is taken in the erect posture.
- ◆ H = hilar region: there is bilateral peri-hilar congestion.

The radiological features are suggestive of chronic obstructive airway disease (COAD).

Define chronic obstructive airway disease

COAD is a disorder that is characterised by reduced maximal expiratory flow and slow forced emptying of the lungs. This limitation in airflow is only minimally reversible with bronchodilators.

What are the differences between emphysema and chronic bronchitis?

Emphysema is a pathological diagnosis in which there is permanent destructive enlargement of the airspaces distal to the terminal bronchioles without obvious fibrosis.

Chronic bronchitis is a clinical diagnosis characterised by increased bronchial secretions, enough to cause cough and expectoration, occurring on most days for a minimum of 3 months of the year for 2 consecutive years. There is mucus hypersecretion secondary to hypertrophy of the glandular elements of the bronchial mucosa. Patients with COAD may have features of both chronic bronchitis and emphysema, although one may be more prominent than the other.

What are the causes of COAD?

Smoking and bronchial hyper-reactivity

Cigarette smoking is a common cause of COAD. Cigarette smoke has been found to attract inflammatory cells into the lungs and stimulates the release of the proteolytic enzyme, elastase, from these cells. Elastase breaks down elastin, a normal structural component of lung tissue. Normally, the lung is protected from the destructive effect of elastase by an inhibitor, alpha-1 antitrypsin (AAT). However, cigarette smoke attracts more cells and stimulates the release of more elastase than can be inhibited by the circulating levels of AAT. In addition, cigarette smoke itself may inactivate AAT therefore swinging the balance in favour of more lung destruction by elastase. The imbalance between the destructive elastase and protective AAT can result in COAD.

Alpha-1 antitrypsin deficiency

This is a rare inherited autosomal recessive disorder probably accounting for less than 5% of all cases of COAD. Low levels of AAT allow the uninhibited action of elastase on the lung parenchyma, giving rise to destruction of the alveoli and the eventual development of emphysema rather than chronic bronchitis. The pattern of emphysema in AAT deficiency differs slightly from that of smoking-induced pure emphysema in that AAT deficiency produces panlobular emphysema affecting predominantly the lower lung fields, whereas smoking-induced emphysema is usually centrilobular, initially affecting the upper lung fields.

Passive smoking

The incidence of respiratory infections is higher in children who live in households where one or both parents smoke. This may increase the risk of COAD.

Infections

Viral infections in the lung enhance inflammation and predispose to bronchial hyper-reactivity, particularly adenovirus and respiratory syncytial virus. Once COAD is established, repeated infective exacerbations of airflow obstruction, either viral or bacterial, may speed up the decline in lung function.

What are the clinical features of COAD?

The two main symptoms of COAD are breathlessness and cough which may or may not produce purulent sputum. A history of persistent productive cough or recurrent infections especially in the winter months is common. The cough is usually worse in the mornings but bears no relationship to the severity of the disease. A large quantity of sputum production is unusual and may suggest bronchiectasis. The presence of haemoptysis should alert to the possibility of carcinoma of the bronchus. Wheeze is often an accompanying feature of breathlessness and may be erroneously attributed to asthma.

In emphysema there is a gradual destruction of alveolar septae and of the pulmonary capillary bed. The body compensates by hyperventilation and a low cardiac output. This results in relatively limited blood flow through a fairly well oxygenated lung with normal blood gases. The rest of the body, however, suffers from tissue hypoxia and pulmonary cachexia due to the low cardiac output. Patients predominantly suffering from emphysema are thin with relatively normal arterial tensions of oxygen and carbon dioxide, and are known as pink puffers.

In chronic bronchitis impaired gas exchange leads to hypoxaemia which stimulates erythropoiesis resulting in polycythaemia. Accompanying hypercapnia and respiratory acidosis cause pulmonary vasoconstriction which may lead to cor pulmonale. Patients with hypoxaemia, hypercapnia and signs of right heart failure are known as blue bloaters.

Clinical examination may reveal the following signs:

- Hyperinflation of the chest suggesting emphysema.
- A barrel-shaped chest (increased anteroposterior diameter).
- Use of the accessory muscles of respiration.
- Reduced cricosternal distance, tracheal tug and paradoxical in-drawing of the lower ribs on inspiration.
- Intercostal recession.
- Hollowing out of the supraclavicular fossae, pursed lip breathing and reduced expansion.

As the disease progresses, signs of right ventricular dysfunction may develop. These include:

- Peripheral oedema.
- Raised jugular venous pressure.
- Hepatic congestion.

What other investigations would you like to perform in this patient?

- Exercise testing such as a 6-minute walk test or stair climbing may give a reasonable estimation of exercise tolerance.
- ECG. Right ventricular hypertrophy or a strain pattern may indicate cor pulmonale.

- Gas transfer studies may give additional information. The transfer factor for carbon monoxide (TLCO) is reduced in emphysema.
- Arterial blood gas analysis. A $PaCO_2$ >5.9kPa or PaO_2 <7.9kPa (on room air) is associated with a poor prognosis.

How would you optimise respiratory function?

During the pre-operative period the following measures should be considered:

- Smoking cessation should be encouraged at least 4-6 weeks prior to surgery.
- Current infection would be a contraindication to elective surgery.
- Treatment of an acute exacerbation includes the use of ß2 agonists, systemic steroids and antibiotics. The cause of expiratory airflow limitation in COAD is narrowing of the small airways caused by chronic inflammation, hypertrophy of the airway smooth muscle and enlargement of the bronchial mucus glands. The bronchoconstriction that accompanies inflammation may be reversed using ß2 adrenoreceptor agonists. Ipratropium, a non-selective competitive muscarinic acetylcholine receptor antagonist, causes bronchodilatation.
- Corticosteroids are used in patients with newly diagnosed COAD to test for reversibility of airflow obstruction. An accepted regimen is 30-40mg of prednisolone per day for 10-14 days, with spirometry measured before and after the end of the course.
- Physiotherapy is an important part of the peri-operative management of patients with COAD. It reduces the incidence of intra-operative bronchial plugging.

What anaesthetic options are available for total knee arthroplasty?

- General anaesthesia with opioid analgesia.
- General anaesthesia with a nerve block, such as femoral and sciatic blocks.
- Spinal anaesthesia with a nerve block.
- Spinal anaesthesia with spinal opioids.
- Combined spinal and epidural anaesthesia.

General anaesthesia with a nerve block provides satisfactory postoperative analgesia. The disadvantages of general anesthesia include postoperative nausea and vomiting, sore throat, shivering, airway trauma, postoperative cognitive dysfunction and impaired respiratory function during the postoperative period.

The benefits of spinal anaesthesia include the fact the patient is awake, there is a reduced risk of venous thromboembolism, reduced blood loss, analgesia during the immediate postoperative period, a reduced incidence of postoperative nausea and vomiting, and a reduced incidence of postoperative cognitive dysfunction.

Combined spinal and epidural anaesthesia offers the benefit of an intense block provided by the spinal, and the opportunity to provide postoperative pain relief with the epidural.

Side effects of spinal anaesthesia with local anaesthetic and opioids (morphine or diamorphine) include failure of the block, pain during insertion of the spinal needle, hypotension, pruritis, urinary retention, post-dural puncture headache, respiratory depression and, rarely, more serious nerve damage.

Which option would you choose in this patient?

As this patient has COAD, he has a risk of developing respiratory complications during the peri-operative period, thus general anaesthesia is best avoided. The other techniques are acceptable, though it may be wise to avoid spinal opioids such as morphine in case there is any respiratory depression.

What intra-operative complications might you anticipate in this patient?

These can be classified as those related to the surgery and those related to the co-existing COAD.

Complications related to surgery

Blood loss may occur after deflation of the tourniquet. Reperfusion drainage systems allow cell salvage and transfusion of salvaged blood back to the patient.

Tourniquet deflation may be associated with a release of acid products into the circulation causing hypercapnia, reduced myocardial contractility and peripheral vasodilatation.

Hypotension and desaturation can occur at the time of insertion of the cement and prosthesis.

Although the risk of pulmonary embolism is less common in total knee arthroplasty compared with total hip arthroplasty, distal calf DVT is more common.

Complications related to the co-existing COAD

If the patient has general anaesthesia, the following may occur:

◆ Sputum plugging. Excessive sputum production can block the bronchi and bronchioles resulting in lobar collapse.
◆ Bronchospasm. Patients with COAD may experience bronchospasm during induction, airway manipulation or during extubation. Avoidance of tracheal intubation, if possible, may reduce the risk of bronchospasm.
◆ Ventilation and perfusion mismatch. General anaesthesia and supine position reduces the FRC which, in combination with atelectasis, can lead to worsening of hypoxaemia.
◆ Pneumothorax. Positive pressure ventilation can cause rupture of emphysematous bullae resulting in pneumothorax. Ventilatory strategy to minimise high airway pressure includes a low respiratory rate, increased expiratory time and avoiding high PEEP.
◆ Patients with COAD may have right ventricular hypertrophy, dilatation or heart failure. Measures should be taken to prevent any further increases in right ventricular pressure due to hypoxic pulmonary vasoconstriction. There is an increased incidence of cardiac arrhythmias in the peri-operative period.

How would you manage postoperative analgesia?

◆ Effective postoperative analgesia facilitates early postoperative mobilisation and recovery.
◆ Simple analgesics. A combination of regular paracetamol and NSAIDs provide analgesia and have an opioid-sparing effect. NSAIDs should

be avoided in patients with aspirin-sensitive asthma, recent gastro-duodenal ulcer and impaired renal function.

◆ Peripheral nerve block. Blocks such as a femoral and sciatic nerve block are effective.

◆ In the absence of nerve block or other form of regional anaesthesia, morphine can be administered in the form of PCA. Morphine PCA provides good pain control and patient satisfaction. Intrathecal opioids such as morphine may be considered if nerve block is not practicable, but there is a danger of respiratory depression.

◆ Non-pharmacological methods such as continuous passive motion or a cooling and compression technique can reduce postoperative pain.

◆ Intra-articular injection of local anaesthetic and wound infiltration with local anaesthetics can reduce the intensity of postoperative pain.

Pulmonary function tests

Pulmonary function tests are performed to evaluate the mechanical and gas exchange functions of the lung. These include:

◆ Spirometry.
◆ Lung volumes and elasticity.
◆ Diffusing capacity.
◆ Exercise testing.
◆ Arterial blood gas analysis.

Spirometry

Spirometry is the measurement of dynamic lung volumes during forced expiration and inspiration. Spirometry measures forced vital capacity (FVC), forced expiratory volume in one second (FEV1), and maximum expiratory flow over the middle 50% of the vital capacity (FEF 25-75%). FEF 25-75% is a sensitive index for small airway obstruction. The presence of airflow limitation occurs when there is a reduction in the ratio of FEV1 to FVC. FEV1 values give a measurement of the severity of COAD which are classified into three stages:

◆ Mild COAD: FEV1 >70% of predicted.
◆ Moderate COAD: FEV1 is 50-69% of predicted.
◆ Severe COAD: FEV1 is <50% of predicted.

Most patients with COAD will show a small increase in FEV1 or FVC in response to bronchodilator therapy. A response greater than 15% of the baseline value indicates a significant reversibility with bronchodilators which suggests asthma.

Total lung capacity (TLC) and residual volume (RV) are characteristically increased in COAD.

In obstructive airway disease (asthma and COAD), FEV1 is reduced markedly in relation to FVC resulting in a low FEV1/FVC ratio (<70%). The flow-volume loop has a characteristic shape with a scooped out appearance (concave to x axis) in the expiratory part of the curve with a reduced maximal flow rate.

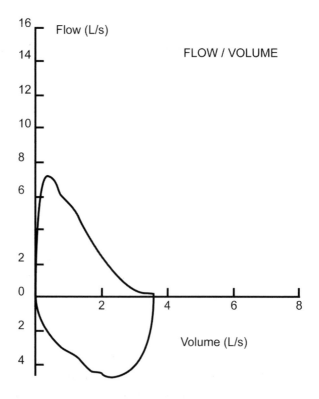

Figure 10.2 Normal flow-volume loop.

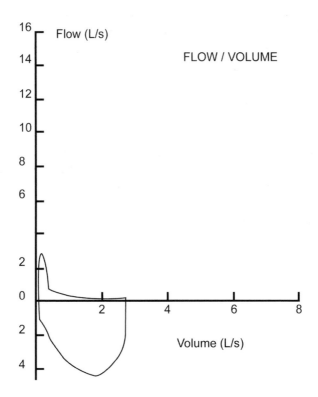

Figure 10.3 Flow-volume loop in obstructive airway disease.

Gas exchange

TLCO capacity measures the integrity and functioning of the gas exchange surface of the lung. It is reduced in emphysema. The transfer factor is a good indicator of the presence and severity of emphysema.

Arterial blood gases

The relationship between symptoms, FEV1 and hypoxaemia is weak. The combination of FEV1 and gas transfer strengthens the prediction of resting hypoxaemia. Hypoxaemia is more likely when the FEV1 is <1.0L.

Pulse oximetry is a useful tool, and arterial blood gas analysis should be performed in patients with an SpO_2 of less than 94%. An SpO_2 of 94% equates approximately to a PaO_2 of 8kPa.

Key points

◆ Cigarette smoking is a common cause of COAD.
◆ Smoking cessation should be encouraged at least 4-6 weeks prior to the surgery.
◆ Spinal anaesthesia with nerve block provides satisfactory postoperative analgesia.
◆ Transfer factor for carbon monoxide (TLCO) measures the integrity and functioning of the gas exchange surface of the lung.

Further reading

1. Fischer HBJ, Simanski CJP, Sharp C, *et al.* Procedure-specific systematic review and consensus recommendations for postoperative analgesia following total knee arthroplasty. *Anaesthesia* 2008; 63: 1105-23.
2. Respiratory function tests and their applications. http://www.thoracic.org.au/rft.pdf.

Short case 10.1: Aortic stenosis

A 75-year-old female patient is scheduled for a total hip replacement. Clinical examination during pre-operative assessment reveals a systolic murmur; further investigations reveal that she has aortic stenosis.

What are the causes of aortic stenosis?

The common causes include senile calcification, a bicuspid aortic valve (congenital) and rheumatic fever.

What are the signs and symptoms of a patient with aortic stenosis?

Symptoms:

◆ Angina.
◆ Syncope - dizziness and fainting spells.
◆ Dyspnoea.
◆ Congestive cardiac failure.
◆ Sudden death.

Signs:

◆ Slow rising pulse with narrow pulse pressure.
◆ The apex beat is usually undisplaced, sustained or heaving in nature indicating left ventricular hypertrophy.
◆ An ejection systolic murmur is heard at the base of the heart, second intercostal space, left sternal border and radiating to the carotid arteries.
◆ A quiet second heart sound as the stenosis gets worse; the aortic component (A_2) of the second heart sound is increasingly delayed giving first a single second heart sound and then reverse splitting.
◆ A fourth heart sound due to a stiff ventricle.
◆ Ejection click.

Why do these patients develop angina?

Aortic stenosis results in reduced forward flow from the left ventricle. As a result the left ventricular end-diastolic pressure (LVEDP) is increased. Due to reduced forward flow, the mean aortic pressure is decreased. As coronary perfusion pressure depends on the difference between the mean aortic pressure and LVEDP, this leads to a reduction in coronary blood flow, even with normal coronary vessels:

Coronary perfusion pressure = Mean aortic pressure - LVEDP.

As the aortic stenosis progresses, left ventricular hypertrophy can develop. This enlarged muscle mass increases oxygen demand.

These patients may also have concomitant atherosclerosis of the coronary vessels.

What changes might you see on an ECG in a patient with longstanding aortic stenosis?

♦ Left ventricular hypertrophy.
♦ Left anterior hemi-block.
♦ Poor R-wave progression.
♦ LBBB or a complete heart block.

What changes might you see on a chest X-ray?

♦ Heart size is usually normal or small, although at the late stages of the disease in the presence of cardiac failure, there may be cardiomegaly.
♦ Calcified aortic valve.
♦ Post-stenotic dilatation of the ascending aorta.

What further investigations would you do to assess the severity of aortic stenosis?

A continuous wave Doppler echocardiogram is used to grade the severity of the lesion. Cardiac catheterisation has been replaced by the Doppler echocardiogram except when the coronary arteries need evaluation.

A 2-D examination can identify structural valve abnormalities such as valve abnormalities, valve thickening, valve calcification and mobility of the valve leaflets. It can also assess structural ventricular abnormalities such as left ventricular hypertrophy, systolic and diastolic dysfunction and left ventricular dilatation. Short axis views can distinguish between bicuspid and tricuspid valves.

A continuous wave Doppler is obtained from the blood flow in the left ventricular outflow tract. The maximum velocity can be used to calculate the maximum pressure gradient across the valve, using the modified Bernoulli equation. Doppler software can also calculate the mean pressure gradient across the valve.

How would you grade the severity of aortic stenosis?

The pressure gradient across the valve can be used to grade the severity of the stenosis, but this is dependent on the flow across the valve. In high output states the severity is therefore often overestimated, and if the ventricle begins to fail the severity may be underestimated.

The severity of aortic stenosis is graded as mild, moderate, severe and critical based on the actual aortic valve area (AVA).

Table 10.5 The grades of severity of aortic stenosis.		
Severity	**Aortic valve area**	**Mean pressure gradient**
Mild	1.2-1.8cm^2	25-40mm Hg
Moderate	0.8-1.2cm^2	25-40mm Hg
Severe	0.6-0.8cm^2	40-50mm Hg
Critical	<0.6cm^2	>50mm Hg

What factors should be considered when anaesthetising this patient for a total hip replacement?

In aortic stenosis, left ventricular output (stroke volume) is reduced. A normal heart can compensate for reduced systemic vascular resistance (SVR) and reduced preload by increasing the contractility, thus maintaining stroke volume. Aortic stenosis is a fixed output state such that stroke volume and cardiac output fail to increase in these circumstances. Increase in heart rate further increases the myocardial oxygen demand and reduces coronary blood flow. When anaesthetising a patient with aortic stenosis the following principles should be followed:

◆ Preload. Adequate preload is essential to maintain stroke volume; hypovolaemia should be avoided.
◆ Myocardial contractility. Normal contractility should be maintained; drugs causing myocardial depression should be administered by careful titration.

- Afterload (systemic vascular resistance). Reduction in systemic vascular resistance should be avoided. Systemic hypotension must be treated aggressively with vasoconstrictors to maintain the blood pressure at pre-anaesthetic values.
- Heart rate. Sinus rhythm should be maintained, and tachycardia and arrhythmias avoided. Plasma electrolytes (particularly potassium) should be kept at normal levels.

The use of a non-cemented prosthesis for total hip replacement should avoid a cement reaction.

If the patient requests spinal anaesthesia what would you do?

A spinal may reduce systemic blood pressure with a reduction of coronary artery perfusion resulting in myocardial ischaemia. The risks associated with spinal anaesthesia (possible myocardial infarction and sudden death) must be explained to the patient.

A combined spinal and epidural with a catheter technique can be used if the condition is mild to moderate, if the block is established slowly with minimal changes in systemic blood pressure.

Postoperative management

Patients with a moderate to severe aortic stenosis require care in a high dependency unit with invasive monitoring. It is vital to maintain intravascular filling, to prevent hypotension and tachyarrhythmias, and to provide adequate analgesia. Inadequate analgesia increases the demands on the heart with increased morbidity and mortality. Regional block techniques (e.g. lumbar plexus block, possibly with a catheter technique) can be used for analgesia for a hip replacement.

Antibiotic prophylaxis against infective endocarditis

Patients with the following cardiac conditions are at risk of developing infective endocarditis:

- Acquired valvular heart disease with stenosis or regurgitation.
- Valve replacement.

- Structural congenital heart disease.
- Hypertrophic cardiomyopathy.
- Previous infective endocarditis.

An atrial septal defect, a fully repaired ventricular septal defect or a fully repaired patent ductus arteriosus, are not considered to be at risk.

Antibiotic prophylaxis against infective endocarditis is now not recommended for the following procedures:

- Dental procedures.
- Upper and lower gastrointestinal procedures.
- Genitourinary tract; this includes urological, gynaecological and obstetric procedures.
- Upper and lower respiratory tract; this includes bronchoscopy, ear, nose and throat procedures.

Key points

- Aortic stenosis results in reduced forward flow from the left ventricle and increases the end-diastolic pressure of the left ventricle.
- The severity of aortic stenosis can be graded based on the valve area and the pressure gradient.
- Safe management of anaesthesia for a patient with aortic stenosis includes maintenance of preload, a slow heart rate and systemic vascular resistance within normal limits.

Further reading

1. Fleisher LA, Beckman JA, Brown KA, et al. ACC/AHA 2007 guidelines on perioperative cardiovascular evaluation and care for noncardiac surgery. Journal of American College of Cardiology 2007; 50: e159-e242.
2. Christ M, Sharkova Y, Geldner G, et al. Preoperative and perioperative care for patients with suspected or established aortic stenosis facing noncardiac surgery. Chest 2005; 128: 2944-53.

3. Brown J, Morgan-Hughes NJ. Aortic stenosis for non-cardiac surgery. *British Journal of Anaesthesia CEACCP* 2005; 5: 1-4.
4. Prophylaxis against infective endocarditis, CG 64. London: NICE, March 2008. http://www.nice.org.uk/CG064.

Short case 10.2: Laparoscopic Nissen fundoplication

This is a chest X-ray of a 72-year-old female patient. She is a known asthmatic who has presented for pre-operative assessment. Comment on this chest X-ray.

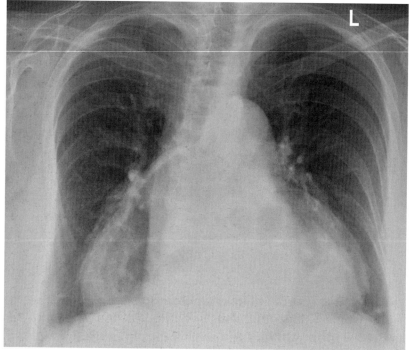

Figure 10.4 Chest X-ray.

This is a postero-anterior view of a chest X-ray. It is adequately penetrated and there is a slight rotation. There is a large hiatus hernia with a stomach shadow occupying the lower part of the lung fields. There is also kyphoscoliosis of the thoracic spine.

What is the differential diagnosis?

◆ Hiatus hernia.
◆ Diaphragmatic hernia.

Can you describe the different types of hiatus hernia?

Hiatus hernia occurs when part of the stomach protrudes through the diaphragmatic hiatus into the thoracic cavity. There are two types of hernia:

◆ Sliding hiatus hernia (80%). In this type, the gastro-oesophageal junction slides up into the chest and interferes with the normal anti-reflux mechanisms. The normal anatomical sphincter mechanism is lost, and regurgitation of gastric contents is more likely to occur. This also results in reflux oesophagitis.
◆ Rolling hiatus hernia (20%). The gastro-oesophageal junction remains in the abdomen but the bulge of the stomach herniates up into the chest alongside the oesophagus.

How would you confirm the diagnosis of hiatus hernia?

The following investigations are useful:

◆ A barium swallow is the best diagnostic test.
◆ Upper GI endoscopy.
◆ A CT scan will rule out the presence of a diaphragmatic hernia.

The patient is scheduled for a laparoscopic repair of her hernia (Nissen fundoplication). What specific history relating to the hiatus hernia would you ask?

◆ Symptomatic gastro-oesophageal reflux or heartburn (e.g. when laying flat or after a meal).
◆ Belching.
◆ Odynophagia (painful swallowing) - from oesophagitis or stricture.
◆ Nocturnal asthma - cough or wheeze at night due to aspiration.

Are there any other investigations that you require prior to anaesthesia?

◆ Full blood count - iron deficiency anaemia is common.
◆ Electrolytes, urea and creatinine - there may be electrolyte disturbances if she is vomiting.
◆ ECG.
◆ Arterial blood gas and lung function tests.

What premedication would you give to this patient?

H_2-receptor antagonists such as ranitidine 150mg orally or protein pump inhibitors, such as omeprazole 20mg or lansoprazole 20mg orally, should be given about an hour prior to induction.

Pro-kinetic drugs such as metoclopramide 10mg orally, about an hour prior to induction facilitates emptying of the stomach. Her bronchodilator therapy should be continued during the pre-operative period.

What anaesthetic technique would you choose for this case?

General anaesthesia with rapid sequence induction, tracheal intubation using a cuffed endotracheal tube and controlled ventilation is the safest option. Invasive arterial blood pressure monitoring may be wise in this patient due to the possible lung function impairment. Controlled ventilation helps to maintain normocapnia and aids the surgical exposure. A gastric tube will be necessary to prevent gastric distension, as gastric distension impairs the surgical view and could increase the risk of gastric perforation from the surgical trocars.

If the patient suddenly desaturated during the intra-operative period what would be your differential diagnosis?

Sudden intra-operative desaturation could be either due to patient or equipment-related factors.

Patient factors

◆ Pneumothorax.
◆ Pneumomediastinum.

- Endobronchial intubation.
- Venous gas embolism.
- Atelectasis due to patient position and CO_2 pneumoperitoneum.

Equipment factors

- Oxygen failure.
- Disconnection.
- Anaesthetic machine or ventilator malfunction.

What other complications are associated with laparoscopic surgery?

- Cardiac:
  - arrhythmias - nodal rhythms and bradycardias are common due to vagal stimulation;
  - cardiac tamponade due to pneumopericardium;
  - myocardial dysfunction.
- Respiratory:
  - respiratory acidosis due to CO_2 absorption.
- Subcutaneous emphysema.
- Surgical trauma:
  - haemorrhage;
  - viscus damage.
- Hypothermia.

What postoperative analgesia would you prescribe for this patient?

Postoperative analgesia should include a multimodal approach: simple analgesia with paracetamol, and additional opioids, supplemented with local anaesthetic infiltration to the port holes and possibly intra/retroperitoneal local anaesthesia.

A thoracic epidural might be considered if pulmonary function is very poor.

This patient will need to be nursed postoperatively in an HDU.

Physiological effects of pneumoperitoneum

The insufflation of a gas into the peritoneal cavity produces an increase in intra-abdominal pressure. Increased intra-abdominal pressure, distension of the peritoneum and absorption of CO_2 can produce cardiovascular, respiratory and renal dysfunction.

Cardiovascular system

The cardiovascular effects are proportional to the increase in intra-abdominal pressure (IAP) caused by the insufflation of CO_2 into the peritoneal cavity. The cardiovascular effects are more pronounced in patients with pre-existing cardiovascular disease and those with hypovolaemia.

With an IAP of <10mmHg there is an increase in the venous return which in turn increases cardiac output. This increase may increase the myocardial wall tension and increase myocardial oxygen demand. An increase in IAP to 10-20mmHg results in compression of the inferior vena cava resulting in reduced venous return and cardiac output. There is also compression of the intra-abdominal organs and an increased release of catecholamines which will increase SVR. As the IAP increases to above 20mmHg these effects are more pronounced and will lead to a reduction in blood pressure. The increase in SVR with the reduction in venous return results in an increased myocardial workload with possible ischaemia.

During Nissen fundoplication there may be increases in the mediastinal and pleural pressures contributing to a significant reduction in cardiac output.

Respiratory system

The increase in IAP results in displacement of the diaphragm upwards, causing a reduction in lung volume, especially functional residual capacity. There is a reduction in total lung compliance which results in basal atelectasis, an increase in airway pressures and a V/Q mismatch. These changes are exacerbated by the changes in position and in the obese patient. The endotracheal tube can also be displaced resulting in endo-bronchial intubation.

Renal system

An increase in the IAP, reduction in cardiac output and increase in renal vascular resistance can reduce the glomerular filtration rate.

Other effects

Regional changes in blood flow occur in the liver reducing the total hepatic blood flow, and in the bowel causing a reduction in gastric intramucosal pH. The intracranial pressure can rise which may result in a reduction in cerebral perfusion pressure.

Key points

◆ In a sliding hiatus hernia, the normal anatomical sphincter mechanism is lost, and regurgitation of gastric contents is more likely to occur.
◆ A patient with a hiatus hernia should receive premedication with a pro-kinetic agent and an H_2-receptor antagonist.
◆ Insufflation of CO_2 into the peritoneal cavity increases intra-abdominal pressure and may reduce cardiac output.

Further reading

1. Perrin M and Fletcher A. Laparoscopic abdominal surgery. *British Journal of Anaesthesia* 2004; 4: 107-10.
2. Joshi GP. Anaesthesia for laparoscopic surgery. *Canadian Journal of Anesthesia* 2002; 49: R1-R5

Short case 10.3: Penetrating eye injury

A 35-year-old male is scheduled for emergency surgery for a penetrating eye injury. He sustained the injury 2 hours ago.

What are the issues involved in the management of this case?

There are two important issues:

- With penetrating eye injury when the globe is perforated, any further increase in intra-ocular pressure (IOP) may cause expulsion of intra-ocular contents and permanently damage the eye.
- This is an emergency procedure and there is a potential risk of aspiration. Succinylcholine is routinely used for rapid sequence induction which can increase the intra-ocular pressure.

What is normal intra-ocular pressure?

IOP normally varies between 10-20mmHg but transient changes occur frequently with posture, during coughing, vomiting and during the Valsalva manoeuvre. In children, crying, eye rubbing and breath holding will cause an increase in IOP.

What anaesthetic factors can affect IOP?

Anaesthetic factors increasing IOP:

- External compression of the globe by a tightly applied face mask.
- Laryngoscopy, through either a pressor response, or from straining in an inadequately anaesthetised patient.
- Succinylcholine increases IOP transiently through its effect on the extra-ocular muscles.
- Large volumes of local anaesthetic solutions placed in the orbit can increase IOP.
- Ketamine can raise IOP.

Anaesthetic factors decreasing IOP:

- Induction agents - propofol and thiopentone.
- Non-depolarising muscle relaxants reduce tone in the extra-ocular muscles.

- Head-up tilt of 15°, which also assists venous drainage.
- Moderate hypocapnia 3.5-4.0kPa reduces choroidal blood volume by vasoconstriction of choroidal vessels.

Could you do this procedure under regional anaesthesia?

No, because of the following reasons:

- Penetrating eye injury will cause distortion of the anatomy and the local anaesthetic solution may not reach its intended site.
- Regional block and deposition of local anaesthetic in the orbit can increase IOP.
- Patients may be anxious and may not be able to stay still for the duration of the procedure.
- There is an added risk of infection because of the open eye wound.

How would you anaesthetise this patient?

General anaesthesia with rapid sequence induction is the preferred choice of anaesthetic technique for this procedure.

Pre-operative management

Pre-operative assessment should include the nature of the injury, details of any other associated injury, duration of starvation and airway assessment. Opioids can cause nausea and vomiting which in turn will increase IOP. Premedication should include ranitidine 150mg orally, or 50mg IV to reduce gastric acidity, and metoclopramide 10mg orally or IV to increase gastric motility.

Intra-operative management

- Standard monitoring including ECG, oxygen saturation, NIBP and $ETCO_2$.
- Pre-oxygenation with 100% oxygen (avoid pressure on the eye with the face mask as it will increase IOP).
- Modified rapid sequence induction using thiopentone and rocuronium (0.8-1mg/kg) with the application of cricoid pressure.

- Pressure response to laryngoscopy can be minimised by using IV lignocaine 1mg/kg or alfentanil 0.5-1mg or lidocaine spray to the vocal cords.
- Intubate with a preformed south facing endotracheal tube (RAE: Ring Adair and Elwyn) and use intermittent positive pressure ventilation (IPPV).
- Maintain oxygenation and normocarbia (hypercarbia can cause an increase in IOP).

Why may succinylcholine cause problems when used for rapid sequence induction?

Succinylcholine increases IOP transiently through its effect on extra-ocular muscles. IV induction agents, however, reduce IOP so that the overall effect may be minimal. The risk of increased intra-ocular pressure associated with succinylcholine should be balanced against the risk of aspiration and anticipated difficult airway on an individual case basis.

How would you manage this patient postoperatively?

The main aim in the postoperative period is to avoid any increase in IOP:

- Avoid patient coughing and bucking on the endotracheal tube during extubation.
- Good postoperative analgesia, if possible avoiding opioids.
- Head-up tilt by 15-20°, which assists venous drainage and decreases IOP.

Key points

- When the globe is perforated, an increase in IOP may cause expulsion of intra-ocular contents and permanently damage the eye.
- The risk of giving succinylcholine should be balanced against the risk of aspiration.
- A head-up tilt by 15-20° assists venous drainage and decreases IOP.

Further reading

1. Khaw PT, Shah P, Elkington AR. Injury to the eye. *British Medical Journal* 2004; 328: 36-8.
2. Seidel J, Dorman T. Anaesthetic management of preschool children with penetrating eye injuries: postal survey of paediatric anaesthetists and review of the available evidence. *Paediatric Anaesthesia* 2006; 16: 769-76.
3. Farmery A. Ophthalmic surgery, In: *Oxford handbook of anaesthesia*, 2nd ed. Allman, KG, Wilson, IH, Eds. Oxford: Oxford University Press, 2006: 662-3.

Applied anatomy 10.1: Arterial system of the hand

Which arteries can you use to establish invasive blood pressure monitoring?

Ideally, the most peripheral artery should be chosen so that if a clot or haematoma forms, it does not compromise the blood supply to the whole arm or limb. Hence, radial and dorsalis pedis arteries are most commonly chosen. In the hand the radial artery has an abundant collateral circulation, therefore this has a low risk of distal ischaemia. Other arteries that can be cannulated are brachial, ulnar, femoral and posterior tibial arteries.

Describe the anatomy of the radial artery

The radial artery originates in the antecubital fossa, as one of the terminal branches of the brachial artery. It runs distally on the anterior part of the forearm. It then winds laterally around the wrist, giving a branch to the superficial palmar arch. It then enters the hand after crossing the anatomical snuff box. It anastomoses with the deep branch of the ulnar artery to form the deep palmar arch.

At the wrist, about 1-2cm proximal to the wrist crease, the radial pulse can be palpated between the distal radius laterally and the tendon of flexor carpi radialis medially. This is used as a landmark for cannulation of the radial artery.

Clinical Science

Describe the collateral supply between the radial and ulnar arteries

The main collateral supply between the radial and ulnar arteries is formed by two arches in the palm, which are called the superficial and deep palmar arches.

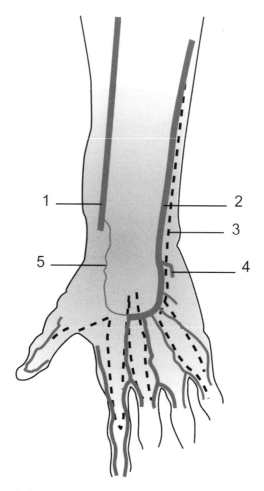

Figure 10.5 Arterial system of the hand.

1. Radial artery; 2. Ulnar artery; 3. Ulnar nerve; 4. Deep palmar branch of the ulnar artery; 5. Superficial palmar branch of the radial artery.

The superficial palmar arch is formed predominantly by the ulnar artery with a contribution from the superficial branch of the radial artery.

The deep palmar arch is formed mainly from the terminal part of the radial artery, with the ulnar artery contributing via its deep palmar branch.

What is Allen's test?

Before attempting radial artery cannulation it is recommended that Allen's test is performed to ensure that there is adequate ulnar collateral circulation in the hand.

To perform the test:

- Elevate the hand and make a fist for 20 seconds and then compress both ulnar and radial arteries.
- Open the fist and note that the hand is blanched white.
- Release the ulnar compression while maintaining the radial occlusion; flushing of the hand should occur within 5-10 seconds. This indicates a normal collateral circulation.
- If it takes longer than 10 seconds, this indicates a poor collateral supply between the radial and ulnar arteries and these should both be avoided.
- The sensitivity of the test to accurately identify the adequacy or inadequacy of the collateral blood flow has been questioned.

Describe how radial artery cannulation should be performed

Positioning

Generally the arm is abducted, the forearm is kept in supine position and the wrist is gently extended. A roll under the wrist can facilitate this position.

Procedure

The skin is prepared in a standard sterile fashion. In an awake patient, the skin and subcutaneous tissue is infiltrated with local anaesthetic at the site of cannulation. The point of maximal impulse is then identified. A good needle entry point can be found just proximal to the flexor retinaculum.

There are two methods of radial artery cannulation: the catheter-over-needle technique or the Seldinger technique.

Catheter-over-needle technique

With the bevel facing up, the catheter-over-needle assembly should be inserted at a 45° angle to the skin, over the arterial pulsation. Once the artery is entered (continuous arterial blood reflux), the angle between the needle and skin is reduced and the catheter (cannula) is advanced over the needle into the artery.

Seldinger technique

The needle is inserted at 45° to the skin, over the arterial pulsation. Once the artery is punctured with the needle, the angle between the needle and skin is reduced to facilitate passage of a guidewire into the artery; it should slide in easily. Once the wire has been inserted, the needle is removed, leaving the guidewire in the artery. Now the catheter is railroaded over the guidewire. Once the catheter is in place, the guidewire is removed. The catheter should be sutured in place to prevent it from being dislodged.

What are the possible complications of invasive blood pressure monitoring?

- Haemorrhage and haematoma.
- Thrombosis and ischaemia.
- Embolism.
- Infection.
- Aneurysm and arteriovenous fistula.
- Accidental injection of drugs.

What are the indications for arterial cannulation?

Peripheral arterial cannulation is performed to obtain an arterial blood sample for blood gas analysis and for continuous monitoring of blood pressure. Femoral artery catheterisation is performed to gain access to the left side of the heart and cerebral arteries for diagnostic and therapeutic purposes.

During the peri-operative period, arterial cannulation is indicated in the following circumstances:

- Where rapid blood pressure changes are anticipated, in patients with cardiovascular disease, hypovolaemia, and those needing inotropic support.
- Where frequent arterial blood gas analysis is required, for instance, in electrolyte disorders and patients with poor gas exchange.
- Where non-invasive blood pressure gives an inaccurate reading, for instance, in morbidly obese patients and patients with arrhythmias.

Inadvertent intra-arterial injection of thiopentone

Intra-arterial injection of thiopentone causes precipitation of acid crystals, which can cause occlusion of the blood vessel and spasm of the vessel. This can lead to critical ischaemia in the limb. Clinically, the arm will go pale and if conscious the patient may complain of severe pain because of the spasm. The main aim in the management is to dilute the drug, induce vasodilatation and prevent thrombosis. The following measures should be taken:

- Stop injecting any more thiopentone.
- Keep the arterial line *in situ* in order to administer treatment medication for the spasm.
- 500ml-1L of warmed sodium chloride fluid can be injected to dilute the thiopentone.
- If the patient is in severe pain because of the spasm, intra-arterial injection of 10ml 1% lignocaine may help.
- Vasodilator drugs such as papaverine (40mg) can be used.
- A stellate ganglion block or brachial plexus block can be used to increase perfusion by producing sympathetic block.
- Heparanise with 500-1000 IU of heparin to prevent thrombus formation.

Key points

◆ The radial artery is most commonly used for arterial cannulation.
◆ In the hand there is a collateral circulation between the radial and ulnar arteries.
◆ Prior to cannulation the adequacy of collateral circulation can be assessed using Allen's test.
◆ The main aim in the management of inadvertent intra-arterial injection is to dilute the drug, produce vasodilatation and prevent thrombosis.

Further reading

1. Patient monitors. In: *Clinical anaesthesiology*, 3rd ed. Morgan GE, Mikhail MS, Murray M. Lange Medical Books, McGraw Hill, 2002.
2. McIndoe A. Intra-arterial injection. In: *Oxford handbook of anaesthesia*, 2nd ed. Allman KG, Wilson IH, Eds. Oxford: Oxford University Press, 2006: 898-9.

Applied physiology 10.2: Postoperative nausea and vomiting (PONV)

A 32-year-old female patient is scheduled to have an elective diagnostic laparoscopy on a gynaecology list. She is normally fit and well. She had a general anaesthetic 2 years ago for removal of a breast lump and experienced severe nausea and vomiting in the postoperative period which lasted for 2 days. She also suffers from motion sickness. She is very concerned that this may recur during the proposed surgery.

What are the adverse consequences of PONV?

Many patients consider PONV as more debilitating than postoperative pain. Besides patient discomfort the other adverse consequences are:

◆ Dehydration and electrolyte imbalance.
◆ Unplanned overnight admissions after the day-case surgery.
◆ Decreased ability to self-care.
◆ Bleeding from the wound.

- Wound dehiscence.
- Aspiration pneumonitis.

What would be your strategy for reducing PONV for this patient?

This patient has a high risk of PONV due to the following factors:

- Female gender.
- Gynaecological and laparoscopic procedure.
- Previous history of PONV.
- History of motion sickness.

The following measures should be taken to prevent PONV:

- At the pre-operative visit, the patient should be reassured that measures will be taken to minimise the incidence of PONV.
- Prolonged pre-operative fasting should be avoided.
- At induction of anaesthesia, gastric insufflation should be avoided by careful and gentle mask ventilation.
- A combination of two anti-emetic agents should be administered for prophylaxis (ondansetron 4mg or granisetron 1mg, and dexamethasone 4mg or cyclizine 50mg).
- Adequate hydration should be ensured during the peri-operative period.
- Nitrous oxide and long-acting opioids such as morphine are best avoided. Analgesia can be provided using a combination of paracetamol, NSAIDs, fentanyl and local anaesthesia infiltration in the laparoscopy ports.

What are the risk factors for PONV?

The risk factors for PONV can be classified into factors related to patients, surgery and anaesthesia.

Patient-related factors

- Gender. The prevalence of PONV is three times higher in women than in men, and not so evident in pre-pubertal children or the elderly.
- Age. Children are twice as likely to develop PONV than adults - the highest incidence is in children between the ages of 6 and 16 years.

- Obesity. Fat-soluble anaesthetics may accumulate in adipose tissue and continue to be released for an extended period resulting in prolonged side effects, including PONV.
- Pre-operative eating patterns. Adequate pre-operative fasting reduces the risk of PONV, whereas excessive starvation appears to increase the risk. In emergency surgery where there has not been an adequate fast the risk is increased.
- A past history of PONV or motion sickness. These patients may have a lower threshold for nausea and vomiting than the rest of the population. Anxiety, due to a previous experience of PONV, may add to the risk.
- Gastroparesis. Patients with delayed gastric emptying secondary to an underlying disease may be at increased risk.
- Patients presenting with intestinal obstruction have an increased risk.
- Smoking. Chronic smokers have a reduced incidence of PONV.

Surgery-related factors

- Intra-abdominal, intracranial, middle ear and squint surgery, and laparoscopic and gynaecological procedures have an increased incidence of PONV.
- Pain. Surgical procedures causing moderate or severe postoperative pain increase the incidence of PONV.
- Duration of surgery. Each 30-minute increase in duration increases PONV risk by 60%, so that a baseline risk of 10% is increased to 16% after 30 minutes.

Anaesthesia-related factors

The following drugs are associated with an increased incidence of PONV:

- Inhalational anaesthetic agents.
- IV induction agents such as ketamine.
- Opioids.
- Nitrous oxide.

Propofol, when used as total intravenous anaesthesia (TIVA) and even at sub-hypnotic doses has been shown to have an anti-emetic effect.

What are the neural pathways involved in PONV?

Nausea and vomiting are reflexes which are co-ordinated by the vomiting centre. Like any other reflex there is an afferent, an efferent and central co-ordination.

Afferent pathway

♦ Limbic cortex. Pain, fear, anxiety and psychological factors can provoke nausea and vomiting. Olfactory and visual stimuli of a 'nauseating smell' and 'sickening sight' can provoke nausea and vomiting.
♦ Visceral afferents. 5-HT$_3$ receptors are present in the gut wall and myenteric plexus. Any form of irritation or inflammation will send afferents to the vomiting centre.
♦ Chemoreceptor trigger zone (CTZ). This is located in the medulla in the area postrema on the floor of the fourth ventricle. The CTZ is rich in dopaminergic (D$_2$) and 5-HT receptors. It lies outside the blood-brain barrier and receives vestibular and labyrinthine afferents.

Vomiting centre

The vomiting centre is located in the medulla oblongata and receives afferents from a large number of sources including the CTZ, the viscera and cerebral cortex. It contains muscarinic (M$_3$) and histaminic (H$_1$) receptors.

Efferent pathway

The efferent pathway involves the vagus and phrenic nerves and the spinal motor neurones supplying the abdominal muscles.

What receptors are involved in PONV?

There are many receptors (see table).

Table 10.6 Receptors involved in PONV.	
Receptor	**Location**
Histamine (H_1)	Labyrinth, vomiting centre
Dopamine (D_2)	CTZ
Muscarinic (M_3)	Vomiting centre
Serotonin (5-HT_3)	Gastrointestinal tract

Strategy for reducing PONV

Based on the risk factors, prophylactic measures should be taken to reduce the incidence of PONV:

◆ If the patient is known to have a history of PONV on one occasion or any two of the other risk factors, they should receive a single agent to prevent PONV.
◆ If the patient is known to have a history of PONV on one occasion and any other risk factors, or any three of the other risk factors, they should have a combination of two anti-emetic drugs, one of which should be a 5-HT_3 antagonist.
◆ If the patient is known to have had PONV on more than one occasion and has more than one other risk factor, they should have a multimodal approach, with more than two anti-emetic agents and possibly TIVA with propofol, avoiding nitrous oxide and volatile agents.

In addition to the above, general measures include peri-operative fluid therapy, avoiding neostigmine, avoiding opioids, a high inspired oxygen concentration, acupuncture, and the use of a multimodal approach to postoperative analgesia.

Anti-emetic drugs

Table 10.7 Anti-emetic drugs.

Class	Drug	Common side effects
Anti-cholinergic	Hyoscine	Dry mouth, sedation
Anti-histamine	Cinnarizine Cyclizine Promethazine	Dry mouth, sedation
Dopamine antagonists	Domperidone Haloperidol Prochlorperazine	Sedation, hypotension, dystonic reactions and extrapyramidal side effects
Cannabinoid	Nabilone	Sedation, dry mouth, postural hypotension
Corticosteroid	Dexamethasone	Steroid psychosis, metabolic derangement
5-HT$_3$ receptor antagonist	Granisetron Ondansetron Tropisetron	Headache, constipation (or less commonly, diarrhoea)

Key points

- Risk factors for PONV are multifactorial.
- Nausea and vomiting are reflexes which are co-ordinated by the vomiting centre. Like any other reflex there is an afferent, an efferent and a central co-ordinator.
- If the patient has any risk factors for PONV, consideration should be given to regional blocks, and the avoidance of emetogenic anaesthetic agents.

Further reading

1. Guideline for management of postoperative nausea and vomiting. Society of Obstetricians and Gynaecologists of Canada, July 2008. http://www.sogc.org/guidelines/documents/gui209CPG0807.pdf.
2. Consensus guidelines for managing postoperative nausea and vomiting. *Anaesthesia and Analgesia* 2003; 97: 62-71. http://www.anesthesia-analgesia.org/cgi/reprint/97/1/62.
3. Guidelines for prevention of postoperative vomiting in children. Association of Paediatric Anaesthetists of Great Britain and Ireland, 2008. http://www.apagbi.org.uk/docs/Final%20APA%20POV%20Guidelines%20ASC%2002%2009%20compressed.pdf.

Applied pharmacology 10.3: Conscious sedation

You have been fast bleeped to assess a 62-year-old male who has collapsed in the endoscopy suite. He has had an elective upper gastrointestinal endoscopy for a suspected gastric ulcer. During the procedure he received 8mg of midazolam.

How would you manage this patient?

Immediate resuscitation involves an airway, breathing and circulation approach. 100% oxygen should be administered via a face mask if breathing is adequate.

If the patient is unconscious with a risk of aspiration, the airway should be protected by tracheal intubation using a cuffed endotracheal tube.

Intravenous access should be secured with a wide-bore peripheral cannula.

Flumazenil 200µg should be given as an IV bolus over 15 seconds, then 100µg IV every minute if required, up to a maximum dose of 2mg.

The BP, HR, and continuous ECG, oxygen saturation, respiratory rate and consciousness level should be monitored.

The most likely cause of collapse in this patient is an overdose of midazolam. If there is no response to flumazenil, he needs to be investigated further for the cause of collapse.

Assuming that this patient became unconscious due to the midazolam overdose, how could this have been avoided?

While administering sedation in titrating doses, the systemic effects of a sedative drug should be closely monitored. In this case, the level of consciousness, respiratory rate and vital parameters should be constantly monitored. A technique of conscious sedation should be used to prevent overdose of a sedative drug.

What do you understand by conscious sedation?

Conscious sedation can be defined as a technique in which the use of a drug or drugs produces a state of depression of the central nervous system enabling treatment to be carried out, but during which verbal contact with the patient is maintained throughout the period of sedation. (Also refer to SOE5, short case 5.3.)

How would one ensure safe provision of conscious sedation?

To provide conscious sedation safely, the following components are essential:

- Appropriate premises and equipment.
- Appropriately trained staff with experience in conscious sedation.
- Minimum standards of monitoring.

What are the indications for using oral or intranasal sedation with midazolam?

The indications for using oral and intranasal sedation include circumstances where IV cannulation cannot be achieved due to a patient phobia or learning difficulties, and circumstances where inhalation sedation with nitrous oxide does not produce adequate sedation.

In what settings is conscious sedation used?

Conscious sedation is used in dental practice, in endoscopy suites for anxious patients and for awake fibreoptic intubation along with local anaesthetic.

What is the most commonly used agent for conscious sedation?

Midazolam is the most commonly used drug for conscious sedation. It can be used in intravenous, oral or nasal routes.

Describe the pharmacology of midazolam

Midazolam is a benzodiazepine. It causes anxiolysis, amnesia, hypnosis and sedation. It is presented as a clear solution in concentrations of 1mg/ml, 2mg/ml and 5mg/ml. It can be administered by oral, nasal and intravenous routes.

Mechanism of action

At a pH of 3.5, midazolam's ring structure is open, making it ionised and water-soluble. At a pH of >4, its ring structure closes making it non-ionised and lipid-soluble. The pH of the solution used is 3.5, but once injected into the blood, as the pH rises to about 7.4, it becomes lipid-soluble. Midazolam acts on the benzodiazepine binding site of $GABA_A$ receptors. It enhances the binding of GABA to the $GABA_A$ receptor which results in inhibitory effects on the central nervous system (CNS).

Pharmacodynamics

It primarily acts on the CNS and causes CNS depression. Because of its anxiolytic properties it will help to reduce sympathetic drive, and in turn cause a reduction in BP and heart rate.

Pharmacokinetics

It has a bioavailablity of 40% when taken orally. It is metabolised in the liver by hydroxylation into an active compound, 1α hydroxymidazolam, and excreted by the kidneys.

The following are clinical uses of midazolam:

◆ Conscious sedation.
◆ As an anxiolytic premedication.
◆ As sedation in ventilated patients in intensive care units.
◆ Acute management of aggressive or delirious patients.

Dosage

◆ For conscious sedation: incremental bolus doses of 0.5-1mg IV should be given, titrated to the desired effect, to a maximum of 5-7mg (the dose should be reduced in elderly patients).
◆ As a premedication: 10-20mg orally 1-1½ hrs, or 70-100μg/kg IM 20-60 minutes prior to induction. In children it can be given at a dose of 0.5mg/kg orally, 30-60 minutes prior to induction.
◆ In the intensive care unit: for sedation it is used at a dose of 30-200μg/kg/hour as a continuous infusion.

Side effects

◆ Residual effects include sleepiness and impaired psychomotor and cognitive functions.
◆ When used in pregnancy, especially the last trimester, it carries a risk to the neonate, including benzodiazepine withdrawal syndrome.

Flumazenil

Flumazenil is an imidanezodiazepine used as a reversal agent for the sedative effect of benzodiazepines. It has a relatively short duration of action (30-45 minutes) compared with the prolonged effects of benzodiazepines; hence, at times it may need to be given as a continuous infusion to overcome the long-acting benzodiazepine effects.

The initial bolus dose is 200μg IV over 15 seconds, then 100μg every minute if needed, up to a maximum total of 2mg. Following an initial response, continuous infusion of 100-400μg/hour may be required.

Side effects of flumazenil include nausea, vomiting, flushing, agitation, convulsions (rare and especially noted in epileptics), and anaphylaxis.

Ramsay Sedation Scale

The Ramsay Sedation Scale scores sedation at six different levels, and measures how arousable the patient is. It is used in intensive care units to assess the level of sedation:

- 1 - patient is anxious and agitated/restless, or both.
- 2 - patient is co-operative, oriented, and tranquil.
- 3 - patient responds to commands only.
- 4 - patient exhibits a brisk response to a light glabellar tap or loud auditory stimulus.
- 5 - patient exhibits a sluggish response to a light glabellar tap or loud auditory stimulus.
- 6 - patient exhibits no response.

One disadvantage of the Ramsay Sedation Scale is that it relies on the ability of the patient to respond, therefore, it cannot be used for patients in intensive care receiving neuromuscular blocking drugs.

Benzodiazepine withdrawal syndrome

Benzodiazepine withdrawal syndrome occurs when a patient who is taking benzodiazepine for a prolonged period, abruptly discontinues the drug. Long-term benzodiazepine use causes tolerance and physical dependence. The withdrawal symptoms include muscular cramps, spasms, blurring of vision, dry mouth, hot and cold flushes, impaired memory, agitation, anxiety, nausea and vomiting, mood swings and convulsions. It is treated using a multimodal approach with pharmaceutical agents (diazepam or chlordiazepoxide, gradually weaning off) and psychological support.

Key points

- During conscious sedation, verbal contact with the patient is maintained throughout the period of sedation.
- Benzodiazepeine overdose can be reversed using flumazenil.
- Midazolam produces anxiolysis, amnesia, hypnosis and sedation.
- The level of sedation can be measured using the Ramsay Sedation Scale.

Further reading

1. Standards for conscious sedation in dentistry: alternative techniques. A report from the Standing Committee on Sedation for Dentistry, 2007. http://www.rcseng.ac.uk/fds/docs/SCSDAT%202007.pdf.
2. Conscious sedation in the provision of dental care. Report of an expert group on sedation for dentistry. Standing Dental Advisory Committee (SDAC), 2003. http://www.advisorybodies.doh.gov.uk/sdac/conscious_sedationdec03.pdf.

Equipment, clinical measurement and monitoring 10.4: Physics of ultrasound

A 65-year-old male patient is admitted to the intensive care unit with a possible diagnosis of pneumonia and sepsis. He is hypotensive despite rapid administration of 2L of crystalloids and has a low urine output.

What invasive monitoring would you like to establish in this patient?

This patient requires monitoring of central venous pressure to ensure adequate preload. Invasive blood pressure monitoring is essential to monitor blood pressure continuously and to assess the response to inotropic therapy. It will also allow serial blood samples to be taken.

What route would you choose to establish central venous access?

The right internal jugular vein (IJV) is more commonly used as it has a straight course to the superior vena cava.

What are the complications of IJV cannulation?

The immediate complications due to needle or catheter placement include arterial puncture, haemorrhage, pneumothorax, haemothorax, air embolism, nerve damage, extravascular catheter placement and chylothorax. Delayed complications include infection, thrombosis of the vein, perforation of the superior vena cava, perforation of the right atrium and possible cardiac tamponade.

Are you aware of any national guidelines regarding the insertion of central lines?

In 2002, NICE (National Institute for Clinical Excellence) published a document regarding the use of ultrasound devices in the placement of a central line, and recommended that the use of two-dimensional (2-D) imaging ultrasound guidance should be considered in most clinical circumstances where central venous cannulation insertion is necessary either electively or in an emergency situation.

What is ultrasound and how is it generated?

Ultrasound waves are a form of acoustic energy which exceeds the threshold of human hearing (above 20kHz). Typical ultrasound machines operate in the frequency range of 2-18MHz which is hundreds of times greater than the limit of human hearing. Ultrasound waves are generated by a piezo-electric crystal transducer encased in a probe. A high frequency alternate voltage is applied to the crystal. The change in the shape of the crystal generates oscillations which are propagated as ultrasound waves.

These waves penetrate the tissues and are reflected at tissue interfaces. These reflected waves are converted into an electrical signal using the piezo-electric crystal as a transducer. Ultrasound waves do not penetrate bone and air.

Highly reflective tissues are termed hyperechogenic and appear white (e.g. bone), weakly reflective tissues are hypoechogenic and appear grey /dark (e.g. muscle). Anechogenic tissues do not reflect at all and appear black (e.g. blood, air).

What is the relationship between the frequency of sound waves and the resolution of the image?

There is a direct relationship between the frequency of sound and resolution of the image produced. A higher frequency ultrasound sound wave produces a better resolution. But if higher frequency waves are used they will not penetrate the deep tissues so the deeper structures will not be identified. A balance must be made with regard to the frequencies used in ultrasound so that there is best resolution and a good depth of penetration.

What are the different modes of ultrasound?

There are four different modes used in ultrasonography:

- A-mode. This is the simplest type of ultrasound. A single transducer scans a line through the body and the beam passes through objects of different consistency and hardness and the reflected echoes are plotted on a screen as a function of depth.
- B-mode. Same as the A-mode but instead of just one transducer a linear array of transducers simultaneously scans a plane through the body that can be viewed as a two-dimensional image on screen.
- M-mode. The M in M-mode stands for motion. This mode also uses an array of transducers, like a B-mode, but here it does this in quick succession to produce motion. Structures such as heart valves can be depicted in a wave-like manner.
- 2D-real time. Most modern ultrasound devices are 2D-real time imaging systems. It produces a constantly updated, two-dimensional view which then becomes a 3D image with height, width and time.

What is the Doppler principle?

The Doppler principle is based on the principle of change in the frequency of reflected signals from moving objects. The difference between the emitted and reflected frequency (frequency shift) is directly proportional to the speed of movement (velocity) of the objects. The flow rate can be calculated by estimating the cross-sectional area of the vessel and integrating it with the velocity. This principle is used in transcranial Doppler, foetal blood flow monitoring, Doppler plethysmography and in cardiac output measurements using a transoesophageal Doppler.

In a colour flow Doppler, flow towards the probe is red and away from the probe is blue.

What are the uses of ultrasound in the anaesthesia and intensive care setting?

- To locate vascular structures for central venous cannulation or arterial cannulation.
- To locate peripheral nerves for nerve blockade.
- To identify fluid collections using thoracic or abdominal ultrasound (pleural effusion, ascites).
- Transthoracic echocardiography/transoesophageal echocardiography is used to assess left ventricular and valvular function.
- Oesophageal Doppler is used to monitor cardiac output.
- Transcranial Doppler is used to monitor flow in the middle cerebral artery during carotid endarterectomy.
- To detect flow in the peripheral vasculature when diagnosing peripheral vascular disease.

Transoesophageal echocardiography (TOE)

TOE provides 180° views of the heart, and is especially good for viewing heart valves and the aorta. It is useful in the diagnosis of bacterial endocarditis, assessment of valve disease (especially mitral valve disease), investigation of congenital heart disease, identification of aortic dissection and assessment of paracardiac masses. During the intra-operative period it can be used to assess left ventricular preload and regional wall motion abnormalities.

The presence of an oesophageal stricture or tumour, and cervical spine instability are absolute contraindications for the use of TOE. It is relatively contraindicated in the presence of oesophageal varices.

Complications associated with TOE include bleeding, oesophageal perforation, microshock and arrhythmias.

Cardiac output monitoring

There are many invasive and non-invasive methods to monitor cardiac output. One of the commonest methods is the transoesophageal Doppler, whereby a Doppler probe is inserted either orally or nasally into the oesophagus. It measures the velocity of blood in the descending aorta and a flow-velocity graph is obtained from which cardiac output and other indices can be continuously derived.

Cardiac output measurement by the thermodilution technique using a pulmonary artery catheter has been used in the past as the gold standard technique. As this technique is invasive and can cause potential risks to the patient because of this, non-invasive methods have gained more popularity.

Table 10.8 Cardiac output monitoring.

Non-invasive methods	Invasive methods
Transoesophageal Doppler	Thermodilution technique
Arterial pulse contour analysis (PiCCO)	Dye dilution technique
Transoesophageal echocardiography (TOE)	Fick's principle

Table 10.9 Measured haemodynamic variables.

Cardiac output (CO)	HR x SV/1000 = 4-8L/min
Cardiac index (CI)	CO/BSA = 2.5-4L/min/m^2
Stroke volume (SV)	CO/HR x 1000 = 60-100ml/beat
Stroke volume index (SVI)	CI/HR x 1000 = 33-47ml/m^2/beat
Systemic vascular resistance (SVR)	80 x (MAP - RAP)/CO = 1000-1500 dynes/cm^5
Systemic vascular resistance index (SVRI)	80 x (MAP - RAP)/CI = 1970-2390 dynes/cm^5/m^2
Pulmonary vascular resistance (PVR)	80 x (MPAP - PAWP)/CO = <250 dynes/cm^5
Pulmonary vascular resistance index (PVRI)	80 x (MPAP - PAWP)/CI = 255-285 dynes/cm^5/m^2

BSA=body surface area
RAP=right atrial pressure
PAWP=pulmonary artery wedge pressure
MPAP=mean pulmonary artery pressure

Key points

♦ Use of two-dimensional (2-D) imaging ultrasound guidance should be considered in most clinical circumstances where central venous cannulation insertion is necessary either electively or in an emergency situation.

♦ Ultrasound waves are generated by a piezo-electric crystal transducer encased in a probe to which a high frequency alternating voltage is applied.

◆ Ultrasound is used in a wide variety of settings in anaesthesia and intensive care, from locating vessels to transoesophageal echocardiography.

Further reading

1. Guidance on the use of ultrasound locating devices for placing central venous access devices, TA 49. London: NICE, 2002. http://www.nice.org.uk/nicemedia/pdf/Ultrasound _49_GUIDANCE.pdf.
2. Marhofer P, Willschke H, Greher M, et al. New perspectives in regional anesthesia: the use of ultrasound - past, present, and future. Canadian Journal of Anesthesia 2005; 52: R1-R5.

Section index